DRUG-INDUCED NUTRITIONAL DEFICIENCIES

Other AVI Books

ALCOHOL AND THE DIET
  Roe
CARBOHYDRATES AND HEALTH
  Hood, Wardrip and Bollenback
DIETARY NUTRIENT GUIDE
  Pennington
ELEMENTARY FOOD SCIENCE
  Nickerson and Ronsivalli
ELEMENTS OF FOOD TECHNOLOGY
  Desrosier
ENCYCLOPEDIA OF FOOD SCIENCE
  Peterson and Johnson
ENCYCLOPEDIA OF FOOD TECHNOLOGY
  Johnson and Peterson
EVALUATION OF PROTEINS FOR HUMANS
  Bodwell
FOOD AND BEVERAGE MYCOLOGY
  Beuchat
FOOD AND THE CONSUMER
  Kramer
FOOD CHEMISTRY
  Aurand and Woods
FOOD FOR THOUGHT
  2nd Edition   Labuza and Sloan
FOOD PROTEINS
  Whitaker and Tannenbaum
FOOD SCIENCE
  2nd Edition   Potter
FUNDAMENTALS OF FOOD FREEZING
  Desrosier and Tressler
IMMUNOLOGICAL ASPECTS OF FOODS
  Catsimpoolas
MENU PLANNING
  2nd Edition   Eckstein
NUTRITIONAL EVALUATION OF FOOD PROCESSING
  2nd Edition   Harris and Karmas
PHOSPHATES IN FOOD PROCESSING
  deMan and Melnychyn
PRACTICAL FOOD MICROBIOLOGY AND TECHNOLOGY
  2nd Edition   Weiser, Mountney and Gould
PRINCIPLES OF FOOD CHEMISTRY
  deMan
PROGRESS IN HUMAN NUTRITION
  Vol. 1   Margen   Vol. 2   Margen and Ogar
PROTEIN RESOURCES AND TECHNOLOGY
  Milner, Scrimshaw and Wang
THE STORY OF FOOD
  Garard
THE TECHNOLOGY OF FOOD PRESERVATION
  4th Edition   Desrosier and Desrosier

DRUG-INDUCED NUTRITIONAL DEFICIENCIES

by DAPHNE A. ROE, M.D.

Professor
Division of Nutritional Sciences
Cornell University
Ithaca, New York

THE AVI PUBLISHING COMPANY, INC.

WESTPORT, CONNECTICUT

Library of Congress Catalog Card Number: 76-12727
ISBN-0-87055-205-8

Printed in the United States of America
by Eastern Graphics Inc., Old Saybrook, Connecticut

Foreword

The widespread use of drugs in contemporary society poses challenging problems for the practicing physician and other health professionals. Patients frequently receive therapy with more than one drug, and the side effects of these agents are varied and complicated. When faced with an ailing patient who is taking several medications, it is often difficult for the physician to determine whether he is dealing with the disease itself, or with the treatment for it. At the present time untoward reactions to drugs constitute significant causes of hospitalization in the United States, and often prolong the duration of hospital stay.

In the day-to-day practice of medicine, drug reactions in many instances are recognized readily. Such signs and symptoms as pruritic rash, leukopenia, nausea and vomiting, general malaise, or fever, may be identified easily, and the offending agent promptly discontinued. Drug toxicity may be dramatic in its presentation, e.g. anaphylaxis, and constitute a medical emergency. Toxicity may be observed within minutes or hours after the initiation of drug treatment. In other instances, a longer time is required. It is often impressive to note the extent to which the most striking features of a patient's illness are often related in some measure to the use of pharmacological agents. For example, in certain patients with prolonged fever and rash, discontinuation of all drugs restores body temperature to normal and results in disappearance of the eruption.

Together with the widespread use of drugs has come the gradual but increasing recognition of the significance of interactions between drugs. One drug may interfere with the intestinal absorption or renal excretion of another drug, or block its binding to plasma proteins and tissue receptor sites. Drugs have been reported both to accelerate and to retard the metabolic transformations of other drugs. The finding that certain drugs, such as phenobarbital, are potent inducers of hepatic drug-metabolizing enzymes, has many implications for the practical use of pharmacological agents. It is apparent that the pharmacologist and the clinician must consider drug interactions in order to gain maximal therapeutic effectiveness as well as to minimize the incidence and severity of untoward reactions.

There has also been increasing recognition of the many physiological variables which influence the body responses to drugs. Such

v

factors as (1) individual differences in the rates of removal of drugs from the body, (2) the presence of alterations of hepatic or renal function, or of acid base balance, (3) the presence of extremes of body weight and fat stores, (4) the status of endocrine function, particularly thyroid, and (5) individual differences in the rates of intestinal absorption or of binding of drugs to plasma proteins, have profound effects upon the results of drug administration. Attention to these matters requires that drug therapy be individualized, and that the special problems posed by each patient be examined separately and carefully. The rapid growth of knowledge and complexity about drug usage has resulted in clinical pharmacology coming into its own as a distinct discipline in internal medicine.

One consequence of the widespread use of drugs is an increase in the diversity of reactions to them. A bewildering array of clinical findings involving virtually every organ system may be attributable to drug therapy. The more subtle manifestations of drug toxicity, particularly those which are not associated with specific symptoms or signs, or those which occur only after extremely prolonged periods of drug administration, may escape notice by the physician. Metabolic complications of drug usage, such as osteoporosis, frequently arise only after long term use of pharmacological agents, and are particularly difficult to detect in the early stages.

An entire category of reactions to drugs which has received only scant attention in clinical practice is the multiplicity of effects upon the nutritional status of the patient. One rarely considers the many ways in which drugs may influence the dietary intake of nutrients, their disposition in the body, and their rates of elimination. The nutritional status of the patient, in turn, may have profound influence upon the therapeutic efficacy of drugs and the likelihood of developing drug toxicity.

As physicians, we often tend to be too simplistic and casual in our approach to evaluating the nutritional status of our patients. In a typical description at the bedside, the patient is considered to be either "well-nourished" or "poorly nourished." This opinion is usually based upon a rapid glance at the patient, and knowledge of the extent to which weight loss or dehydration has occurred during the course of the illness. Because overt signs of certain vitamin deficiencies, such as cheilosis, glossitis, hyperkeratosis and petechial hemorrhages, are only rarely encountered, vitamin status is presumed to be normal. If no specific etiology for anemia can be determined, it is frequently labelled as a "nutritional anemia," with little thought given to its pathogenesis or treatment. Rarely is any aspect of the patient's nutritional status carefully scrutinized or quantitated.

Much of the thinking we do about the nutrition of patients is superficial, largely because our education in this subject has also been superficial. Few medical schools properly focus on nutrition in their curricula, and many treat the subject with disdain. Nutrition is considered appropriate material for nurses and dieticians, but not for medical students. Under these circumstances, it is not difficult to understand why the physician tends to shed his responsibility for nutritional management to supporting medical personnel, and why he often remains unaware of the implications of drug therapy for nutrition. The need for upgrading the education of physicians in nutrition at the undergraduate and post-graduate levels is urgent.

The present volume is devoted to a systematic examination of the multiplicity of mechanisms by means of which drugs influence the nutritional status of the patient. Some of these mechanisms, such as nausea and vomiting, are obvious ones, but their full significance has often not been appreciated. Nausea and vomiting are such common sequelae of drug ingestion that one tends to focus attention nearly exclusively on what appear to be the critical problems: loss of water and electrolytes, shifts in acid-base balance, and maintenance of blood pressure. The consequences of nausea and vomiting, particularly on a chronic basis, are much more complicated than these, and often lead to depletion of a number of important nutrients. Anorexia due to drugs is a less dramatic symptom than vomiting but may be equally important in reducing dietary intake and thereby producing various nutritional deficiencies.

In addition to influencing dietary intake, drugs affect the metabolism of nutrients at a wide variety of sites, including intestinal absorption, plasma-binding and transport, peripheral utilization, transport across cell membranes, intracellular reactions, storage in tissues, turnover, and elimination and excretion. Knowledge of the multiplicity of these effects should help the physician to provide more appropriate drug therapy. It is evident that drugs are important causes of malnutrition, in addition to their other side effects. This problem must be considered particularly with respect to older individuals, who constitute the largest group of drug users. The economic deprivation of the elderly in our population and their social isolation compound the problem of their already impaired drug-metabolizing and excreting abilities. The enormous physiological changes in organ functions which occur with aging must always be kept in mind when prescribing drugs to older patients.

Suggestions for evaluating and monitoring the nutritional hazards of drugs, and for initiating new research programs are also made in this volume. The issues raised are serious ones, and must be dealt with by various governmental agencies as well as by the medical profession and allied fields. The basic problems remain those of developing awareness of the side effects of drugs, encouraging education about clinical pharmacology and nutrition, and coordinating the activities of industry, medicine and government.

RICHARD S. RIVLIN, M.D.
Associate Professor of Medicine
Member, Institute of Human Nutrition
College of Physicians and Surgeons
Columbia University

February 1976

Preface

This book deals with nutritional disorders caused by drugs, a subject of growing importance as new drugs are produced and established drugs are given to larger groups of people either for the prevention and treatment of disease or for population control.

Diverse drug groups, including such widely used medications as anticonvulsants, antimalarials, antituberculous drugs, and contraceptive steroids have been shown to increase nutrient requirements. These drugs, as well as certain antibiotics, sedatives and cholesterol-lowering agents, can cause specific vitamin deficiencies, if the increased vitamin requirements imposed by drug intake are not met by diet or by oral and parenteral vitamin supplements. Stimulants, such as dextroamphetamine, given to control behavioral problems in hyperactive children, have been shown to impair growth. Diuretics and also antacids can produce mineral depletion. Certain drugs given to pregnant women can induce fetal malnutrition which can lead to malformations.

These side effects are brought about because drugs can impair absorption, increase excretion, or decrease nutrient utilization. Certain drugs can also lead to decreased nutrient intake because of attendant anorexia. The risk of drug-induced nutritional deficiencies varies, being highest in those on marginal diets, and in those whose nutritional status is compromised by physiological stress such as pregnancy, or by pre-existent disease. Alcoholics are prone to develop drug-induced malnutrition because their nutritional status is impaired prior to the initiation of therapy using drugs that further deplete the body of specific nutrients.

The reader will be introduced to the subject by a review of basic concepts including nutrient and drug metabolism and drug-nutrient interactions. A survey of the literature pertaining to drug-induced hypovitaminoses and other drug associated nutritional problems in man is given. The bibliography, however, is selective, because the author believes that it is more important to explain the circumstances in which drug-induced malnutrition or drug-induced nutrient depletion occurs, rather than to include very large numbers of case reports extracted from published literature. Discussion of the diagnosis of drug-induced deficiencies has necessitated appraisal of biochemical tests which may not always be available in hospital laboratories.

While it is hoped that biochemical evaluation of nutritional status will soon become generally available to the medical profession, at the present time it is still possible to detect the majority of cases where drugs are causing nutrient depletion through an increased awareness of the risk, and by the performance of such laboratory tests as are presently feasible. Whenever a physician is considering the institution of therapy with a drug known to be capable of impairing nutritional status, appropriate nutrient supplementation should be considered; more especially, if the patient's diet has been inadequate or if he has some disease which has already interfered with nutrient absorption or utilization. If the patient has been on a drug or drug group for a period of time and signs or symptoms develop which are not referable to the primary disease, nor to direct toxic effects of the drug or drugs in use, then the possibility of drug-induced malnutrition should be considered. This book has been written because the author believes that nutritional side effects of drugs are preventable, and that most of them occur because physicians are unaware that they exist.

While the present work is intended primarily for use by physicians, it is hoped that it may also be used as a work of reference by nutritionists, clinical pharmacologists, nurses, and medical students.

The author wishes to acknowledge her indebtedness to associates in the Division of Nutritional Sciences at Cornell University, and more particularly to Dr. Donald B. McCormick who has offered advice and assistance in interpretation of biochemical studies and evaluation of biochemical publications pertinent to the subject. Thanks go also to Mrs. Catherine Brashear who prepared most of the figures for publication. Special thanks go to my secretary, Mrs. Beverly Hastings, who prepared drafts and final copy of the manuscript. Further I would like to express my thanks to Dr. D. K. Tressler and Mr. J. J. O'Neil of the AVI Publishing Company.

My deepest thanks go to my husband, Shad, and to my children, David, Laura and Adrian, without whose support this book could not have been written.

DAPHNE A. ROE, M.D.

February 1976

Contents

CHAPTER   PAGE

1. BASIC CONCEPTS 1

2. FACTORS AFFECTING NUTRITIONAL
   REQUIREMENTS 70

3. VARIABLES DETERMINING INCIDENCE AND RISK .. 92

4. DIAGNOSIS OF DRUG-INDUCED MALNUTRITION ... 102

5. DRUG-INDUCED MALABSORPTION 129

6. IATROGENIC HYPEREXCRETION AND TISSUE
   DEPLETION OF MINERALS AND VITAMINS 145

7. ANTIVITAMINS 154

8. FETAL MALNUTRITION, ABNORMAL DEVELOP-
   MENT, AND GROWTH RETARDATION 187

9. ALCOHOL AND ALCOHOLISM 202

10. NUTRITIONAL EFFECTS OF ANTICONVULSANTS ... 211

11. NUTRITIONAL EFFECTS OF ORAL
    CONTRACEPTIVES 222

12. NUTRITIONAL EFFECTS OF ANTITUBERCULOUS
    DRUGS 239

13. NUTRITIONAL EFFECTS OF ANTI-PARKINSON
    DRUGS: L-DOPA 247

14. SAFETY AND PREVENTION 253

INDEX 263

CHAPTER 1

Basic Concepts

NUTRIENTS AND THEIR INTERACTIONS WITH DRUGS

In order to understand the mechanisms involved in the development of drug-induced nutrient depletion, it is necessary for the reader to review current concepts of nutrition and malnutrition. This exercise is essential to the interpretation of such questions as why drugs interact with certain nutrients more than others, why particular groups of drugs create a limited number of deficiency states, and why patterns of malabsorption occur when specific drugs are taken. Whereas drugs can interfere with the endogenous synthesis of nutrients, or impair the digestion and absorption, or affect nutrient metabolism or excretion, the types of malnutrition so produced are circumscribed. It can be generalized that with the exception of certain vitamin antagonists, drugs in therapeutic dosage interfere to a limited extent with nutrient utilization, having least effect over short periods of time or where the intake of a nutrient exceeds demand, or when nutrient stores are ample. When the effects of drugs on nutritional status are viewed in this light, it is predictable that for any given population, drugs will have most effect in chronic drug users. Within this group, the drugs will emphasize pre-existing nutrient lack, incurred by marginal intakes of nutrients or by disease.

If, for example, we limit our consideration to drug-induced malabsorption, certain drugs will decrease the absorption of macronutrients including sugars, fats, and amino acids, fat- and water-soluble vitamins, and minerals. Whether or not a particular nutritional deficiency supervenes depends not only on the residual absorptive capacity of the small intestine, but also on the prior nutrition of the patient or population. While it is probably true to say that drugs can affect the utilization of any nutrient, whether or not deficiency or depletion results is determined by nutrient availability and the economy of physiological systems concerned with nutrient metabolism. Girdwood (1971) commented that the precise amount of each of the vitamins that is believed to be required by the human male and female at different ages should not concern us as much as the various factors that may affect the actual amount of these vitamins available to the body. Similar comments to those of Girdwood could be made with respect to nutrients other than vitamins.

Causes of Nutrient Depletion

In the United States and in all other parts of the world in which the food supply is adequate for the needs of most people, the risks of nutrient depletion are related to 1) socioeconomic factors, 2) nutrient losses due to food processing and preparation, 3) food habits, 4) decreased food intake associated with restrictive diets, 5) lack of interest in food, or anorexia, 6) failure to increase nutrient intake with respect to physiological needs, 7) alcoholism, 8) drug addiction, 9) disease, and 10) medications. In western countries, a major factor determining a balanced diet is the proper choice of foods. Since foods vary markedly one from another in their ability to supply essential nutrients, a balanced diet becomes almost synonymous with a varied diet. This does not mean, of course, that a diet containing 20 kinds of crackers would be desirable, but rather that a wide range of foods should be taken, so that the nutrient content of one will complement that of another with respect to requirements of different nutrients. Hansen (1973) has pointed out that foods with a substantial number of important nutrients without excessive calories are of good quality. He suggests a classification of foods according to the nutrient: calorie ratio, those foods having such a ratio greater than 1 being particularly desirable in a population which tends to consume excessive calories. Deliberate omission of certain key sources of nutrients from the diet, such as milk (supplying vitamin A, D and calcium as well as protein), green leafy vegetables (supplying folic acid, vitamin K and carotene), and liver (providing a major source of fat-soluble and B vitamins as well as iron), contributes to the incidence of nutrient depletion in this country. Blood levels of nutrients, particularly vitamins, have been used in recent years as a measure both of dietary intake and of nutritional status.

In the Canadian Nutrition Survey (Nutrition Canada 1973), it was found that in people of all age groups low serum folate values were prevalent. The preliminary data presently available from this study also suggest that in special subgroups of the Canadian population there is a significant incidence of iron deficiency, calcium and vitamin D deficiency, thiamin depletion, and among pregnant women protein depletion. Data derived from nutrition surveys carried out in the last ten years show that malnutrition including avitaminosis is uncommon in industrialized countries except among special groups of the population such as the elderly and those in hospitals (Brocklehurst *et al.* 1968; Leevy *et al.* 1965).

Among hospital patients, hypovitaminemia is far more common than clinical vitamin deficiencies. In the study by Leevy *et al.* (1965) the most common vitamin deficiency encountered was that of folic acid and this occurred most frequently in alcoholic persons. There was also a frequent occurrence of low-circulating levels of vitamins A, C and B_6 in this hospital group.

From available information it can be predicted that prevalent forms of nutrient depletion, especially hypovitaminoses, will be those most accentuated by drug ingestion. This may be a partial explanation for the fact that drug-induced folate deficiency is the most frequent form of vitamin depletion due to pharmacological agents which is found in those developed countries from which reports have been published. However, it may be anticipated, in developing countries where endemic malnutrition exists, that ingestion of drugs would also exacerbate other dietary deficiencies.

In order to understand the mechanisms involved in the development of drug-induced nutrient depletion, this review of nutrient sources—their absorption, metabolism and excretion—has been compiled. Detailed discussion of particular nutrients is justified, either on the basis of frequent drug interactions, or because in the clinical sense they are most commonly affected by drug intake. It is important not only to realize how nutritional deficiencies are incurred through drug action, but also how the body is defended against the occurrence of such deficiencies. Varied and multiple nutrient sources, accessory systems of nutrient absorption, as well as metabolic adaptation, contribute to the economy of the body in preserving nutritional status at a reasonable level.

Water-Soluble Vitamins Significantly Affected by Drugs

Vitamin B_6.—Sources of B_6 vitamers include the pyridoxine present in plant materials and pyridoxal and pyridoxamine, coming from foods of animal origin. The vitamin is present in many foods and the richest sources are liver (beef, calf and pork), herring, salmon, nuts such as walnuts and peanuts, wheat germ, and yeast. While the vitamin is present in significant amounts in meats, fish, fruits, cereals and vegetables, it is present to a lower extent in milk and other dairy products. Since pyridoxal and pyridoxamine are decomposed rapidly at high temperatures and are broken down by autoclaving, there is concern that modern food processing may diminish dietary sources of the vitamin. Evidence presently available suggests that vitamin B_6 vitamers are absorbed by simple diffusion across the cells of the small intestinal mucosa (Booth and Brain 1962; Brain and Booth 1964).

Utilization of vitamin B_6 depends on conversion of the various forms of the vitamin to a metabolically active coenzyme, pyridoxal phosphate (Fig. 1.1). Pyridoxine and pyridoxamine are phosphorylated by pyridoxal kinase with ATP. Then the resultant pyridoxine

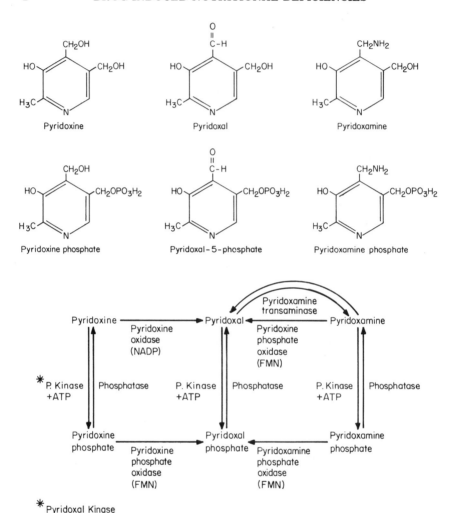

From Wada and Snell (1961)

FIG. 1.1. VITAMERS OF B_6 AND THE FORMATION OF PYRIDOXAL PHOSPHATE

or pyridoxamine phosphate react with oxidases to form pyridoxal phosphate (Wada and Snell 1961). The latter compound can also be formed directly by phosphorylation of pyridoxal. McCormick *et al.* (1961) showed that the brain, liver and kidney contained the highest concentrations of pyridoxal phosphokinases. Anderson *et al.* (1971) demonstrated that in man pyridoxine can be converted to pyridoxal phosphate in circulating erythrocytes. In an editorial (Nutrition Reviews 1972) discussing the work by Anderson *et al.* (1971) and by others in the same field, it is pointed out that there is evidence that pyridoxal phosphate can also be converted to pyridoxal in the red cell, and that the pyridoxal passes out into the plasma. Indeed, there is strong evidence that pyridoxal is the major transport form of the vitamin. The editor of this review questions whether pyridoxal in the plasma may enter other tissue cells so that it could be converted to the active coenzyme, pyridoxal phosphate, and also whether pyridoxal can be taken up by the liver cells before conversion to the end product, pyridoxic acid, which can be excreted in the urine.

Pyridoxal phosphate is the key coenzyme in many reactions involving amino acid metabolism. In such reactions an amino acid condenses with pyridoxal phosphate on an enzyme surface and a Schiff base is thus formed. When the Schiff base intermediate is bound to a particular enzyme, the bonds at a specific carbon atom are labelized and reactions are then possible involving a number of different bonds (Larner 1971). Specific enzyme proteins are responsible for particular rearrangements within the Schiff base.

There are three important classes of B_6 dependent reactions which will concern us in discussion of the effects of drugs:

1. B_6 is necessary to the metabolism of the amino acid, tryptophan, and is required at several steps along the pathway leading from tryptophan to the formation of niacin. It is for this reason that drugs that are vitamin B_6 antagonists are capable of inducing frank niacin deficiency (Fig. 1.2).

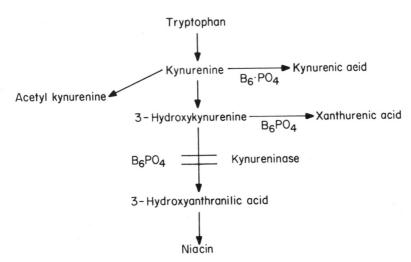

FIG. 1.2. ENDOGENEOUS PATHWAY FOR NIACIN BIOSYNTHESIS FROM TRYPTOPHAN SHOWING VITAMIN B_6-DEPENDENT REACTIONS AND STEP PREFERENTIALLY BLOCKED BY B_6 ANTAGONISTS

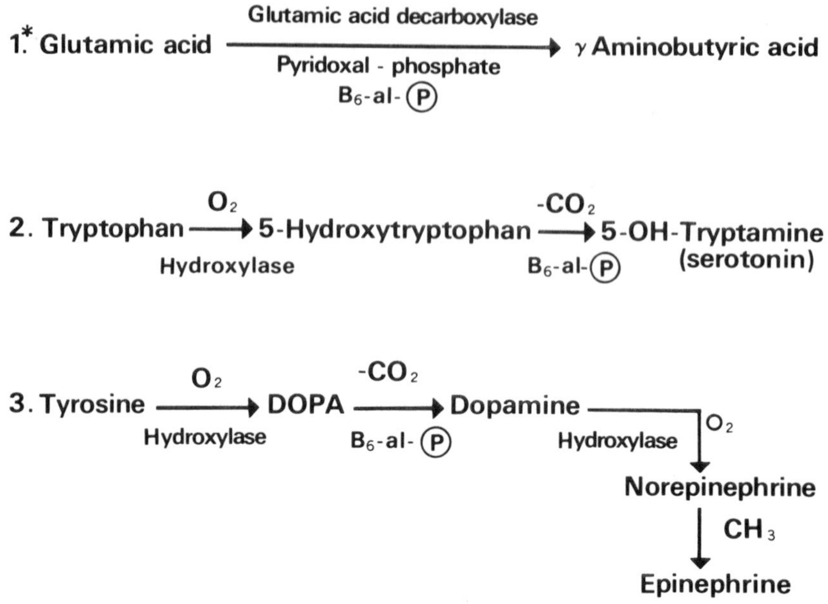

1.* Glutamic acid $\xrightarrow[\substack{\text{Pyridoxal - phosphate} \\ B_6\text{-al-}\textcircled{P}}]{\text{Glutamic acid decarboxylase}}$ γ Aminobutyric acid

2. Tryptophan $\xrightarrow[\text{Hydroxylase}]{O_2}$ 5-Hydroxytryptophan $\xrightarrow[B_6\text{-al-}\textcircled{P}]{-CO_2}$ 5-OH-Tryptamine (serotonin)

3. Tyrosine $\xrightarrow[\text{Hydroxylase}]{O_2}$ DOPA $\xrightarrow[B_6\text{-al-}\textcircled{P}]{-CO_2}$ Dopamine $\xrightarrow[\text{Hydroxylase}]{}$ $\Big] O_2$

Norepinephrine

$\Big| CH_3$

Epinephrine

*Convulsions in drug induced B_6 deficiency may be associated with decreased function of B_6 dependent, glutamic acid decarboxylase

FIG. 1.3. VITAMIN B_6 AND THE SYNTHESIS OF NEUROTRANSMITTERS

2. B_6 is necessary for the synthesis of a number of neurotransmitters and neurohormones including serotonin, gamma-aminobutyric acid and epinephrine. The fact that these compounds are necessary to neuronal function at many levels explains neurological symptoms associated with drug-induced B_6 deficiency (Fig. 1.3).

3. Vitamin B_6, in the form of pyridoxal phosphate, is a necessary factor in the synthesis of delta-aminolevulinic acid. The activity of the enzyme Δ-aminolevulinic acid synthetase, which allows condensation of succinyl coenzyme A and glycine to form Δ-aminolevulinic acid, requires B_6 for its activity and this synthetase is the rate-limiting enzyme in heme synthesis. Vitamin B_6 is also required for globin formation (Fig. 1.4).

It is important to remember that when one speaks of the syndromes of vitamin B_6 deficiency caused by drugs, one may refer to an actual deficiency caused by hyperexcretion of the vitamin, or to a lack of

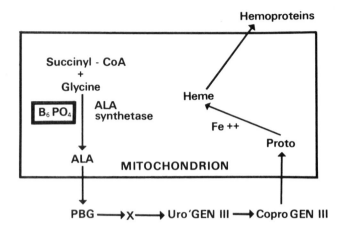

ALA aminolevulinic acid
PBG porphobilinogen
Uro'GEN III uroporphyrinogen III
Copro'GEN III coproporphyrinogen III
Proto protoporphyrin IX
X intermediates
Enzymes catalyzing heme biosynthesis omitted
except ALA synthetase

FIG. 1.4. ROLE OF PYRIDOXAL PHOSPHATE IN HEME BIO-
SYNTHESIS

conversion of the vitamers to the coenzyme form, or to specific defects in B_6 dependent apoenzymes (Fig. 1.5).

Syndromes of vitamin B_6 deficiency can then be divided into three important groups:

1. Neuropathic, in which there is a sensory neuritis. In this condition there also may be evidence of involvement of the central nervous system and convulsions can occur. In the milder forms of B_6 depletion, depression is a common symptom.

2. Anemic, in which hypochromic, sideroblastic anemia develops.

3. Pellagrous, in which cutaneous, gastrointestinal and central nervous system signs and symptoms occur which are identical with those of pellagra. The evolution of these syndromes in patients made B_6 deficient by administration of a B_6 antagonist were described by Vilter *et al.* (1953).

Folic Acid (Folacin).—Folic acid and its derivatives are found in a number of foods, the richest sources being liver, yeast, dark green, leafy vegetables, broccoli, asparagus, legumes, and fruits, more espe-

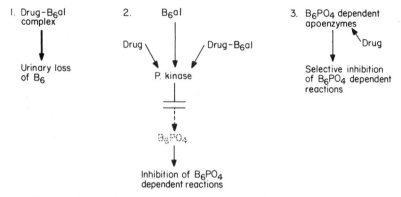

P. kinase = pyridoxal kinase

FIG. 1.5. MODE OF ACTION OF DRUGS CAUSING FUNCTIONAL DEFICIENCY OF VITAMIN B_6

cially oranges or orange juice. Food folate from plant and animal sources consists of several methyl and formyl derivatives of the vitamin including 5-methyl, 10-formyl and 5-formyltetrahydrofolate. In uncooked foods, the reduced form of the vitamin exists as polyglutamates (Brown *et al.* 1973). It has been demonstrated by several authors that folate present in milk is protein bound (Ghitis 1967; Metz *et al.* 1968). Folate in foods is unstable on exposure to air and light, thus accounting for loss of the vitamin in storage. Folate is also lost from food through elution into cooking fluids or canning fluids, and through cooking procedures. Relative stability of folate in fruits and citrus fruits may be due to the presence of ascorbic acid, which protects folate from degradation.

Folate is absorbed by an active transport mechanism, absorption being possible in all segments of the small intestine but maximal in the jejunum (Fig. 1.6). A gamma-glutamylcarboxypeptidase (conjugase) has been shown to be present in a number of tissues including the small intestinal mucosa (Baugh *et al.* 1975). Rosenberg *et al.* (1969) studied the absorption of polyglutamic folate using everted gut sac preparations, and showed that in this process intestinal conjugase is necessary so that smaller preferentially absorbed peptides of folic acid can be formed. Bayless (1969) has suggested that a deficiency of conjugase could cause nutritional folate deficiency. Burnstein *et al.* (1970) found that certain unconjugated bile acids inhibit intestinal conjugase activity and they suggest that it might be the activity of these bile acids which caused nutritional folate deficiency in the manner suggested by Bayless. Melikian *et al.* (1971) showed that when monoglutamic folate was administered to human

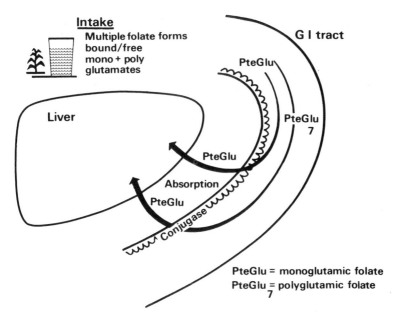

Intake
Multiple folate forms
bound/free
mono + poly
glutamates

Liver

G I tract

PteGlu

PteGlu
7

PteGlu

Absorption
PteGlu

Conjugase

PteGlu = monoglutamic folate
PteGlu$_7$ = polyglutamic folate

FIG. 1.6. DIETARY FOLACIN AND ITS ABSORPTION

subjects it appeared in the portal blood unaltered, and that conversion of the free folate to its metabolically active form, 5-methyltetrahydrofolate, occurred mainly in the liver.   Conjugation of monoglutamic folate to form polyglutamates also takes place in the liver (Cawthorne and Smith 1973; Whitehead 1973).

It has been shown by Johns *et al.* (1965) that folic acid present in plasma is partly free and partly combined with plasma proteins. Some controversy exists as to the nature of folate binding to serum proteins. Elsborg (1972) only demonstrated albumin as a carrier protein. In a series of studies Markkanen *et al.* (1974) showed that bound folate in the plasma existed in three forms, folate being bound to alpha-2-macroglobulin, transferrin and albumin.   Changes in the binding of folate to serum proteins were demonstrated by this group to occur during various phases of the menstrual cycle and during pregnancy.

Folate is widely distributed in the body, both in cells and in extracellular fluids.   Folate concentration is highest in the liver, kidney, and cells of the hemopoietic system including erythrocytes and leukocytes (Chanarin 1960A). Since the publication of a report by Herbert and Zalusky in 1961, it has been known that the folate content of cerebrospinal fluid is higher than that of the serum. There is a continuous exchange of folate between cells and tissue fluids. Folate levels in erythrocytes and/or in liver biopsy samples reflect tissue stores of the vitamin.

Folate is excreted by two routes: into the bile, and via the urine. There is an enterohepatic circulation of folate, some of the folate, probably most of it, being reabsorbed from the duodenum in normal subjects (Baker *et al.* 1965). In studies of the urinary excretion of folate carried out by McLean and Chanarin in 1966, it was shown that between ¼ and ⅓ of the folic acid activity in the urine, following an intravenous dose of tritium labeled folate, was due to 5-methyltetra-hydrofolate, and it was found that this compound was present due to tissue displacement and not because of the administered dose of labeled folic acid (Fig. 1.7).

Pteroylmonoglutamic acid is the precursor of various coenzyme forms of the vitamin that function in single carbon transfer reactions. The coenzyme form of the vitamin which acts as an acceptor of one carbon unit is tetrahydrofolic acid, which is formed by the activity of the folate reductase system. Tetrahydrofolates are necessary for the biosynthesis of purines and the biosynthesis of the pyrimidine, thymidylate, which is required in the formation of DNA (Blakley 1969). Tetrahydrofolate is also required for the synthesis of the methyl group of methionine and choline and in histidine degradation.

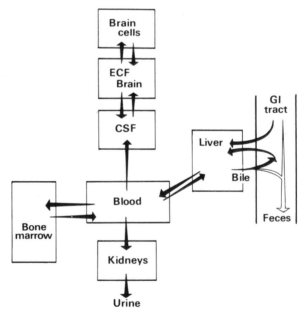

FIG. 1.7. MAJOR DISTRIBUTION OF AN EXCRETION
OF FOLATE

It has been shown in mammalian and avian tissues that methyltetrahydrofolic acid mediates the methylation of biogenic amines including
serotonin (Banerjee and Snyder 1973). Tetrahydrofolate also plays a
role in collagen formation. *In vitro* it is known that this coenzyme
form of the vitamin participates in the hydroxylation of collagen
proline (Hautvast and Barnes 1974). At the cellular level, major
functions of the coenzymes of folate include the maturation of
erythrocytes and leucocytes and the maintenance of tissue integrity,
particularly in relation to epithelia which are rapidly turning over.
Interrelationships exist functionally between cobalamins derived from
vitamin B_{12} and folate (Fig. 1.8).

Clinical features of folate deficiency which may be due to drugs
include megaloblastic anemia, glossitis, diarrhea, and weight loss.
Other symptoms and signs may include hyperpigmentation of the skin,
hepatomegaly, splenomegaly, ankle edema and such non-specific
signs of anemia as palpitations, angina, light-headedness and faintness

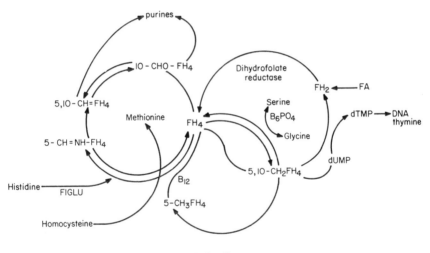

FA = Folic acid (PGA)
FH_2 = Dihydrofolate
FH_4 = Tetrahydrofolate
$5,10-CH_2FH_4$ = 5,10-methylenetetrahydrofolate
$5-CH_3FH_4$ = 5-methyltetrahydrofolate
$5,10-CH=FH_4$ = 5,10-methenyltetrahydrofolate
$10-CHO-FH_4$ = 10-formyltetrahydrofolate
$5-CH=NH-FH_4$ = 5-formiminotetrahydrofolate
dUMP = deoxyuridylate
dTMP = thymidylate

FIG. 1.8. INTERCONVERSION AND MAJOR ROLES OF FOLATE COENZYMES,
SHOWING FUNCTION OF VITAMIN B_{12} IN REGENERATION OF TETRAHYDRO-
FOLATE

(Sullivan 1970). In the development of folate depletion the following hematologic and biochemical changes occur successively: (1) The serum folate levels are decreased. (2) There is a steady and progressive fall in erythrocyte folate levels. (3) The urinary excretion of formiminoglutamic acid is increased. (4) Morphological changes appear in the bone marrow with the development of megaloblastosis and in the peripheral blood hypersegmentation of neutrophils is first seen. Thereafter if depletion continues, macrocytic anemia develops with a fall in the erythrocyte count and markedly increased mean corpuscular volume of erythrocytes (Chanarin 1969B).

Acute folate deficiency, due to blocking of the folate reductase enzyme by folate antagonists, results in severe reactions which may be fatal unless the patient receives folinic acid (Fig. 1.9). Symptoms include ulcerative stomatitis, diarrhea often of considerable severity and intestinal ulceration (Calabresi and Welch 1965).

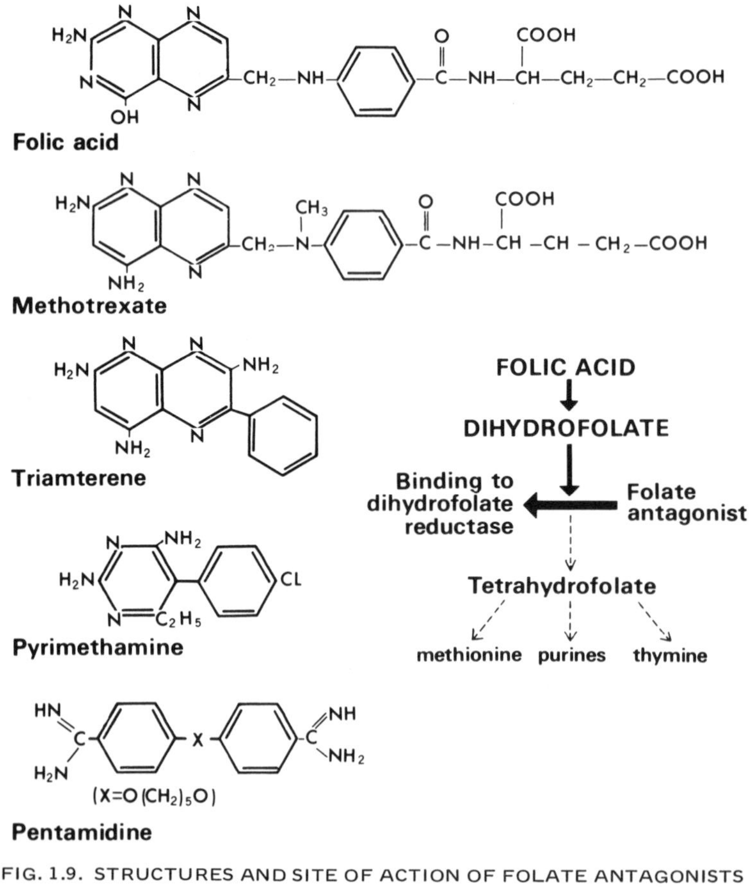

Folic acid

Methotrexate

Triamterene

Pyrimethamine

Pentamidine
(X=O (CH₂)₅O)

FOLIC ACID
↓
DIHYDROFOLATE
↓
Binding to dihydrofolate reductase ← Folate antagonist
↓
Tetrahydrofolate
methionine purines thymine

FIG. 1.9. STRUCTURES AND SITE OF ACTION OF FOLATE ANTAGONISTS

Vitamin B_{12}.—Sources of vitamin B_{12} for man include all animal protein foods including meat, fish, shellfish, milk and eggs. Liver, kidney and other animal foods derived from viscera contain more vitamin B_{12} than muscle meats. Shellfish is rich in vitamin B_{12} because these invertebrates ingest microorganisms which are able to synthesize the vitamin. Vitamin B_{12} is unstable at an alkaline pH and losses may occur during cooking procedures. The vitamin, as it occurs in animal products, is protein-bound. The combined effects of pepsin in the stomach and the locally acid pH split off vitamin B_{12} from its protein-binding sites. The acidity of the stomach also enhances the transfer of vitamin B_{12} from the food protein to its binding with gastric intrinsic factor. The vitamin B_{12} intrinsic factor complex passes through the small intestine to the site for absorption in the terminal ileum. It appears that intrinsic factor, a glycoprotein, has binding sites both for vitamin B_{12} and for a protein acceptor present on the microvillar membrane of the terminal ileum. In the absence of the intrinsic factor as, for example, in pernicious anemia, or with loss of integrity of the ileal binding site, vitamin B_{12} cannot be absorbed. Absorption of vitamin B_{12} is calcium dependent. Once vitamin B_{12} passes across the microvillar membrane it is separated from intrinsic factor and becomes localized to the mitochondria within the cells. The vitamin is partially converted to a coenzyme form, $5'$-deoxyadenosylcobalamin in the epithelial cells of the ileum. For absorption into the circulation, vitamin B_{12} must become attached to the transport protein, Transcobalamin II (TC II). TC II stimulates uptake of vitamin B_{12} by cells of the hemopoietic system, including reticulocytes, as well as into liver cells. The other transport protein for vitamin B_{12}, Transcobalamin I, may be derived from the protein that binds vitamin B_{12} in the tissues (Toskes and Deren 1973) (Fig. 1.10).

The vitamin is widely distributed in human tissues and tissue fluids where it exists in a bound state. The liver contains large amounts of vitamin B_{12}. Toohey and Barker in 1961 found that in human livers, as in the livers of other mammalian and avian species, the major coenzyme forms of the vitamin is deoxyadenosylcobalamin-B_{12}. As discovered by Cohn *et al.* in 1949, vitamin B_{12} in the liver is protein-bound.

The functions of vitamin B_{12} as a coenzyme are two-fold: as $5'$-deoxyadenosyl-B_{12} it is needed for the isomerization of methyl-malonyl-coenzyme A to succinyl-coenzyme A, and secondly, as methyl-cyanocobalamin it is needed for the methylation of homo-cysteine to form methionine (Gurnani *et al.* 1960; Sakami and Ukstin 1961). Tisman and Herbert (1973) found that cells from the bone marrow in patients with a vitamin B_{12} deficiency took up less methyl-

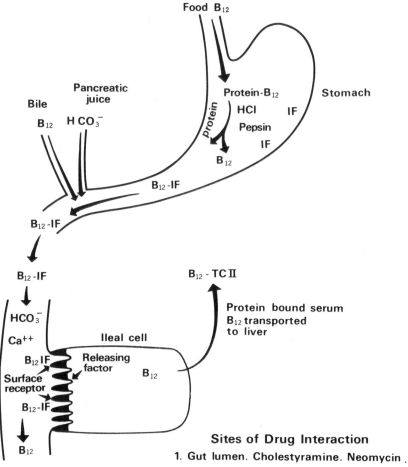

Sites of Drug Interaction
1. Gut lumen. Cholestyramine. Neomycin.
2. Ileal surface receptor. PAS. Colchicine. Neomycin. Ethanol. KCI. Biguanides.

FIG. 1.10. ABSORPTION OF VITAMIN B_{12}

tetrahydrofolate than the cells from normal bone marrow. Addition of vitamin B_{12} to their *in vitro* preparations enhanced the cell uptake of methyltetrahydrofolate in the vitamin B_{12} deficient patients. These data suggest that there is a vitamin B_{12} requirement for the cell uptake of the coenzyme form of folate.

Severe vitamin B_{12} deficiency results in a megaloblastic anemia with symptoms and hematologic changes identical with those of folate deficiency. Characteristic vitamin B_{12} neuropathy associated with sub-acute combined degeneration of the spinal cord is found with vitamin B_{12} deficiency in pernicious anemia or following gastrectomy or partial gastrectomy. Such a neuropathy has not been found in cases of drug-induced vitamin B_{12} malabsorption. Biochemical changes characteristic of vitamin B_{12} depletion or deficiency include a reduced serum vitamin B_{12} level (Herbert 1963). Increased methylmalonic acid excretion is a good indicator of vitamin B_{12} dysfunction. Hyperexcretion of this compound occurs because in the absence of deoxyadenosylcobalamin, methylmalonyl-coenzyme A cannot be converted to succinyl coenzyme A, but instead is broken down by hydrolysis and excreted in the urine as the free acid (Gompertz and Hoffbrand 1970). Levels of serum folate may be high in vitamin B_{12} deficiency, because of a block in the conversion of methyltetrahydrofolate to tetrahydrofolate which requires a B_{12}-containing enzyme (Herbert and Zalusky 1962). Low dietary intake of vitamin B_{12} such as may occur in vegans and/or vitamin B_{12} malabsorption induced by drugs, or by disease, may continue for a long time before hematologic evidences of vitamin B_{12} deficiency are manifest.

Interactions Between Vitamin B_{12} and Folate.—Metabolic interactions exist between vitamin B_{12} and folate. Megaloblastosis, common to deficiency of both these vitamins, has been explained on the basis of these relationships. In order that methyltetrahydrofolate can be converted to other folate coenzymes, the vitamin B_{12}-dependent methyltransferase reaction must be intact, and in vitamin B_{12} deficiency the activity of this enzyme is diminished. This results in diminished tissue levels of certain folate coenzymes which are necessary to purine and pyrimidine biosynthesis and hence normal DNA biosynthesis (Buchanan 1964). In both folate and vitamin B_{12} deficiency, abnormal DNA synthesis is believed to result in the formation of megaloblastic cells which are unable to enter mitosis or to mature in the normal manner (Hoffbrand *et al.* 1974). Silber and Moldow (1970) have stated that a failure in folate utilization is the final cause for decreased (or abnormal) DNA synthesis in megaloblastic anemia. However, there may be a more direct cause for impairment of DNA synthesis in vitamin B_{12} deficiency, in that synthesis of thymidylate synthetase is impaired (Hurani 1973).

Functional Deficiencies of Vitamin B_6, Folate and Vitamin B_{12} Induced by Drugs.—Effects of drugs on vitamin B_6, folate and vitamin B_{12} absorption or utilization account for the largest proportion of all drug-induced nutritional deficiencies. Drugs in five major groups have been shown either to function as vitamin B_6 antagonists, or to increase the turnover of vitamin B_6 in the body. These include isonicotinic acid hydrazide and cycloserine as well as certain other antituberculous drugs; hydralazine used in the treatment of hypertension; penicillamine, a metal chelator; L-dopa, used in the treatment of Parkinson's disease; and the oral contraceptives (Fig. 1.11). Drugs in ten major groups have been shown to affect the absorption of folate to act as folate antagonists or to increase the turnover or loss of folate from the body. These include the cytotoxic agent, methotrexate, the antimalarial, pyrimethamine, anticonvulsants such as diphenylhydantoin, phenobarbital and primidone, and the diuretic, triamterene. Other drugs known to affect folate utilization include oral contraceptives, the antituberculous drug cycloserine, anti-inflammatory agents such as salicylazosulfapyridine, aspirin, and

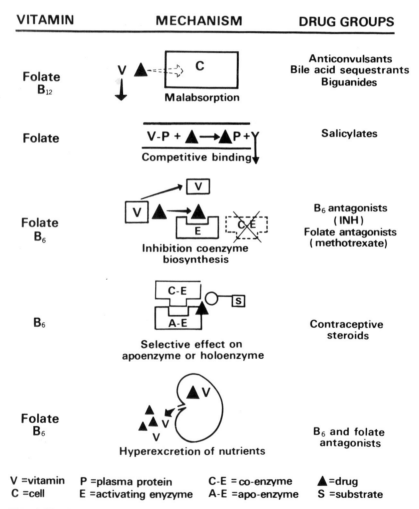

VITAMIN	MECHANISM	DRUG GROUPS
Folate B_{12}	Malabsorption	Anticonvulsants Bile acid sequestrants Biguanides
Folate	Competitive binding	Salicylates
Folate B_6	Inhibition coenzyme biosynthesis	B_6 antagonists (INH) Folate antagonists (methotrexate)
B_6	Selective effect on apoenzyme or holoenzyme	Contraceptive steroids
Folate B_6	Hyperexcretion of nutrients	B_6 and folate antagonists

V =vitamin   P =plasma protein   C-E = co-enzyme   ▲=drug
C =cell   E =activating enyzyme   A-E =apo-enzyme   S =substrate

FIG. 1.11. COMPARISON OF MECHANISMS FOR PRODUCTION OF VITAMIN B_6, FOLATE AND VITAMIN B_{12} DEPLETION BY DRUGS

pentamidine, an anti-infective aromatic diamidine. Drugs in four groups have been shown to affect the absorption of vitamin B_{12}. These include the biguanides, metformin and phenformin; paraamino-salicylic acid, an antituberculous drug; the bile acid sequestrant, cholestyramine; and potassium chloride. Further, alcohol, the most commonly used drug of all, affects the absorption and/or utilization of these vitamins, primarily because it induces a direct toxic effect on the gastrointestinal tract, on the hemopoietic system and on the liver, whereby normal metabolism of these vitamins may be interrupted. The frequency and diversity of drug effects on these vitamins can be explained in relation to the many drug-nutrient interactions between absorption sites and subsequent loci of metabolism (Fig. 1.12).

Deficiencies of pyridoxine or folate may co-exist with other hypovitaminoses. When this fact is considered in the context of the effect of drugs on these vitamins, it need not be assumed that the drug primarily affects the metabolism of several vitamins, but rather that depletion of one vitamin affects the requirement for another. Niacin deficiency can be secondary to a vitamin B_6 deficiency induced by pyridoxine antagonists, endogenous synthesis of niacin from tryptophan being a B_6-dependent reaction. If this reaction is inhibited by drugs, due to their effect on vitamin B_6 metabolism, and at the same

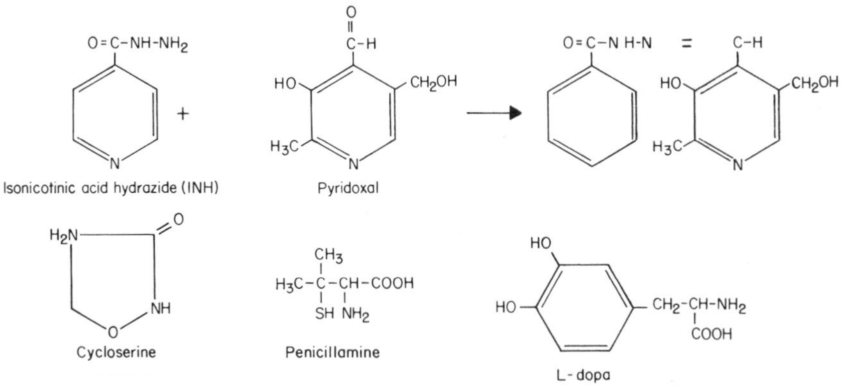

O=C-NH-NH₂

Isonicotinic acid hydrazide (INH)

Pyridoxal

Cycloserine

Penicillamine

L-dopa

1. Formation of hydrazones or Schiff bases of B_6al causes tissue depletion of B_6 with or without excretion of free B_6 and hydrazone in urine. (INH, L-dopa)

2. Inhibition of pyridoxal kinase by a) drug, b) condensation product of drug and B_6al (INH, CS)

3. Direct competition of phosphorylated analogs or antagonists with natural coenzymes for apoenzyme surface (penicillamine forms thiazolidine compound with B_6-al-(P))

FIG. 1.12. VITAMIN B_6 ANTAGONISTS AND MECHANISMS WHEREBY THEY INDUCE DEFICIENCY OF THIS VITAMIN

time there is a marginal intake of dietary niacin, then niacin deficiency associated with pellagra may develop (Goldsmith 1964; DiLorenzo 1967).

Riboflavin depletion which may coexist with impairment of vitamin B_6 metabolism can be explained because it has been shown by Wada and Snell (1961) that riboflavin is involved in the oxidation of pyridoxine phosphate to pyridoxal phosphate. Plasma ascorbic levels have been found to be decreased in both folate and vitamin B_{12} deficiency (Vilter 1963).

Kahn and Brodsky (1966) have suggested that vitamin B_{12} is needed for the maintenance of normal plasma ascorbic levels.

Niacin.—Niacin is derived from the diet both directly and indirectly. The vitamin is consumed in coenzyme form in animal and plant products including liver, yeast, lean meats, poultry and legumes. The pyridine nucleotides include nicotinamide adenine dinucleotide (NAD) and nicotinamide adenine dinucleotide phosphate (NADP). Niacin is added to enriched breads and cereals. In addition, niacin is produced endogenously through the metabolism of the amino acid tryptophan derived from dietary protein. Pyridine nucleotides from food sources as well as dietary proteins are digested in the intestinal tract yielding niacin (nicotinic acid) and tryptophan. These compounds are then absorbed and reach the liver via the portal circulation. Resynthesis of pyridine nucleotides occurs in the liver after the conversion of tryptophan to niacin and, hence, the utilization of niacin for pyridine nucleotide synthesis. Intracellular synthesis of pyridine nucleotides can occur in many tissues of the body, utilizing nicotinamide. In the liver, nicotinamide, derived from pyridine nucleotides, is readily converted to N^1-methylnicotinamide which is excreted as an end product in the urine. The 6-pyridone derivative of N^1-methylnicotinamide is also excreted (Dietrich 1971).

In the conversion of tryptophan to niacin, the first step is the formation of N-formylkynurenine which is mediated by the enzyme tryptophan pyrrolase. This enzyme is inducible, being increased after the administration of tryptophan. Tryptophan pyrrolase activity is also stimulated by administration of glucocorticoids (Goodwin 1963). Estrogens also affect the activity of tryptophan pyrrolase, and it has been suggested that the observed effects of oral contraceptives on tryptophan metabolism are not entirely due to interference with pyridoxal phosphate-dependent reactions that may additionally be related to the inducing effects of the estrogens on the enzyme determining the initial step in the conversion of tryptophan to niacin (Wolf et al. 1970; Lumeng et al. 1974).

The conversion of tryptophan to niacin shows some individual variation as well as some variation with the ratio of niacin to tryptophan in the diet (Nakagawa *et al.* 1969). Large doses of tryptophan are effective in the treatment of niacin deficiency or pellagra. On the other hand, pellagra is precipitated in people on a marginal niacin intake when the conversion of tryptophan to niacin is also impaired (Vilter *et al.* 1949).

The coenzymes NAD and NADP are concerned with hydrogen transport at the substrate level. Very many dehydrogenases require one or the other of these two coenzymes for activity. Coupling with oxidation-reduction sequences is necessary for NAD- and NADP-dependent reactions. The coenzymes NAD and NADP are important in carbohydrate metabolism, i.e., anaerobic and aerobic metabolism of glucose, in the TCA cycle; in lipid metabolism including fatty acid oxidation and synthesis, triglyceride synthesis, and steroid synthesis; in protein metabolism, in the degradation and synthesis of amino acids and in the pentose pathway (Kroger and Klingenberg 1970).

Among the NAD-dependent dehydrogenases, alcohol dehydrogenase, which catalyzes the conversion of ethanol to acetaldehyde is important in the present context. The question has been asked whether niacin deficiency or deficiency of NAD might decrease the rate of metabolism of ethanol and conversely whether administration of niacin would potentiate ethanol metabolism. In the rat, niacin treatment prevents the accumulation of fats in the liver, but keeps blood alcohol elevated. Indeed, it has been postulated that niacin blocks alcohol dehydrogenase activity when it is given in pharmacological amounts (Baker *et al.* 1973). However, physiological doses of niacin do not have a significant effect on alcohol metabolism via the alcohol dehydrogenase pathway. Disulfiram inhibits aldehyde dehydrogenase which normally oxidizes acetaldehyde to acetic acid, this effect being apparently due to a competition with NAD^+ (Graham 1951).

Nicotinamide coenzymes are necessary for mitochondrial and microsomal mixed function oxidations. For example, in the adrenal cortex, NADPH is required for reactions concerned with steroidogenesis, i.e. 11β-hydroxylation, cholesterol side chain cleavage, and 18-hydroxylation (Simpson and Estabrook 1969). NADPH is also necessary to microsomal drug oxidation reactions (Gillette *et al.* 1957).

Specific inactivating enzymes have been isolated for NAD-dependent apoenzymes and inactivation of these enzymes is protected by addition of the respective coenzyme. The activity of NAD-dependent enzymes decreases with niacin deficiency, because of effects of the degradative enzyme on the apoenzyme (Katunuma 1972).

Niacin deficiency may not only affect multiple and diverse endogenous metabolic systems, but may also impair drug metabolism through inactivation of biotransformation systems.

Niacin deficiency manifests itself clinically as pellagra, with the well known triad of dermatitis, diarrhea and dementia. The disease is slowly progressive with an initial phase of malaise followed by photosensitivity of the light-exposed skin, digestive disturbances including sore tongue, gastritis, and diarrhea, severe neurological disturbances, a confusional psychosis, depression, and wasting (Roe 1973). Drug induced pellagra has been associated with the intake of isonicotinic acid hydrazide, a vitamin B_6 antagonist, which interferes with the conversion of tryptophan to niacin (DiLorenzo 1967). It has been reported that antimetabolites, including 6-mercaptopurine and 5-fluorouracil may also cause pellagra (Barrett-Connor 1967) (Fig. 1.13).

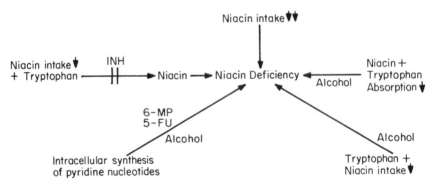

FIG. 1.13. CAUSAL FACTORS AND MECHANISMS OF PRODUCTION OF NIACIN DEFICIENCY INCLUDING THE ROLE OF DRUGS

Riboflavin.—Riboflavin is an essential dietary component. Its sources include milk, cheese, eggs, meats, whole grains and enriched cereals, green leafy vegetables and legumes such as peas and lima beans. The richest source is yeast. Most of the flavin present in food other than milk is in the form of the two flavin coenzymes, flavin mononucleotide (FMN) and flavin adenine dinucleotide (FAD). During the process of digestion the major part of these coenzymes is converted to free riboflavin. FAD is poorly absorbed but both FMN and free riboflavin are well absorbed at the levels usually ingested in the diet. Free riboflavin, present in breads and certain cereal products, is added as a part of the enrichment process (Aurand and Woods 1973).

There is evidence that riboflavin is absorbed from the proximal part of the small intestine. Enteric-coated or sustained release preparations of riboflavin are less well absorbed than other sources, presumably because they pass the optimal area in the intestine for absorption (Stripp 1965; Campbell and Morrison 1963).

Riboflavin absorption is increased in the presence of food within the intestinal tract. Levy and Jusko (1966), who made this observation, considered that this food-enhanced absorption of riboflavin might be due to a decrease in the intestinal transit rate so that the vitamin was retained in the neighborhood of the absorption sites. It has also been suggested by Levy and Hewitt (1971) that the potentiating effect of food on riboflavin absorption can be explained as being due to a food stimulation of bile output. These authors developed this hypothesis on the basis of an observation that persons with biliary obstruction show decreased riboflavin absorption (Jusko et al. 1971).

Riboflavin is phosphorylated in the intestinal mucosa during absorption. Absorption of the coenzyme form of riboflavin, riboflavin-5′-phosphate (FMN) shows the same saturation kinetics as riboflavin. It appears that in the process of absorption the coenzyme is dephosphorylated and then rephosphorylated (Stripp 1965; Jusko and Levy 1967).

There is reason to believe that riboflavin absorption is decreased by hypermotility of the intestinal contents and vice-versa. Hyperthyroidism or the administration of thyroxine decrease riboflavin absorption and hypothyroidism is associated with increased riboflavin absorption. Levy et al. (1972), who studied the effects of thyroid dysfunction in children on riboflavin absorption, concluded that the observed changes were due to alterations in the intestinal propulsive rate. It may be predicted that any drug which increases the rate of passage of intestinal contents, particularly those causing severe diarrhea, would decrease riboflavin absorption.

After riboflavin and FMN are absorbed from the intestinal tract, a large fraction of the vitamin and coenzyme are bound to plasma proteins, particularly albumin (Jusko and Levy 1969). Riboflavin may be displaced from plasma protein binding sites by drugs such as boric acid which complex with the ribityl side chain of the vitamin. Absorbed boric acid induces hyperexcretion of riboflavin either as the free vitamin, or as the borate complex (Roe et al. 1972).

Riboflavin is excreted in the urine and in the feces. Not only is the vitamin filtered in the glomerulus and reabsorbed in the proximal renal tubule, but also renal tubular secretion of riboflavin occurs in man (Levy and Jusko 1966). Riboflavin in the feces may be derived from nonabsorbed sources or from biliary secretions (Christensen 1969).

Riboflavin is stored mainly in the liver and the kidney. In the liver, free riboflavin is converted to FAD and FMN and very small amounts of free riboflavin are present in this tissue (Rivlin 1970). The enzymatic phosphorylation of riboflavin to form FMN involves ATP and the presence of the enzyme flavokinase. FMN is transformed to FAD by another reaction involving ATP and an enzyme FAD pyrophosphorylase. Thyroxine increases the activity of flavokinase (Rivlin and Langden 1969).

Hypothyroidism, whether associated with pathology or removal of the thyroid gland, or induced by administration of radioactive iodine or possibly thyroid antagonists, causes decreased tissue levels of FMN and FAD and also a reduced flavokinase activity. These changes in flavin coenzyme levels are similar to those found in riboflavin deficiency, as also is the reduction in flavokinase activity (Rivlin et al. 1968; Rivlin 1970).

FMN and FAD combine with specific apoenzymes to form the flavoprotein holoenzymes which participate in electron transport. From substrate, hydrogen atoms are transferred to flavoproteins either directly or through pyridine nucleotide intermediates. Flavin coenzymes are involved in many processes of intermediary metabolism including lipid metabolism, the biosynthesis of sterols in the adrenal gland, the intermediary metabolism of amino acids, certain pyrimidines, purines and pteridines (Horwitt and Witting 1972). The reduced forms can then be reoxidized with proton release. Pyridoxine phosphate oxidase, which is necessary to the conversion of pyridoxine phosphate to pyridoxal phosphate is also a flavoprotein (Goodwin 1963). The flavin coenzymes FMN and FAD are active components of the microsomal mixed function oxidase systems necessary to drug metabolism (Kamin 1969).

The classical signs of riboflavin deficiency include angular stomatitis, cheilitis, glossitis and localized dermatitis which may be limited to the face or extend to other parts of the body, more particularly the scrotum. Vascularization of the cornea and keratitis represent specific ocular signs (Sydenstricker 1941; Kruse et al. 1940).

Correlation between these clinical signs and biochemical evidence of riboflavin deficiency has not been good, and it has frequently been suggested that many of the signs previously attributed to riboflavin deficiency may either be non-specific or due to a deficiency of other B vitamins such as pyridoxine and folic acid. In a study by Rosenthal *et al.* (1973), riboflavin deficiency was identified in 50% of a group of alcoholic patients who were hospitalized for complicating diseases. Whereas these patients showed an increased erythrocyte glutathione reductase activity, indicative of a riboflavin deficit, classical physical signs of riboflavin deficiency were absent. Riboflavin deficiency in chronic alcoholism may be due to deficient intake of the vitamin, to defective absorption or, in the case of patients with cirrhosis, to impaired coenzyme synthesis. Unfortunately, there is no definitive work on this subject.

During nutritional rehabilitation of African children with marasmus and kwashiorkor, a condition of bone marrow hypoplasia affecting the red cell series has been identified. This is associated with an anemia with a response to the parenteral administration of riboflavin or prednisone (Foy *et al.* 1961; Kondi *et al.* 1963). The syndrome of red cell hypoplasia has been reproduced in baboons by feeding a riboflavin deficient diet. The deficient animals showed structural and functional changes in the adrenal cortex, as well as the erythroid hypoplasia. ACTH stimulation in the riboflavin deficient animals gave a very low or no response, indicating adrenal failure, which was confirmed by the histological finding of adrenal atrophy and hemorrhage at autopsy. Some of the baboons were given prednisone which reversed the erythroid hypoplasia but did not affect signs of riboflavin deficiency such as ulcerating dermatitis. These latter symptoms were reversed, as was the erythroid hypoplasia, by the administration of parenteral riboflavin. It is assumed, therefore, that marrow changes and resultant inhibition of erythropoiesis in riboflavin deficiency is due to secondary adrenal failure (Foy *et al.* 1972). A question which should be explored is whether drugs that induce erythroid hypoplasia or aplastic anemia act by causing adrenal atrophy secondary to riboflavin depletion.

Lane and Alfrey (1965) produced an anemia in human subjects by coadministration of a riboflavin deficient diet and the riboflavin antagonist galactoflavin. The anemia developed rapidly and was normochromic and normocytic. Reticulocytopenia was marked and there was selective erythroid hypoplasia of the bone marrow with maturational failure of the pronormoblasts. Incorporation of iron into the red cells was very markedly reduced during the period of riboflavin deficiency. These effects were reversed by the administration of riboflavin. It has been suggested that riboflavin deficiency causes an inhibition of activity of erythropoietin. On the basis of the primate studies and also the observed effects of prednisone on erythroid hypoplasia in riboflavin deficient children, it would appear that riboflavin deficiency interferes with the synthesis of adrenal glucocorticoids and that this, in turn, may impair the production or release of erythropoietin by the kidney.

In the rat, riboflavin deficiency induces changes in the hepatocytes with fragmentation of the endoplasmic reticulum. It has also been shown in these experimental animals that chronic riboflavin deficiency decreases the activity of drug-metabolizing enzymes, a condition which is reversed by the feeding of riboflavin (Tandler et al. 1968; Patel & Pawrr 1974). These findings suggest that chronic drug intake, which requires increased activity of drug-metabolizing systems in the liver, may possibly increase riboflavin requirements (Fig. 1.14).

Thiamin.—Significant food sources of thiamin include whole cereal grains, nuts, pork and eggs. Milk and potatoes furnish important quantities of this vitamin when they are used extensively. Legumes are a fairly good source of thiamin. Thiamin losses occur with food preparation, particularly with respect to beans and baked products (Aurand and Woods 1973). Foods enriched with thiamin include breakfast cereals, white flour, corn meal, breads, pasta and milk modifiers.

Thiamin, at least in the rat, is absorbed from the small intestine by active transport. Thiamin analogs, such as pyrithiamine and chloro-ethylthiamine, inhibit the active transport of thiamin and it has been

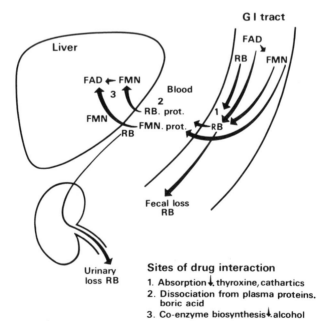

Sites of drug interaction
1. Absorption ↓ thyroxine, cathartics
2. Dissociation from plasma proteins. boric acid
3. Co-enzyme biosynthesis ↓ alcohol

FIG. 1.14. FLAVIN ABSORPTION, TRANSPORT, BIOTRANS-FORMATION AND EXCRETION IN MAN

suggested that the structure of the thiamin molecule conditions inter-action with a specific intestinal carrier (Komai *et al.* 1974; Komai and Shindo 1974).

Amprolium, which is used in the prophylaxis of coccidiosis in poultry, prevents thiamin absorption, and it has been suggested that this is why this drug prevents the development of coccidial infections (Polin *et al.* 1963). Although thiamin is synthesized by intestinal bacteria, it appears that little if any of this source of the vitamin is available to man (Friedemann *et al.* 1948).

Phosphorylation of the vitamin is necessary to the formation of the coenzyme form of thiamin, thiamin pyrophosphate. The principal sites of phosphorylation are the liver, the erythrocytes, and the cells of the cerebral cortex (Rindi *et al.* 1962; Deus and Blum 1970; Sharma and Quastel 1965). It has been suggested by Fennelly *et al.* (1967) that in alcoholics with severe cirrhosis there is a failure of the liver to convert thiamin to the metabolically active form.

Thiamin functions in the enzymatic catabolism of pyruvic acid and in the decarboxylation of alpha-ketoglutaric and other α-keto acids. In severe thiamin deficiency, blood pyruvate levels are elevated, as are blood levels of α-ketoglutarate. Elevation of blood pyruvate concentrations in thiamin deficiency can be emphasized by carrying out the test after a glucose load. Thiamin pyrophosphate is required by the enzyme transketolase which participates in oxidative carbo-hydrate metabolism. Transketolase functions in relation to ribulose-5-phosphate metabolism and catalyzes the production of ribose from glucose, ribose synthesis being necessary for nucleotide formation. Erythrocyte transketolase activity is now used as a functional test of thiamin status. It is a particularly useful test to detect minor degrees of thiamin deficiency (Sauberlich 1967).

Severe dietary deficiency of thiamin causes the development of the disease beri-beri and, in alcoholics, thiamin deficiency is associated with the development of Wernicke's encephalopathy. Thiamin defi-ciency in alcoholics may be due to deficient intake of the vitamin, impaired absorption or, as already discussed, to impaired formation of the coenzyme form of the vitamin. A delayed therapeutic response of alcoholic subjects with Wernicke's encephalopathy to administra-tion of thiamin may be due to hepatic injury or to slow recovery of neurons (Fennelly *et al.* 1967; Cole *et al.* 1969).

Alcoholics with thiamin deficiency may show a characteristic peripheral neuropathy (Fennelly *et al.* 1967). The requirement for thiamin may be increased in patients receiving digitalis alkaloids. Increased serum pyruvate levels have been found in patients with digitalis intoxication (Zbinden 1962).

Ascorbic Acid.—Rich sources of vitamin C in the diet include citrus fruits and fruit juices, other fresh fruits, especially black currants, green peppers, tomatoes, cabbage, cauliflower, broccoli, green beans and peas, as well as breakfast cereals and fruit beverages fortified with the vitamin. Massive intake of vitamin C may have certain deleterious effects, although it has recently been advocated and popularized for the prevention and treatment of the common cold (Pauling 1970). A small group of paraplegics taking 1 gm of vitamin C daily to keep their urine acid were shown by Murphy and Zelman (1965) to have low serum vitamin B_{12} levels. Vitamin C in high dosage reduces serum vitamin B_{12} levels as measured microbiologically (Herbert 1964). Massive amounts of ascorbate also destroy vitamin B_{12} in food, and it has therefore been suggested that large amounts of the vitamin should not be taken with meals (Herbert and Jacob 1974). An inhibitory effect of high vitamin C intake on beta-carotene utilization has been demonstrated (Mayfield and Roehm 1956; Bieri 1973). The vitamin is readily absorbed from the small intestine, and readily excreted into the urine when the tissues are saturated (Burns 1965).

High concentrations of vitamin C are found in the pituitary gland, the adrenal cortex, the corpus luteum, the thymus, liver, brain, testes, ovaries, thyroid, pancreas, kidney and also in the leukocytes and platelets. ACTH administration causes a depletion of adrenal ascorbic acid but this does not have an adverse effect on the synthesis of adrenal steroids (Pirani 1952). In rats, cortisone and dihydrocortisone have been shown to decrease the ascorbic acid content of the liver (Nathani and Nath 1972). Cortisone also increases plasma ascorbic acid levels in rats fed an adequate diet, but not in riboflavin-deficient animals (Chatterjee and Ghosh 1970). The ascorbic acid concentration of the plasma and leucocytes is decreased by intake of contraceptive steroids (Rivers and Devine 1970; McLeroy and Schendel 1973). McLeroy and Schendel (1973) have suggested that contraceptive steroids may decrease the intestinal absorption of ascorbic acid, or that they may stimulate the metabolism of the vitamin. Harris *et al.* (1973) obtained experimental evidence that ascorbic acid is metabolized more quickly by women taking oral contraceptives.

Ascorbic acid functions in relation to the oxidation-reduction reactions of the body. It plays a major role in biological hydroxylation reaction. It is essential for the normal synthesis of collagen, and elastin. During the formation of collagen, ascorbic acid is required for the enzymatic hydroxylation of peptide-bound proline to form hydroxyproline. The vitamin also participates in the hydroxylation of lysine as it occurs in protocollagens. Hydroxylation of elastin proline is vitamin C dependent. It has been suggested but not confirmed that the vitamin is necessary to normal collagen protein synthesis (Barnes and Kodicek 1972).

Ascorbic acid may also function in mixed function oxidase systems. In animals such as the rat, which synthesize ascorbic acid, drugs that stimulate drug-metabolizing enzymes also promote the synthesis of this vitamin. The vitamin influences the metabolism of drugs, and in guinea pigs metabolism of zoxazolamine is impaired by ascorbic acid deficiency (Conney et al. 1961). Conney and Burns (1962) have shown that ascorbic acid-deficient animals metabolize many drugs inadequately.

According to Coffey and Wilson (1975), many drugs are capable of inducing tissue desaturation of ascorbic acid, including alcohol, anorectic agents, anticonvulsant drugs as well as tetracycline. Among the drugs shown to cause tissue depletion of ascorbic acid, aspirin is the most important. Aspirin is known to cause a reduction in platelet levels of ascorbic acid.

Vitamin C deficiency is associated with the development of scurvy. In experimental scurvy production in human subjects, the first changes were biochemical, with decreased urinary excretion of ascorbic acid and decreased plasma values for the vitamin. The initial clinical signs of deficiency include follicular hyperkeratosis of the thigh, buttocks, calves and backs of the arms. These are followed by perifollicular hemorrhages, conjunctival hemorrhages, and oozing or bleeding-and-swollen gums (Hodges et al. 1969).

Subclinical vitamin C deficiency has been reported to be frequent among drug addicts (Davis and Rose 1973); presumably the etiology is multifactorial.

Fat-Soluble Vitamins Significantly Affected by Drugs

Vitamin D.—Numerous drugs have been shown to affect the absorption or metabolism of vitamin D. These drugs include laxatives, antacids, anticonvulsants, and certain sedatives such as glutethimide, diphosphonates and corticosteroids. Among these drugs the anticonvulsants, glutethimide, aluminum hydroxide, and laxatives such as mineral oil and phenolphthalein have been shown to produce clinical signs of vitamin D deficiency with the development of rickets or osteomalacia.

Vitamin D or derivatives of vitamin D are necessary for the uptake of calcium from the intestinal tract, and the normal mineralization of bone. In the light of recent investigations, it can be stated that sterols, within the vitamin D class, function in an analogous manner to steroid hormones. Whenever or however vitamin D deficiency is produced in children, rickets results; in adults, a similar deficiency causes osteomalacia. All substances which prevent or cure rickets and osteomalacia are deemed antirachitic. Certain sterols of plant or animal origin, when irradiated with ultraviolet light, acquire antirachitic potential (Olson and DeLuca 1973). The most widely distributed sterol with provitamin D properties, in vertebrates, is 7-dihydrocholesterol. This sterol, which is closely related to cholesterol, has been isolated from the epidermis and sebaceous glands of many mammals, and there is evidence for its biosynthesis within sebaceous tissue (Windaus and Bock 1937; Wheatley and Reinertson 1958; Gaylor 1962). Conversion of 7-dihydrocholesterol to vitamin D (cholecalciferol) apparently occurs in the human epidermis, since cholecalciferol or vitamin D_3 has been isolated from epidermal extracts (Rauschkolb et al. 1969).

Ergosterol is the main provitamin D in plants, and its synthesis follows the same general pathway as that of cholesterol. Vitamin D_2 is formed from ergosterol through a pathway involving photochemical intermediates. Irradiated ergosterol is used to fortify foods, and as a source of vitamin D_2 in nutrient supplements (Olsen and DeLuca 1973).

Most common foods are poor natural sources of vitamin D. It is present in certain species of fish, in egg yolk, in liver from fish, bird and mammalian sources, in butter and milk. Milk, though an inferior natural source, is fortified with this vitamin in a number of countries. In the United States, liquid whole and skim milk, evaporated milk, and non-fat dried milk are fortified either with vitamin D_2 or D_3. Certain breakfast cereals and infant formulas are similarly fortified. In eggs, vitamin D is confined to the yolks and its concentration in this portion is variable, being dependent on the amount of vitamin D supplied in chicken feed and the amount of sunlight to which the birds are exposed. Fish liver oils are the most concentrated natural sources of vitamin D (Kutsky 1973).

While it has been stated that normal adults do not require a dietary source of vitamin D, this may be misleading since the conclusion assumes exposure to sunlight—a condition which may not be achieved by those living in urban communities or those who are, by custom, heavily clothed, or those who are house-bound. Field studies, as well as the reports of monitored ultraviolet light exposure on people on a vitamin D deficient diet, have indicated that the amount of vitamin D produced in the skin varies with the degree of actinic conversion of this provitamin at wavelengths between 290 and 320 nm. This actinic conversion depends, in turn, on climatic conditions, air pollution, skin pigmentation, the mode of dress, area of skin exposed, and duration of exposure, as well as the use or otherwise of light barriers (Allende 1972; Hodgkin et al. 1973). Adults who, for one reason or another, are screened from the sun require dietary sources of vitamin D to prevent osteomalacia. Exogenous vitamin D is also indispensible to infants and children as well as pregnant and lactating women whose requirements are higher due to bone growth or skeletal mineral replacement under physiological stress (Yendt et al. 1969).

Vitamin D_3, formed in the skin of man, is probably absorbed via the cutaneous lymphatics. Ingested vitamin D is absorbed preferentially from the duodenum and jejunum and, to a lesser extent, from the ileum. Intestinal absorption is promoted by dietary lipids, and there is a requirement for the intraluminal presence of bile salts to achieve optimal uptake (Thompson et al. 1969). Absorbed vitamin D from the diet is secreted into the lacteals, and it can be recovered from the intestinal lymph with the chylomicra (Avioli and Haddad 1973). In studies using tritiated vitamin D_3, Blomstrand and Forsgren (1967) showed that in normal human subjects absorption of the vitamin is maximal four hours after administration. These workers were able to recover the labeled vitamin from lymph samples collected through a thoracic cannula. In a patient with biliary obstruction they found that only a very small amount of tritiated D_3 could be recovered from the lymph. Vitamin D from both the cutaneous and intestinal sources may be taken up into the liver directly from the lymphatic system, or may reach the general circulation via the thoracic duct, and thereafter pass to the liver. Endogenous and exogenous vitamin D are mixed after absorption and either metabolized in the liver or passed to storage depots in adipose tissue and muscle (Rosenstreich et al. 1971; Mawer and Schaefer 1969). Vitamin D is transported in the plasma, bound to a specific protein having the characteristics of an alpha-globulin (Peterson 1971).

The initial step in the metabolism of vitamin D is hydroxylation in the 25 position by the liver (Suda et al. 1970; Blunt et al. 1968). This reaction is regulated by the activity of the hepatic enzyme, calciferol-25-hydroxylase. There is evidence from animal studies that the levels of this enzyme are regulated by the concentration of vitamin D_3 at the site of hydroxylation. The 25-hydroxylation system is also conditioned by negative feedback of the reaction product, 25-hydroxycholecalciferol (25-HCC) (Bhattacharyya and DeLuca 1973). Vitamin D_2 is hydroxylated in the liver to form 25-hydroxyergocalciferol (25-HEC). Like the parent vitamins, 25-HCC and 25-HEC are transported in the plasma, bound to a globular protein or proteins (Smith and Goodman 1971).

The hepatic metabolite of vitamin D_3, 25-HCC, is metabolized in the kidney to yield several distinctive hydroxylation products, including 1,25-dihydroxycholecalciferol (1,25-DHCC). The controlling factor determining the type of metabolite produced may be the intracellular calcium concentration.

In the vitamin D-deficient animal on low calcium and phosphate intake, 1,25-DHCC is the most active form of vitamin D_3 in both the intestinal mucosa and bone. Under more normal circumstances of vitamin D and mineral intake, or in conditions of hypercalcemia, another renal metabolite of 25-HCC, 24,25-dihydroxycholecalciferol (24,25-DHCC) is the usual dihydroxy metabolite of vitamin D_3 in the plasma. When 24,25-DHCC is administered at low dosages over a period of time, there is stimulation of intestinal calcium transport, but mobilization of bone calcium does not occur. Delayed effects of 24,25-DHCC have been attributed to the further conversion of this vitamin D metabolite to 1,24,25-trihydroxycholecalciferol (1,24,25-THCC) which may act to promote calcium uptake at the intestinal site. While formation of the renal metabolites of vitamin D occurs as long as the existent mitochondrial system is intact, 1-hydroxylation is critical for the intestinal binding of active metabolites, i.e. 1,25-DHCC or presumably 1,24,25-THCC (Avioli and Haddad 1973; Haussler 1974).

The intestinal mucosal sites of action of the renal metabolites of vitamin D have been investigated. After administration of 1,25-DHCC, intestinal binding initially involves a cytoplasmic receptor protein, and this is followed by association of the steroid with the chromatin fraction of the intestinal mucosal cells (Chen and DeLuca 1973; Tsai and Norman 1973). Patrick (1973) has also shown that 1,25-DHCC is bound to the microvillar membrane of the intestine where it causes structural reorganization of this brush border to effect calcium absorption.

While a number of renal metabolites of vitamin D have been demonstrated, only the function of 1,25-DHCC is well understood. This metabolite exerts primary control of calcium transport in the intestine. Calcium transport across the mucosal epithelial cell involves passage across the brush border and exit from the basal membrane. It has been shown in animal experiments that passage of calcium across the intestinal mucosal cell is mediated by a calcium-binding protein which is synthesized or released in response to the presence of this active form of vitamin D. Evidence suggests that this calcium-binding protein acts to provide an effective carrier system (Wasserman 1969). In the intestine, active vitamin D metabolites stimulate mucosal growth as well as protein synthesis (Urban and Schedl 1969). It is suggested that several metabolites of vitamin D may stimulate intestinal calcium absorption but that none are as effective as 1,25-DHCC.

Bone calcium mobilization activity is manifested by 1,25-DHCC and, to a lesser extent, by 24,25-DHCC. It seems likely that the vitamin D metabolite which primarily causes bone calcium resorption in mammals, including man, may be 1,25-DHCC, though its exact site or mode of action has not been established (Raisz et al. 1972).

The interrelationships between vitamin D metabolites, parathyroid hormone, and calcitonin in calcium homeostasis are complex. The hypocalcemic action of calcitonin is due to inhibition of bone resorption and calcium release, but this hormone also may have a selective function in determining which of the renal metabolites of vitamin D will be produced. Parathyroid hormone acts on the kidney and gut to regulate plasma calcium by controlling its absorption and excretion. At the renal site of action, parathyroid hormone reduces calcium clearance and enhances phosphate excretion, while on the gut it increases calcium absorption, apparently through stimulated renal synthesis of 1,25-DHCC (Garabedian et al. 1972).

Inactivation and excretion of vitamin D metabolites have been studied. Biliary and, to a lesser extent, urinary excretion occurs. Glucuronides are formed, these being the terminal inactive metabolites of vitamin D which are eliminated in the urine. The rate of production of these inactive metabolites appears to be dependent on the activity of a hepatic microsomal enzyme system (Avioli et al. 1967; Hahn et al. 1972).

While the statement is still valid that the development of rickets and osteomalacia is dependent on an absolute deficiency of vitamin D sterols or, ultimately, on a deficient availability of calcium and phosphate for bone mineralization, such deficiency is known to be brought about by numerous mechanisms. It should be clear from the foregoing account that vitamin D-dependent calcium deficiency with osteopenia will arise not only when there is inadequate synthesis of cholecalciferol in the skin, or when dietary intake of plant or animal sources of the vitamin are low, but also if there is inadequate absorption of vitamin D, or if formation of the active metabolites is impaired, or the inactive metabolites are formed to excess. Rickets or osteomalacia can also result from severe phosphorus depletion.

Drugs can cause vitamin D deficiency in a number of different ways, which can be explained on the basis of present knowledge of the synthesis and metabolism of this vitamin (Fig. 1.15). Physical and chemical ultraviolet light barriers, used as topical medications to protect photosensitive persons, could impair the cutaneous synthesis of vitamin D_3. Absorption of dietary sources of vitamin D is diminished by pharmacologic agents which bind bile acids, because, as previously stated, bile acids are necessary to the optimal absorption of vitamin D_2 and D_3. Glucocorticoids in high and prolonged dosage may inter-

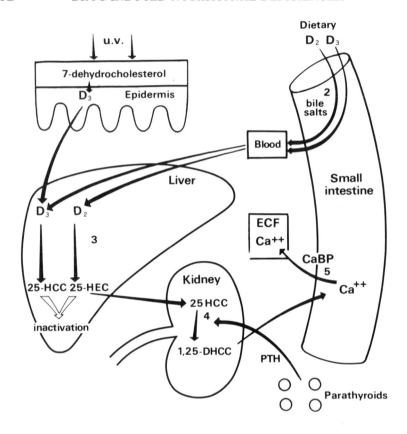

Sites of drug interaction

1. Light barriers   3,5. Anticonvulsants
2. Bile acid sequestrants   4. Diphosphonates

FIG. 1.15. VITAMIN D SOURCES, ABSORPTION, MAJOR METABOLIC
PATHWAYS AND EFFECT ON CALCIUM ABSORPTION

fere with the hepatic metabolism of vitamin D and reduce the plasma levels of 25-HCC. Drugs and other foreign compounds which function as microsomal enzyme inducers in the liver cause an accelerated degradation of vitamin D_3 and 25-HCC to more inactive polar metabolites. Drug-stimulated hepatic microsomal enzyme activity is caused by a variety of compounds including sedatives, anticonvulsants, muscle relaxants, and certain oral antidiabetic agents. Four such drugs, phenobarbital, diphenylhydantoin, primidone, and glutethimide, have already been shown to accelerate the degradation of 25-HCC and to cause either rickets or osteomalacia. Another group of drugs, the diphosphonates, which have been used to treat Paget's disease, block the production of 1,25-DHCC in the kidney and have been shown to be capable of inducing osteomalacia. There is also evidence that medications such as mineral oil, which impair vitamin D-dependent calcium transport at the brush border of the intestinal mucosa, can cause vitamin D deficiency. Whether or not clinical vitamin D deficiency is the outcome of drug administration depends not only on the mechanism of action of the particular drug or drug group, but also on the dosage, duration of intake, exposure of the skin to sunlight or artificial sources of ultraviolet light, and dietary intake and storage of vitamin D sources. Insofar as drug-induced vitamin D deficiency has been identified in clinical practice, it is described in this text together with the relevant bibliography.

Clinical, Radiological and Biochemical Features of Vitamin D Deficiency.—Rickets is characterized by abnormal development of the skeleton and teeth. Clinical signs vary with the age of onset. In the infant under eight months of age, ossification of the skull is slow and irregular. The anterior fontanelle remains membranous for longer than normal; that is, instead of closing at the 18th month, it remains open until the second, third, or even the fourth year of life. Thickening of the bone around the centers of ossification of the frontal and parietal bones is the cause of the characteristic bosses on the skull known as "Parrot's nodes." The rounded elevations on the frontal and parietal bones, separated by the depressions formed by the sutures, may give the head a fanciful resemblance to a hot cross bun. In other areas of the skull such as along the occipitoparietal sutures, the bone is thin, and craniotabes is manifested. This sign, which is present in severe early rickets, is elicited by pressure over the thinned areas of the skull which indent and then snap back into position like a ping-pong ball. Thoracic signs develop early and may lead to respiratory difficulties. Inward bending of the lower ribs along the attachment of the diaphragm coupled with outward flowing of the lower ribs causes a circular depression of the chest known as "Harrison's Sulcus." Excess osteoid forming at the costo-chondral junctions produces localized enlargements, easily recognized on palpation, and constituting the "rickety rosary." Multiple rib fractures are common. Secondary respiratory disease is due to decreased thoracic capacity and mechanical function. Recurrent pulmonary infection, emphysema, and cor pulmonale may develop. Kyphoscoliosis and pelvic deformities occur in the child whose rickets is active after he or she has learned to sit up. The pelvic changes which tend to occur in the first year of life include forward projection of the sacrum and narrowing of the lateral walls. Bending deformities of the long bones occur in several cases, but the most constant change in the long bones is enlargement of the epiphyses, which is best seen at the ankle and wrist. Radiological changes at the lower end of the ulna and radius are present before other bony abnormalities develop. The ends of these bones are widened, the termination of the shaft becomes blurred and irregular, and rarifaction occurs behind the epiphyseal line. As the disease advances the spreading out of the ends of the long bones increases, and the shafts assume a crater like appearance. Radiological changes, in severe cases, involve the shaft with lamellated thickening of the cortex and then subperiosteal bone formation. The eruption of teeth is delayed and the teeth of the first dentition may be poorly formed and subject to early caries. Weak musculature is a common feature. Tetany is a rarer complication.

In classical rickets due to the combined effect of poor musculature and bony changes, the normal milestones of physical development are delayed. Indeed, retarded physical progress may alert the parents to seek medical advice (Sheldon 1943).

Owing to the reduced incidence of endemic rickets, the diagnosis may be missed. Further, since the drugs known to induce rickets are unlikely to be given in early infancy, it is uncommon to see drug-induced rickets with cranial changes unless the drug effects are super-imposed on rickets caused by the inadequate intake of vitamin D or inadequate exposure to sunlight.

Biochemical indicators of rickets include combined hypocalcemia, hypophosphatemia, and increased serum alkaline phosphatase activity. Isolated finding of any one of these biochemical abnormalities is in-sufficient evidence on which to base a diagnosis of vitamin D defi-ciency (Sauberlich 1974).

Normally the product of serum calcium $\times$ serum phosphorus, each expressed in mg/100 ml serum, is about 60. In rickets, this product is often 40 or less, but there are cases in which the serum calcium is re-duced to tetany levels and yet the serum phosphorus is normal. Ele-vation of serum alkaline phosphatase levels above 13 King-Armstrong units, followed by or coexisting with a decreased product of serum calcium and serum phosphorus, is highly suggestive of a diagnosis of rickets. Confirmation of this diagnosis requires radiological evidence of distal ulnar epiphyseal changes and/or decreased bone mineral mass, estimated by photon absorptionometry.

As in the case of other vitamin deficiencies, it is usually stated that the diagnosis is proven by therapeutic trials; i.e., the clinical, radiologic and biochemical signs of the disease should be reversed by administra-tion of vitamin D in adequate dosage. Assumption that cure can be affected by vitamin D therapy requires qualification. Whether the vitamin D can be absorbed, whether it can be metabolized to form active products, and whether induction of calcium transport can be affected thereby, all require consideration. In drug-induced vitamin D deficiency, as in genetically determined vitamin D deficiency, the dose level of the vitamin required to counteract the disease may exceed the levels recommended for the cure of classical rickets.

The cause and even the diagnosis of drug-induced deficiency of vitamin D are likely to be overlooked, because its major occurrence is within institutionalized groups of patients receiving anticonvulsants who might be prone to vitamin D depletion because they have a poor diet or because they are kept indoors. Moreover, within such a group there will be a high incidence of children having bony abnormalities due to prenatal causes, so that a diagnosis of rickets goes unsuspected. Vitamin D deficiency in patients on anticonvulsants has only been recognized in very recent times, and this is probably due to confusion with other diagnoses. Drug-induced vitamin D deficiency can also be superimposed upon cases of depletion of this vitamin associated with malabsorption syndromes.

Osteomalacia differs from rickets in clinical signs and radiographic appearances, the variations in the two syndromes of vitamin D deficiency being due to the age factor only. Unlike rickets, osteomalacia occurs after the completion of bony growth. Therefore, the typical rachitic changes of the provisional zones of ossification are lacking. Pain is a common symptom, being localized as a rule to the back and thighs, shoulder region or ribs. Widespread softening of bones occurs but cases vary one from another in the portions of the skeleton which are most involved. Deformities of the pelvis, thorax and long bones may be present. In severe cases, kyphoscoliosis may reduce height and cause the head to sink forward onto the chest. Bones tend to bend rather than fracture, though pathological fractures are not uncommon, particularly of the ribs. A waddling gait is brought about by pelvic and femoral deformities together with moderate to severe muscular weakness. As in rickets, tetany may develop. Incomplete fractures of the pubic rami, femoral neck or the border of the scapula or the upper end of the humerus (Looser's zones) are diagnostic.

Osteomalacia should be suspected in drug users when the presenting symptoms are those of bone pain, progressive difficulty in walking, and weakness of the proximal limb muscles. Evidence of generalized decalcification of the skeleton, with or without more specific radiologic signs, such as Looser's zones, rib fractures and long bone deformities, would support the diagnosis. Biochemical findings are entirely similar to those of rickets, and include changes in the serum calcium and phosphorus levels, together with elevated serum alkaline phosphatase.

A reliable method of diagnosis is the iliac crest bone biopsy which reveals osteoid seams with absorption and atrophy of the bone trabeculae (Bartter, 1963; Hodgkin *et al.* 1973; Christiansen *et al.* 1973; Nordin 1973).

Vitamin K.—Vitamin K has been known as the antihemorrhagic factor, because it is necessary to the normal coagulation of the blood. At least two naturally-occurring forms of the vitamin are found and, of these, vitamins K_1 and K_2 have been shown to be capable of preventing hemorrhagic states due to lowering of prothrombin levels. Vitamin K_1 is found in green leafy vegetables such as spinach, kale, cabbage and collard greens. This form of the vitamin, also known as phylloquinone, is produced by the photosynthetic portions of plants. Vitamin K_2, or menaquinone, is synthesized by intestinal bacteria in man as well as in other animals. Vitamin K is found in high concentrations in liver, particularly pork liver, and eggs and milk contain small amounts. The vitamin K in these latter food sources may be derived from green plants or from bacterial synthesis (Aurand and Woods 1973). Vitamin K_3, a synthesized form of the vitamin, is used therapeutically. It is closely related in structure to menaquinone (Matshiner 1969).

All three forms of vitamin K are lipid soluble.[1] Vitamin K_1 is absorbed, at least in the rat, in the upper part of the small intestine as an active, energy-mediated process. Uptake of vitamin K_1 is as a micellar solution, potentiated by the presence of bile salts (Hollander 1973). Vitamin K_3 is absorbed by the distal portion of the small intestine and this has been shown to consist in a passive transport mechanism. Absorption of vitamin K_3 is not affected by the presence or otherwise of bile salts. The structural resemblance of vitamin K_2 to vitamin K_3 would suggest that the former may also be absorbed by passive transport and that this may take place in the lower portion of the small intestine (Hollander and Truscott 1974).

Vitamin K deficiency in man has not been produced by administration of a vitamin K free diet. It is therefore assumed that the intestinal synthesis of vitamin K_2 can supply the human needs for vitamin K, and therefore this form of the vitamin must be absorbed, perhaps as with vitamin K_3, in the lower part of the small intestine, though it would seem likely that the colon can absorb vitamin K_2 also by a passive transport process. However, at present there is no proof for this hypothesis.

---

[1] Water soluble derivatives of vitamin K_3 (menadione) are available for clinical usage.

In man, vitamin K_1 is transported by the lymphatic system (Blomstrand and Forsgren 1968). Presumably vitamin K in its different forms can reach the liver either via the lymphatic circulation or directly through the portal system.

An adequate supply of vitamin K is necessary in order to maintain physiological levels of the clotting factors II, VII, IX and X in the blood. These factors, i.e. prothrombin (II), proconvertin (VII), Christmas factor (IX) and Stuart-Prower factor (X) are collectively known as the vitamin K-dependent clotting factors. When their concentrations are abnormally low in the plasma, vitamin K deficiency is indicated (Olson 1970). Seegers et al. (1968) proposed that prothrombin is an aggregate protein consisting of different vitamin K-dependent clotting factors, which are separately synthesized and then combined together. The mechanism whereby vitamin K activates prothrombin has now been elucidated. In the liver, vitamin K_1 exists in at least two forms, as phylloquinone, and as phylloquinone-2,3-epoxide (Matschiner et al. 1970). Oxidation of vitamin K_1 to this epoxide through the activity of phylloquinone epoxidase has been studied in rats by Willingham and Matschiner (1974). They found that epoxidase activity is stimulated if plasma prothrombin levels are lowered either by anticoagulants or by vitamin K deficiency. The activity of this enzyme is restored to normal when vitamin K is administered. At least in the rat, in which these studies were conducted, it appears that conversion of the vitamin K epoxide to vitamin K under the influence of a reductase enzyme is necessary to vitamin K activity. Vitamin K is necessary for the post-ribosomal modification of the K-dependent clotting factors, allowing biological activity and calcium binding of prothrombin. A peptide has been isolated from bovine prothrombin that contains the vitamin K-dependent portion of the molecule. The properties of this peptide apparently account for the differences between prothrombin and its inactive precursor (Nelsestuen and Suttie 1973). Peptides have now been isolated both from prothrombin and from factor X which contain at least a portion of the vitamin K-dependent part of the molecule (Nelsestuen et al. 1974).

Vitamin K deficiency is manifested by an increased bleeding tendency. Hemorrhage may take place from epithelial surfaces, causing bleeding from the gastrointestinal tract, the urinary tract, the uterus and the nasal mucosa. Ecchymoses are not uncommon. Hemorrhage may also take place from other sites of injury, surgery, or pre-existing tissue damage. Hypoprothrombinemia and decreased plasma levels of the other active K-dependent clotting factors is frequently drug-

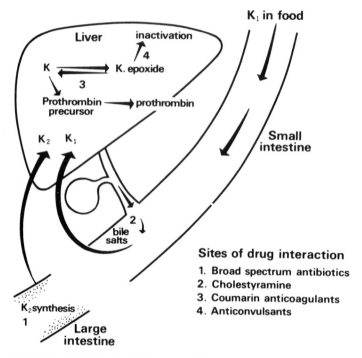

FIG. 1.16. VITAMIN K, SOURCES, ABSORPTION AND METABOLISM

induced. Administration of broad spectrum antibiotics can decrease synthesis of vitamin K_2 by intestinal microorganisms but no untoward effects with respect to vitamin K status result unless vitamin K intake is inadequate. Several drugs have been shown to decrease vitamin K absorption, notably mineral oil and the bile acid sequestrant, cholestyramine. The most common group of drugs to cause vitamin K deficiency are the coumarin anticoagulants. Since 1943 it has been known that aspirin and other salicylates can induce hypoprothrombinemia with a hemorrhagic diathesis. Dicumarol potentiates this hypoprothrombinemic effect, and it can be overcome by administration of vitamin K (Link *et al.* 1943; Quick and Clesceri 1960; Fausa 1970) (Fig. 1.16).

Vitamin A.—The vitamin A content of the diet comprises sources of the preformed vitamin as well as carotenes with vitamin A activity. Forms of vitamin A occurring naturally include retinol, or vitamin A_1 alcohol, dehydroretinol, or vitamin A_2 alcohol, aldehyde derivatives of these two forms, as well as esters of retinol and dehydroretinol. In the human diet retinol esters represent more than 90% of the intake of preformed vitamin A. Rich sources of vitamin A as the retinyl ester include milk and milk products, liver, kidney, and fish. The free retinyl form is the predominant form of vitamin A in eggs (Plack 1965).

Beta-carotene is the most valuable precursor of vitamin A in our diet. Excellent sources of β-carotene in the American diet include carrots, sweet potatoes, and yellow corn. Other substantial sources of carotenes include dark green, leafy vegetables, winter squash, broccoli, apricots, pumpkin and tomatoes (Thompson 1965). Dietary deficiency of vitamin A occurs in people living on a cereal diet lacking both preformed vitamin A and carotene sources. Retinyl esters in the diet are hydrolized to retinol in the small intestine. Retinol is then absorbed in micelle form through the action of bile salts. Inside the mucosal cells, retinol is re-esterified preferentially with palmitic acid. Retinyl palmitate travels in chylomicra via the lymphatic system to the blood and is then stored in the liver. Each molecule of β-carotene is enzymatically cleaved to two molecules of retinal and then the retinal is reduced to retinol in the intestinal mucosa. β-Carotene and other carotenoids are also absorbed without cleavage. Optimal absorption of vitamin A sources requires the presence of dietary fat, the integrity of the exocrine pancreas which can supply lipase to break down retinyl esters, and the availability of bile salts to promote uptake of retinol and carotenes (Roels 1970; Fidge *et al.* 1969).

A number of drugs can impair vitamin A absorption. Mineral oil acts as a solvent for carotene, and to a lesser extent, for vitamin A itself, which then are carried down the intestine and pass out of the body in the feces. Neomycin decreases the absorption of vitamin A by several mechanisms, through inhibition of pancreatic lipase, through inactivation of bile salts, and by causing mucosal damage. Cholestyramine decreases vitamin A absorption by adsorbing bile salts. Other drugs which damage the intestinal mucosa also decrease vitamin A absorption (Fig. 1.17).

In spite of these drug effects on the absorption of carotenes and vitamin A, the risk of clinical deficiency of vitamin A is low in countries such as the U.S. where there are ample dietary sources of vitamin A and vitamin A precursors. In Southeast Asia, the Philippines and in other countries where dietary deficiency of vitamin A is prevalent, it may be predicted that drugs which impair vitamin A absorption can have serious consequences and precipitate clinical manifestations of vitamin A deficiency.

Hepatic stores of vitamin A include retinyl palmitate, stearate, and oleate. These forms are hydrolyzed in the liver and the free retinol is then bound to a specific retinol-binding protein for transport to tissues

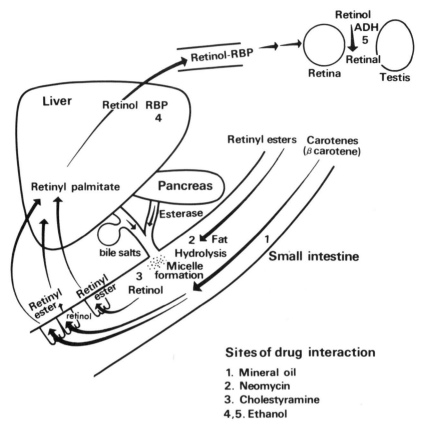

FIG. 1.17. VITAMIN A ABSORPTION, TRANSPORT, STORAGE AND UTILIZATION

requiring vitamin A. Vitamin A is not only required for specific visual function, but also is necessary for the synthesis of mucopolysaccharides and, more especially, for the stabilization of cellular and intracellular membranes. Also, it may be necessary to the synthesis of normal steroid metabolites (Thompson 1965; Fell 1965).

The two major physiological functions of vitamin A require conversion of retinol to retinal through an oxidation process requiring the activity of alcohol dehydrogenase (ADH) and the coenzyme function of NAD (Wald and Hubbard 1960). Retinol-dependent physiological processes include the visual cycle and spermatogenesis. Impaired conversion of retinol to retinal can result from competitive utilization of alcohol dehydrogenase in the metabolism of other substrates including ethanol. Alcohol dehydrogenase metabolizes ethanol preferentially because of its higher affinity for this enzyme (Von Wartberg 1971). Van Thiel *et al.* (1974) have carried out studies which indicate that in alcoholics, as well as in alcohol-treated rat testicular tissue, failure of conversion of retinol to retinal may provide a mechanism to explain sterility. These workers showed that, *in vitro*, testicular tissue can promote retinal formation and that formation of this form of vitamin A is inhibited by ethanol oxidation. The amounts of ethanol necessary to inhibit retinal formation are low and below the range found in alcoholic persons. Based on older studies of male chronic alcoholics with hepatic cirrhosis, and recent unpublished studies of chronic alcoholics with mild liver impairment, these authors suggest that alcoholism is a common cause of male sterility in the U.S. and this may be explained by interference with vitamin A metabolism.

Night blindness has long been accepted as the classical early sign of vitamin A deficiency. Alcoholics may become night blind because of competitive inhibition of retinal formation from retinol by ethanol (Mezey and Holt 1971). Other factors may contribute to signs of vitamin A deficiency in alcoholics, including poor intake of the vitamin, malabsorption, and failure of hepatic synthesis of retinol-binding protein (Fig. 1.17).

Vitamin E.—Tocopherols, which are collectively considered as dietary vitamin E, occur in vegetable oils including soybean oil, nuts, wheat germ oil, eggs, liver, and margarines. It has been pointed out by Bieri and Poukka Evarts (1974) that today, gamma-tocopherol is a more common form of vitamin E than alpha-tocopherol in the daily diets because of increased usage of edible fats and oils made from soybean oil. Vitamin E requirements are increased with intake of polyunsaturated fatty acids.

α-Tocopherol absorption follows fat absorption, and factors that affect the one also affect the other. It has been suggested that a necessity for bile in α-tocopherol absorption might be secondary to the effect of bile salts on the absorption of fat (Gallo-Torres 1970). In the rat, cholestyramine decreases α-tocopherol absorption more especially if the tocopherol is fed with long chain fat diets rather than medium chain fat diets (Losowsky *et al.* 1972). Absorption of α-tocopherol is slightly better than that of δ-tocopherol. Tocopherols are taken up into the lymph vessels of the intestinal mucosa (lacteals) in chylomicra, and reach the general circulation where the tocopherols are transported in association with lipoproteins, particularly the higher density lipoproteins. The level of total tocopherol in the serum is related to the levels of certain lipid fractions and to the total lipid content of the serum. Thus, if the total serum lipids are high, the serum tocopherol levels are high, and vice-versa. Administration of triiodothyronine (T3) to normal subjects produced a fall in vitamin E levels of the plasma as well as plasma cholesterol. While the peroxide hemolysis procedure has been widely used as a test of vitamin E status, the results of the test are directly influenced by serum tocopherol levels, and these in turn are influenced by the serum lipid levels. Therefore, it would appear that the test may be invalidated unless the serum lipid levels are known to be within a moderate range (Horowitz *et al.* 1972).

Weiss and Bianchine (1969) described patients with hyperlipoproteinemia who had raised serum vitamin E levels. Seven patients with hypercholesterolemia and eight with hypertriglyceridemia showed a reduction in their serum lipids when they were given the drug clofibrate, and a functionally related experimental drug, SU-13437. Concurrently serum vitamin E levels were decreased, and returned to pretreatment levels when the drugs were withdrawn. The authors think it is likely that the explanation for these drug effects is that carrier lipoprotein for vitamin E is diminished, with fewer carrier sites available for the vitamin. A vitamin K-dependent coagulation defect has been reported in a patient on Warfarin, who was also taking vitamin E at moderately high dosage and clofibrate (Colligan and Marcus 1974). The appearance of ecchymoses on this patient's skin and excessive prolongation of the prothrombin time followed addition of vitamin E to the treatment regimen. These evidences of vitamin K deficiency were reversed when vitamin E treatment was discontinued, but Warfarin therapy was continued, as well as clofibrate. It is suggested in this report that vitamin E may interfere with vitamin K utilization in man. In laboratory animals, hypervitaminosis E causes a prolongation of the prothrombin time and a hemorrhagic condition that can be reversed by administration of vitamin K (Mellette and Leone 1960).

Various functions have been attributed to vitamin E, but in reality very few functions have been identified. As a lipid antioxidant, vitamin E prevents the production of toxic lipid peroxides in the tissues. Increased knowledge of the selenium-glutathione (Se-GSH) peroxidase system has shown that vitamin E has a highly specific function in many and perhaps all tissues. Inhibition of peroxidation is related to activity of the Se-GSH peroxidase system. Breakdown of lipid peroxides to hydroxy fatty acids by Se-GSH peroxidase protects cell components from the toxic effects of peroxide and also stops a further breakdown of these peroxides to free radicals which can then again initiate peroxidation. Vitamin E works synergistically with the Se-GSH peroxide reduction system, providing a chain-breaking reaction effect against peroxide formation which is additive to the hydroperoxide-reduction effect of the Se-GSH peroxidase (Tappel 1974).

A number of syndromes of vitamin E deficiency have been described in man. However, in most of these conditions the common characteristic is one of steatorrhea and decreased serum lipid levels. Patients believed to have vitamin E deficiency include those with biliary, pancreatic, or intestinal disease characterized by excessive loss of lipids in the feces. Such diseases include chronic pancreatitis, Whipple's disease, and the hereditary disease, abetalipoproteinemia. In these conditions evidence of vitamin E deficiency has been obtained from the hydrogen peroxide hemolysis test, and also low serum tocopherol levels. In view of the previously mentioned association between low serum lipids and decreased serum tocopherol levels, and the further association between low serum tocopherol levels and a positive hydrogen peroxide hemolysis test, it may be questioned whether these subjects with diseases associated with steatorrhea can really be said to have a true vitamin E deficiency (Binder and Spiro 1967).

Binder and his colleagues (1967) observed a few subjects who they considered to have a severe vitamin E deficiency. In these persons there was a focal necrosis of muscle and a severe peripheral neuromyopathy. It has been suggested that these patients show an analogous disease to that seen with vitamin E deficiency in experimental animals. In infants a syndrome of vitamin E deficiency has been described in which there is no gross evidence of steatorrhea. The infants who are premature exhibit edema, anemia, shortened erythrocyte survival time, positive hydrogen peroxide hemolysis tests, and low serum tocopherol levels. The syndrome appears to be associated with a high intake of polyunsaturated fatty acids in formulas. It has been reversed by administration of vitamin E (Ritchie et al. 1968).

It has been shown that absorption of vitamin E is defective in premature infants. Hemolytic anemia associated with vitamin E deficiency in these infants is exacerbated by therapeutic iron administration (Gross and Melhorn 1972).

Aftergood and Alfin-Slater (1974), observing the effects of contraceptive steroids on rats, thought that these resembled vitamin E deficiency. Lowering of plasma α-tocopherol levels was found in rats receiving a contraceptive steroid. It is suggested that this change could be due to an effect of the oral contraceptives on lipoprotein distribution.

Minerals Significantly Affected by Drugs

Iron.—Major sources of iron in the diet include muscle meats, fish, poultry, liver, kidney, heart, and egg yolk. Other dietary sources of iron include shellfish, cocoa, molasses, green vegetables such as spinach, and enriched flour and cereals. Much of the iron ingested is in a complex form either as iron porphyrin or heme, or as iron protein complexes. The iron added to cereals is commonly reduced iron, though in certain instances ferrous sulfate has been used for fortification. Heme iron, present in meats and other animal protein foods, except milk, is split from bound protein by digestion and is absorbed into the mucosal cells of the small intestine as heme (Conrad 1970). Heme iron is better absorbed than other sources of iron in the diet. Ferrous iron sources, either used in fortification of foods or as iron supplements, are absorbed more efficiently than iron from ferric salts or ferric complexes (Bannerman 1965; Brise and Hallberg 1962).

Certain dietary constituents and metabolites present within the intestinal lumen promote the absorption of non-heme iron. These include ascorbic acid, meats including poultry and fish, fructose, sorbitol and certain organic acids including succinic, lactic, pyruvic and citric acids (Brise and Hallberg 1962; Monsen et al. 1974; Jacobs and Miles 1969; Herndon et al. 1958; Pollack et al. 1964). Several amino acids enhance iron absorption (Kroe et al. 1963). Certain dietary constituents depress iron absorption, including phosphate and phytates (Peters et al. 1971; Hegsted et al. 1949).

Certain drugs have been shown to depress iron absorption, both in experimental animals and in man. Benjamin et al. (1967) showed that bicarbonate depresses iron absorption in guinea pigs. This may have significance in patients who habitually take large quantities of bicarbonate as an antacid. Greenberger (1973), using intestinal loops from rats, showed that tetracycline depressed the mucosal uptake or transfer of radioiron. However, changes in iron absorption were only produced when tetracycline was administered in doses far exceeding those used therapeutically in human subjects. It was found by this author that tetracycline treatment caused an inhibition of protein synthesis in the intestinal mucosa and it has been postulated that the impaired iron uptake and this alteration in protein synthesis are associated. In healthy human subjects, serum iron levels have not been found to be decreased by tetracycline administration.

Neuvonen et al. (1970) have shown that inorganic iron preparations depress blood levels of certain antibiotics including tetracycline, oxytetracycline, methacycline, and doxycycline. Greenberger (1973) has also carried out experiments in which it was shown that cholestyramine binds both inorganic and heme iron *in vitro*, and further, that in rats cholestyramine impairs the absorption of inorganic iron. According to this author, long-term cholestyramine treatment in rats results in decreased non-heme iron stores.

Both many intraluminal and extraluminal factors affect iron absorption. Gastric acid potentiates iron absorption, principally by its effect on the digestion of iron compounds in the diet. Iron status affects the uptake of iron by the mucosal cells of the small intestine, the transport across the mucosal cell, and the transport out of the mucosal cell. Van Campen (1974), who has summarized our present knowledge of the effects of iron status on iron absorption, has commented that iron lack activates systems especially designed to increase iron uptake and transport by the mucosal cells of the intestine, and that iron overload causes mechanisms to be activated which depress iron uptake. Iron is preferentially absorbed from the proximal portion of the small intestine and most efficiently in the duodenum (Hastings-Wilson 1952).

Iron losses are by desquamation of cells from the gastrointestinal tract, the urinary tract, as well as from the skin. Iron losses may be by hemorrhage, which may be physiological, as in menstruation and pregnancy losses; pathological, or from the adverse effect of certain drugs (Finch 1969). Aspirin intake in doses of 1-3 gm/day can induce occult bleeding in the gastrointestinal tract in about 70% of normal subjects. Aspirin may also play a role in causing gastric hemorrhage in certain patients with pre-existing gastrointestinal disease, including peptic ulcer, esophageal varices, and alcoholic gastritis (Weiss 1974). A number of authors, including Callender (1973), consider that chronic intake of aspirin or other salicylates is a prominent cause of iron deficiency anemia.

After absorption from the gastrointestinal tract, iron is transported in the plasma bound to transferrin. Levels of transferrin in the plasma are increased by administration of estrogens or contraceptive steroids (Cartei et al. 1970; Horne et al. 1970).

The unsaturated iron-binding capacity of transferrin may determine the rate of transfer of iron from the intestinal mucosa to the serum. Transferrin binds to intestinal epithelial cell membranes, and enhances the release of iron from these cells (Nutrition Reviews 1973).

Based on animal experiments, Levine et al. (1972) have postulated that transferrin performs a shuttle role for iron. Newly saturated transferrin is readily released from intestinal binding; the iron is then transported to the bone marrow where it is released, and the transferrin is once more unsaturated and able to take up more iron, presumably at the intestinal site.

In studies by Norrby et al. (1972) it has been shown that combination oral contraceptives increase iron absorption, and it has been suggested that this occurs because of high transferrin concentrations. Whether or not iron absorption is increased by all oral contraceptives has not been demonstrated and the author has shown that serum iron levels are not necessarily raised in women on contraceptive steroids (Roe *et al.* unpublished).

Transport, utilization, storage and catabolism of iron-containing compounds requires the alternate conversion of ferrous to ferric iron. Oxidation of the ferrous iron which is absorbed is accomplished by ferroxidases, including the copper-containing protein, ceruloplasmin (Osaki *et al.* 1971). Plasma ceruloplasmin values are increased in persons taking estrogens or oral contraceptives (Wallach 1974; Miale and Kent 1974).

Serum iron is mainly derived from iron in the reticuloendothelial system, where it is stored as the polymer, ferritin. It was previously thought that xanthine oxidase catalyzed the detachment of iron from ferritin, but since allopurinol, an inhibitor of xanthine oxidase, does not affect mobilization of iron from storage sites, this theory has been refuted. A ferritin reductase system occurs in the liver which is capable of detaching iron from ferritin; this system requiring NADH and FMN. Iron released from ferritin is picked up by transferrin and delivered to the sites of iron utilization, including the red cell precursors in the bone marrow. The iron must then be reduced so that it is available for hemoglobin synthesis and presumably for synthesis of other iron-containing compounds such as myoglobin and the cytochromes. Insertion of iron into the immediate heme precursor, protoporphyrin IX, requires activity of the enzyme ferrochelatase, which is present in the liver and in the reticulocytes (Frieden 1973). In some way, presently unexplained, vitamin B_6 antagonists, such as INH, impair the uptake of iron into protoporphyrin and are capable of causing sideroblastic anemia (Tanaka and Bottomly 1974).

Prior to the destruction of effete erythrocytes by the spleen, hemoglobin is oxidized to methemoglobin and concomitantly, the ferrous iron is converted into the ferric forms. Normally, iron liberated by physiological hemolysis is either reutilized for heme synthesis or is stored as ferritin. There is evidence, both from rat studies and in man, that acute hemolysis such as that produced by drugs, increases iron absorption (Manis and Schachter 1966; Pirzio-Biroli and Finch 1960), which suggests that depletion of iron stores is not the sole determinant for the uptake of further iron from the intestine (Fig. 1.18).

Zinc.—The best food sources of zinc are animal protein foods including meat, eggs, milk products and fish, especially shellfish. The zinc content of vegetables and cereal grains varies according to the soil on which they are cultivated and the methods of storage and food preparation. Zinc may also be a contaminant in foods coming from galvanized cooking vessels (Osis *et al.* 1972). Limited information is

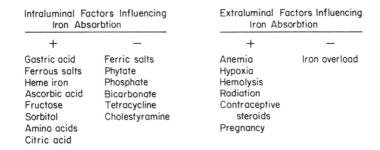

Intraluminal Factors Influencing Iron Absorbtion		Extraluminal Factors Influencing Iron Absorbtion	
+	−	+	−
Gastric acid	Ferric salts	Anemia	Iron overload
Ferrous salts	Phytate	Hypoxia	
Heme iron	Phosphate	Hemolysis	
Ascorbic acid	Bicarbonate	Radiation	
Fructose	Tetracycline	Contraceptive	
Sorbitol	Cholestyramine	steroids	
Amino acids		Pregnancy	
Citric acid			

Drug Determinants of Chronic Excessive Loss of Iron

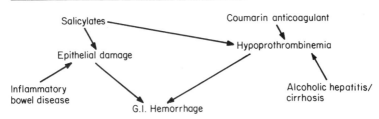

FIG. 1.18. DRUGS AND DIETARY CONSTITUENTS AFFECTING IRON ABSORPTION AND LOSS FROM THE GASTROINTESTINAL TRACT

available on the absorption of zinc, but presently available data from animal experiments suggest that zinc is preferentially absorbed in the proximal part of the small intestine, and that, like iron, only a portion of the ingested zinc may be absorbed (Methsessel and Spencer 1973). In the rat, it appears that zinc absorption is regulated by the zinc content of the duodenal mucosa (Evans and Grace 1973).

A number of dietary constituents may impair the absorption of zinc. The most important of these is the presence of high levels of phytate in the diet, as in some cereal grains. Intake of phytate is high among low income people in Egypt and Iran who habitually eat whole wheat unleavened bread, and it is among these people that symptoms of zinc deficiency have been primarily observed (Reinhold et al. 1973).

Zinc is an essential component of carbonic anhydrase and of a number of other metalloenzymes. Notably, certain enzymes necessary to cellular oxidative processes, such as alcohol dehydrogenase, are zinc dependent (Parisi and Vallee 1969; Mikac-Devic 1970). Zinc is also necessary to normal protein synthesis and is required for the incorporation of sulfur-containing amino acids into certain tissue proteins (Hsu et al. 1969).

A role for zinc in vitamin A metabolism has been identified by Smith et al. (1973). It was found by these workers that vitamin A is not mobilized from the liver in zinc deficiency and it has been suggested that zinc may be involved possibly in the synthesis or function of retinol-binding protein. In pigs it has been shown that zinc deficiency depresses serum vitamin A levels (Stevenson and Earle 1956). There is also evidence that zinc deficiency interferes with vitamin A utilization, probably because the zinc-dependent enzyme, alcohol dehydrogenase, is necessary to retinol oxidation in tissues such as the liver, retina and testes.

Transport of zinc in the blood involves binding of the mineral to several plasma proteins and amino acids. The work of Boyett and Sullivan (1970) indicated that zinc is tightly bound to transferrin and to alpha-2-macroglobulin. Parisi and Vallee (1970) isolated α-2-macroglobulin from serum and showed that it contained 30 to 40% of total serum zinc. For many years, it has been known that zinc is bound to plasma albumin, though it has been suggested that zinc is easily detached from this binding site (Vikbladh 1951). Prasad and Oberleas (1970) studied amino acid binding of zinc in vitro and concluded that binding to specific amino acids may be important in zinc transport. Giroud and Henkin (1972) found that cysteine and histidine are the most important amino acid ligands for zinc in plasma. On the basis of their work and that of others they have concluded that albumin is the plasma component that binds exchangeable zinc and that serum amino acids compete for zinc bound to albumin. A relative increase in the concentration of amino acids that bind zinc may result in a transfer of zinc from albumin and promotion of zinc loss by renal filtration.

Several states and syndromes of zinc deficiency have been described which are reversible or partially reversible by zinc administration. There is, however, a curious diversity of symptoms which is presently not well explained. Zinc deficiency is believed to be the cause of dwarfism, gonadal immaturity and anemia in some Iranian and Egyptian boys and girls; deficiency arising in these youngsters because dietary zinc is bound to phytate and hence is unavailable for absorption. Halsted et al. (1974) have suggested that growth retardation in cystic fibrosis and other malabsorption states may be due to zinc deficiency, presumably because of excessive loss of zinc in the feces.

In alcoholics, evidence of vitamin A deficiency, including impairment of dark adaptation and testicular dysfunction, may be attributed to the utilization of alcohol dehydrogenase for the oxidation of ethanol, or it is possible that there may be an impaired activity of alcohol dehydrogenase due to an associated zinc deficiency (Meazy and Holt 1971; Van Thiel and Lester 1974). Excessive urinary excretion of zinc which occurs in chronic alcohol imbibers with and without cirrhosis (Vallee *et al.* 1959; Sutherland 1962) may be secondary to hypoalbuminemia and decreased binding of zinc to albumin causing a relative increase in glomerular filtration of zinc. Hypoalbuminemia has been associated with reduction in serum zinc levels in cirrhosis patients (Walker *et al.* 1973) and in the dwarfed middle Eastern boys (Caughey 1973).

A syndrome of hypogeusia (decreased taste acuity), dysgeusia (abnormal taste sensation), hyposmia (decreased sense of smell), and dysosmia (abnormal smell sensation) has been found amenable to treatment with zinc supplements (Henkin *et al.* 1971). Interestingly hypogeusia and hyposmia have occurred in certain people receiving the chelating agent, D-penicillamine, perhaps because of excretion of a zinc chelate in the urine (MacFarlane 1974).

There have been a number of reports which have linked zinc deficiency to delayed wound healing (Sandstead and Shepard 1968; Miller *et al.* 1965). Sandstead *et al.* (1970) who studied the effect of zinc depletion in rats on the closure of surgically produced wounds, confirmed that deficiency of this mineral retards healing and they further demonstrated that zinc supplementation of normal animals will not promote healing of incisions. They suggest that the role of zinc in tissue repair is in some way related to zinc's role in nucleic acid or protein synthesis. Delayed wound healing associated with zinc deficiency has been reported in man by Flynn *et al.* (1973).

It is possible that the effects of corticosteroids on zinc status may be related to induced catabolism of lean body mass with the breakdown of zinc-containing or other proteins, the formation of zinc-amino acid complexes in the plasma, and hence increased renal loss of zinc (Fell *et al.* 1973).

Serum zinc (or plasma) levels are depressed in women receiving contraceptive steroids, and it has been demonstrated that it is the estrogen component of these drugs that causes lowering of serum zinc (Halsted *et al.* 1968; McBean *et al.* 1971). This may be a reflection of alterations in levels of transferrin and α-2-macroglobulin, brought about by contraceptive steroids, leading to changes in zinc binding and perhaps secondary hyperexcretion. There has been no evidence of any zinc deficiency in women on these drugs (Fig. 1.19).

Magnesium.—Magnesium is widely distributed in articles of diet, including animal protein foods, cereals and green legumes and green vegetables where it is derived from chlorophyll. Limited intake of magnesium may occur in milk-based diets and also in binge drinking alcoholics whose total food intake is very low (Aurand and Woods 1973). Absorption of magnesium apparently occurs in all portions of the small intestine, although there are some data to indicate that

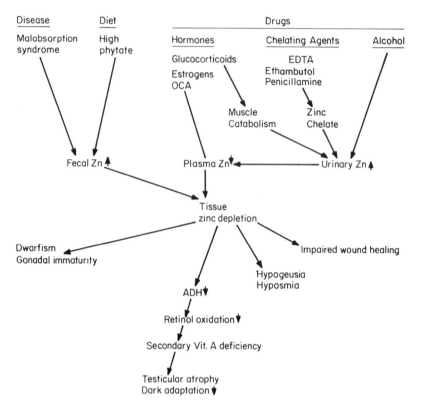

FIG. 1.19. CAUSES AND CONSEQUENCES OF ZINC DEPLETION

maximal absorption occurs in the proximal portion of the small intestine. Vitamin D may influence magnesium absorption (Guenter and Sell 1971; George *et al.* 1962).

Magnesium is predominantly an intracellular component, being concentrated in the mitochondria, and is an important activator of many enzyme systems including ATPase, coenzyme A and enzymes that are concerned with ribosomal protein synthesis. In man, magnesium deficiency is associated with neuromuscular dysfunction, characterized by tetany, seizures, ataxia, muscle weakness, tremors, behavioral disturbances and lowered magnesium levels in the serum. Deficiency occurs usually as a result of excessive gastrointestinal loss or renal loss of this mineral (Wacker and Parisi 1968). Intracellular magnesium depletion and hypomagnesemia occur commonly in chronic alcoholics and appears to arise through the combined effects of a poor diet and hyperexcretion of magnesium in the urine (Lim and Jacob 1972A). Hypomagnesemia combined with alkalosis are believed to be the factors which induce seizures and other symptoms of delirium tremens associated with alcohol withdrawal (Victor 1973).

Fankushen *et al.* (1964) have indicated that profound hypomagnesemia in alcoholics may not only be due to their poor diet and to the renal losses of magnesium, but also to gastrointestinal losses brought about by vomiting and sometimes diarrhea. These authors have noted a slow response in alcoholics to magnesium supplementation.

Numerous diuretics increase the urinary excretion of magnesium including chlorothiazide, hydrochlorothiazide, ammonium chloride and mercurial diuretics (Wacker and Parisi 1968). Smith *et al.* (1962), while studying magnesium depletion caused by various diuretics, noted that this depletion caused an increased sensitivity to digoxin induced arythmias.

Hypomagnesemia has been commonly associated with malabsorption syndromes which may be drug-induced. Wacker and Parisi (1968) have suggested that the steatorrhea may be the main cause of magnesium loss because of the excretion of large quantities of magnesium soaps.

A lowering of serum magnesium associated with hemodilution has been observed in patients with acute intermittent porphyria. Abnormal electrolyte and water metabolism in these patients is associated with an inappropriate secretion of antidiuretic hormone. Attacks of acute intermittent porphyria are frequently drug-induced, more particularly when barbiturates are administered (Hellman *et al.* 1962) (Fig. 1.20).

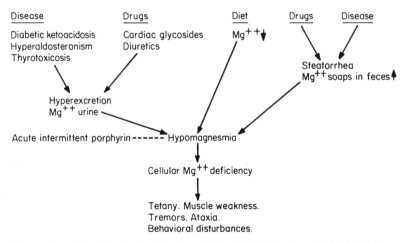

FIG. 1.20. DETERMINANTS, CONSEQUENCES AND EFFECTS OF HYPOMAG-NESEMIA

CLASSIFICATION OF DRUG-NUTRIENT INTERACTIONS

A very large number of drug-nutrient interactions have been proposed, but only a few of these actually lead to nutrient depletion or deficiency. Effect of drugs on nutrients can be divided into several categories according to whether the pharmacologic agent affects nutrient synthesis, absorption, transport, storage, metabolism, or excretion.

Effects of Drugs on Nutrient Synthesis

Physical and chemical ultraviolet light barriers may decrease synthesis of vitamin D in the skin. Broad spectrum antibiotics can decrease endogenous microbial synthesis of vitamin K_2 in the colon. Limited use of light barriers as well as the availability of vitamins D and K from other sources accounts for the fact that these drug effects are rare or insignificant causes of nutrient depletion.

Effects of Drugs on Nutrient Absorption

Drug-induced impairment of nutrient absorption can be divided into several categories. The drug may provide a vehicle for nutrient solution. For example, mineral oil can dissolve dietary carotene, which is then lost to the normal absorptive process and passes out in the feces. Drugs can adsorb or interfere with the physiological activity of bile salts so that fats and fat-soluble vitamins requiring bile salts for their optimal absorption are taken up inefficiently from the intestinal tract. Drugs can induce cellular damage of the intestinal mucosa, nutrient loss being dependent on the site, extent and duration of the cellular injury. Selective interference with transport mechanisms for nutrients can be drug-induced. Drugs can produce damage to the exocrine pancreas, causing decreased production and/or release of pancreatic enzymes and consequent maldigestion of fat, protein and starch (Fig. 1.21).

Effects of Drugs on Nutrient Distribution and Excretion

Displacement of nutrients from plasma protein- or tissue-binding sites may be effected by pharmacologic agents. The drug may complex with the nutrient which is then detached from the binding site, it may replace the nutrient on a protein-binding site, or produce a combined effect. Examples include the formation of Schiff bases between hydrazides such as isonicotinic acid hydrazide and pyridoxal, drug chelates formed with minerals such as zinc or copper, and complexes formed between borate and the ribityl side chain of riboflavin. Results of these drug-nutrient interactions are to promote renal excretion of the affected nutrients, either free or in a complex with

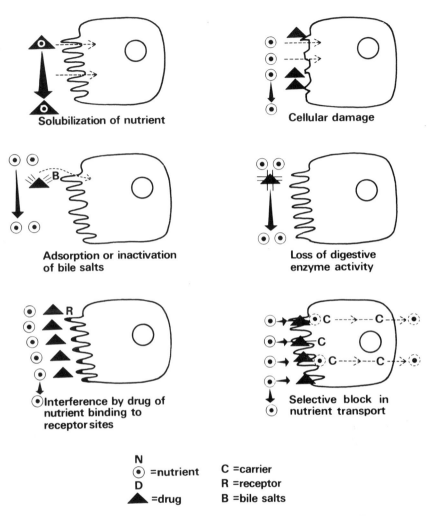

Solubilization of nutrient

Cellular damage

Adsorption or inactivation
of bile salts

Loss of digestive
enzyme activity

Interference by drug of
nutrient binding to
receptor sites

Selective block in
nutrient transport

N
⊙ =nutrient   C =carrier
D   R =receptor
▲ =drug   B =bile salts

FIG. 1.21. EFFECTS OF DRUGS ON NUTRIENT ABSORPTION

the drug. In either circumstance nutrient depletion may supervene
(Fig. 1.22).

Effects of Drugs on Nutrient Metabolism

Drugs can function as antivitamins by combining with or inhibiting
enzyme systems required for the conversion of vitamins to their
coenzyme or active forms. Interference with the physiological functions of active vitamins can also be brought about by drug-induced

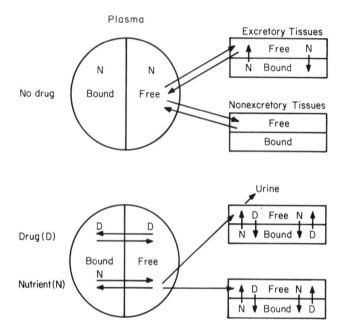

Competitive protein binding by drug increases free nutrient and promotes its excretion.

FIG. 1.22. TRANSFER OF NUTRIENTS (N) FROM PLASMA TO TISSUES AND EFFECT OF DRUGS

inhibition of enzyme systems, dependent on coenzyme function (Fig. 1.23).

Structurally unrelated drugs that stimulate the activity of microsomal drug-metabolizing enzymes can also stimulate the catabolism and reduce the body stores of fat-soluble and perhaps certain water-soluble vitamins (Roe 1974). It has been suggested that vitamin K deficiency, occurring in the infants of women receiving phenobarbital during pregnancy, occurs on this basis. Similarly, vitamin D deficiency and folate deficiency in people taking anticonvulsant drugs known to be hepatic microsomal-inducing agents are believed to occur because they increase nutrient turnover. The rate of metabolism of these vitamins in the body is believed to be increased with subsequent depletion (Fig. 1.24).

Nutrient Depletion from Drug-Nutrient Interactions

Clinical syndromes of nutrient depletion attributable to pharmacological agents arise most frequently on the following circumstances: 1) when drugs cause massive malabsorption; 2) when drugs affect nutrients participating in numerous metabolic functions, e.g. vitamin

1) Conversion of vitamin to coenzyme blocked

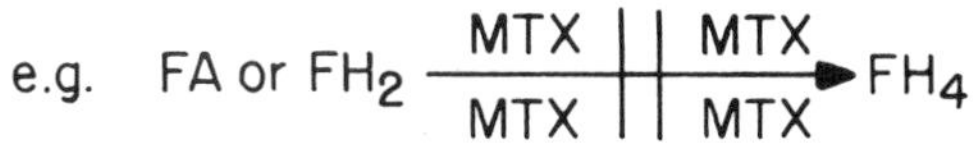

$$\text{e.g.} \quad \text{FA or FH}_2 \xrightarrow[\substack{\text{MTX} \quad \text{MTX} \\ \text{MTX} \quad \text{MTX}}]{} \text{FH}_4$$

2) Synthesis of active vitamin metabolite inhibited

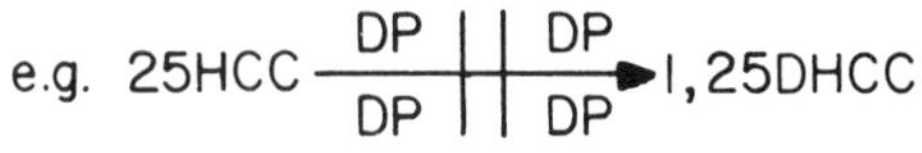

$$\text{e.g.} \quad \text{25HCC} \xrightarrow[\substack{\text{DP} \quad \text{DP} \\ \text{DP} \quad \text{DP}}]{} \text{1,25DHCC}$$

3) Retention of inactive form of vitamin promoted

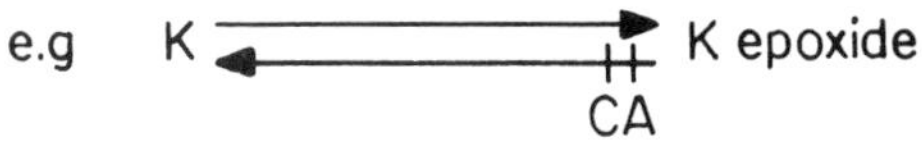

$$\text{e.g} \quad \text{K} \underset{\text{CA}}{\overset{\longrightarrow}{\longleftarrow}} \text{K epoxide}$$

$$
\begin{aligned}
\text{FA} &= \text{folic acid} \\
\text{FH}_2 &= \text{dihydrofolate} \\
\text{FH}_4 &= \text{tetrahydrofolate} \\
\text{MTX} &= \text{methotrexate} \\
\text{25HCC} &= 25 \cdot \text{hydroxycholecalciferol} \\
\text{1,25DHCC} &= 1,25 \cdot \text{dihydroxycholecalciferol} \\
\text{DP} &= \text{diphosphonate} \\
\text{CA} &= \text{coumarin anticoagulant}
\end{aligned}
$$

FIG. 1.23. DRUGS AS ANTIVITAMINS

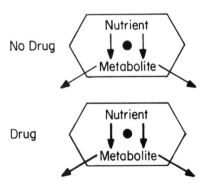

FIG. 1.24. CELLULAR CATABOLISM OF NUTRIENTS PROMOTED BY DRUGS FUNCTIONING AS MICRO-SOMAL ENZYME INDUCERS

B_6 or folate; 3) when drugs function as vitamin antagonists; 4) when drugs causing nutrient depletion are given for extended periods of time; and 5) when the drug-nutrient effects accentuate pre-existing subclinical malnutrition of dietary or disease origin.

Drug Absorption

It has been shown that most drugs are absorbed from the gastrointestinal tract by passive non-ionic diffusion. Active transport of drugs only operates in cases where drugs are substituted-purines, pyrimidines, or unusual amino acids. Drugs may also be absorbed by facilitated transport, apparently by passage through pores in the epithelial membranes, and also by pinocytosis, though these mechanisms do not appear to play a prominent role.

It has been generally accepted that a lipid membrane such as the gastrointestinal tract is permeable to lipid-soluble compounds and that highly ionized water-soluble substances will not get through as well. It is true that the drugs that are strong organic acids or bases are not well absorbed. However, the earlier viewpoint that weakly acidic drugs are mainly absorbed from the stomach and weakly basic drugs from the small intestine is not supported by fact. The small intestine has the greatest capacity for absorption of drugs as well as nutrients due to the very great extent of the mucosal surface area (Prescott 1974). The fact that most drugs, as well as most nutrients, are absorbed from the small intestine may explain why this is the major site of interaction. The idea that drug-induced malabsorption might commonly arise because of competition between drugs and nutrients for absorptive processes is not born out by fact, because of the lack of evidence of substrate competition for active transport processes between drugs and nutrients. There is, however, some evidence that drugs can inhibit the absorption of nutrients by interference with carrier systems, and, more particularly, by decreasing the availability of sodium necessary to the transport of many nutrients. Adverse effects of drugs on the absorption of water-soluble nutrients may be explained by the creation of cellular damage by those drugs. It has been shown that whenever a drug creates injury to the intestinal epithelium, there is an adverse effect on absorption. This, however, does not mean that drug-induced malabsorption is always due to cell damage (Levine 1971).

Drugs that interfere with the absorption of fats or fat-soluble vitamins do so mainly by creating a state of maldigestion. Thus, for example, drugs such as neomycin, which can inhibit pancreatic lipase, prevent the hydrolysis of long chain triglycerides. Similarly drugs that impair the availability of bile salts will diminish fat absorption as well as the absorption of fat-soluble vitamins that are dependent for their optimal absorption on the presence of bile salts. Increased gut motility, due for example to cathartic agents, may decrease nutrient absorption, though evidence presently available suggests that the changes in motility alone rarely induce malabsorption (Faloon 1970).

Effects of Antimetabolites

Advances in modern chemotherapy can be attributed in large part to the development of drugs which function as antimetabolites either in microorganisms or in mammalian cell systems. Control of metabolic diseases, infections, neoplastic processes, and thromboembolic disease has been made increasingly possible through the development of drugs which are amino acid analogs inhibitors of protein synthetase, purine and pyrimidine analogs, as well as antagonists to the water- and fat-soluble vitamins. Antimetabolite drugs which have been shown to have therapeutic efficacy are highly specific in their functions. Drugs which have been designed for antivitamin function may 1) inhibit the growth of microorganisms; 2) inhibit the growth or diminish the turnover of cells in malignant processes such as cancer, or benign processes such as psoriasis; 3) depress the clotting mechanism. Most antivitamins are structural analogs of vitamins functioning as essential nutrients. Certain antivitamins function as growth suppressants in bacterial systems because they interfere with the nutrient requirements of the microorganism. Whereas sulfa drugs behave as folate antagonists for microorganisms, they have no such effect in man. These drugs suppress the bacterial biosynthesis of folic acid by preventing incorporation of paraaminobenzoic acid into the pteridine moiety of the molecule. Human subjects are not at risk because they obtain their folate from exogenous sources.

Antivitamins either block coenzyme synthesis or inhibit enzymatic reactions dependent on coenzyme function. Effects of antivitamins may be reversed by the end products of the inhibited reactions, but only in some instances by an excess of the normal substrate (Woolley 1963; Goldstein et al. 1968).

Variability in Drug Metabolism

Whether or not a drug actually causes vitamin or other nutrient depletion may depend on the duration of drug activity within the body. The duration of drug activity depends upon its rate of metabolism as well as on the integrity of routes of drug elimination. The rate of drug metabolism depends upon both genetic and acquired factors. Genetic variability in the rate of metabolism of lipid-soluble drugs may not only influence their therapeutic action, but also their retention in the body so that they exert an adverse effect on nutritional status. Thus, for example, slow inactivators of isonicotinic acid hydrazide are more liable to develop vitamin B_6 deficiency than other persons.

The metabolism of one drug may be inhibited by another. For example, bishydroxycoumarin inhibits the metabolism of diphenylhydantoin. Prolonged administration of one drug may reduce the activity of another, because the first drug stimulates production of drug-metabolizing enzymes which cause inactivation of the second drug. On the other hand, if a drug, such as a coumarin anticoagulant, is first given independently at levels to establish therapeutic control, and then another drug, itself a stimulator of drug metabolism, such as phenobarbital, is added, the activity of the coumarin anticoagulant is reduced because of its increased rate of inactivation. If the phenobarbital is then withdrawn and treatment with the anticoagulant is continued without an appropriate decrease in dose, hemorrhage may follow due to the sudden increase in anticoagulant activity (Nies 1974).

Drugs functioning as microsomal enzyme-inducers not only stimulate the metabolism of other drugs, but also of normal body constituents, including vitamins. Individual variability in the rate and magnitude of vitamin depletion through this mechanism may reflect differences in the rate of drug biotransformation (Conney 1969).

Impaired renal or hepatic function may not only alter and slow the rates of metabolism of pharmacologic agents capable of causing nutrient depletion, but may also diminish the rate of elimination of such drugs (Reidenberg 1974).

BIBLIOGRAPHY

AFTERGOOD, L., and ALFIN-SLATER, R. B. 1974. Oral contraceptive-α-tocopherol interrelationships. Lipids 9, 91–96.

ALLENDE, M. F. 1972. The enigmas of pigmentation. J. Am. Med. Assoc. 220, 1443–1447.

ANDERSON, B. B. et al. 1971. Conversion of vitamin B_6 compounds to active forms in the red blood cell. J. Clin. Invest. 50, 1901–1909.

ANON. 1972. Conversion of vitamin B_6 compounds in human red cells. Nutr. Rev. 30, 119–121.

ANON. 1973. The role of transferrin in iron absorption. Nutr. Rev. 31, 131–132.

ANON. 1973. National Survey. Nutrition: A national priority. Information Canada, Ottawa.

AURAND, L. W., and WOODS, A. E. 1973. Food Chemistry. Avi Publishing Co., Westport, Conn.

AVIOLI, L. V. et al. 1967. Metabolism of vitamin D_3-^{3}H in human subjects: Distribution in blood, bile, feces and urine. J. Clin. Invest. 46, 983–992.

AVIOLI, L. V., and HADDAD, J. G. 1973. Vitamin D: current concepts. Metabolism 22, 507-531.
BAKER, H. et al. 1973. Inhibition by nicotinic acid of hepatic steatosis and alcohol dehydrogenase in ethanol-treated rats. Exp. Molec. Path. 19, 106-112.
BAKER, S. J., KUMAR, S., and SWAMINATHAN, S. P. 1965. Excretion of folic acid in bile. Lancet 1, 685.
BANERJEE, S. P., and SNYDER, S. H. 1973. Methyltetrahydrofolic acid mediates N- and O-methylation of biogenic amines. Science 182, 74-75.
BANNERMAN, R. 1965. Quantitative aspects of hemoglobin-iron absorption. J. Lab. Clin. Med. 65, 944-950.
BARNES, M. J., and KODICEK, E. 1972. Biological hydroxylations and ascorbic acid with special regard to collagen metabolism. In Vitamins and Hormones 30, Academic Press, New York and London.
BARRETT-CONNOR, E. 1967. The etiology of pellagra and its significance in modern medicine. Am. J. Med. 42, 859-867.
BARTTER, F. C. 1963. Osteomalacia. In Cecil-Loeb Textbook of Medicine, 11th Edition, P. B. Beeson, and W. McDermott (Editors). W. B. Saunders Co., Philadelphia and London.
BAUGH, C. M. et al. 1975. Absorption of folic acid poly-α-glutamates in dogs. J. Nutr. 105, 80-89.
BAYLESS, T. F. 1969. Intestinal deconjugation of dietary folate. New Eng. J. Med. 280, 1019.
BENJAMIN, B. I., CORTELL, S., and CONRAD, M. E. 1967. Bicarbonate-induced iron complexes and iron absorption: One effect of pancreatic secretion. Gastroenterology 53, 389-396.
BHATTACHARYYA, M. H., and DeLUCA, H. F. 1973. The regulation of rat liver calciferol-25-hydroxylase. J. Biol. Chem. 248, 2969-2973.
BIERI, J. G. 1973. Letter. Effect of excessive vitamins C and E on vitamin A status. Am. J. Clin. Nutr. 26, 382-383.
BIERI, J. G., and POUKKA EVARTS, R. 1974. Gamma-tocopherol: Metabolism, biological activity, and significance in human vitamin E nutrition. Am. J. Clin. Nutr. 27, 980-986.
BINDER, H. J., and SPIRO, H. M. 1967. Tocopherol deficiency in man. Am. J. Clin. Nutr. 20, 594-601.
BLAKLEY, R. L. 1969. The Biochemistry of Folic Acid and Related Pteridines, North Holland Publishing Co., Amsterdam and London.
BLOMSTRAND, R., and FORSGREN, L. 1967. Intestinal absorption and esterification of vitamin D_3-1,2^{3}H. Acta Chem. Scand. 21, 1662-1663.
BLOMSTRAND, R., and FORSGREN, L. 1968. Vitamin K_1-^{3}H in man. Its intestinal absorption and transport in the thoracic duct lymph. Intern. Abstra. Vitamin Forsch. 38, 45-64.
BLUNT, J. W., DeLUCA, H. F., and SCHNOES, H. K. 1968. 25-Hydroxycholecalciferol: a biologically active metabolite of vitamin D_3. Biochem. 7, 3317-3322.
BOOTH, C. C., and BRAIN, M. C. 1962. The absorption of tritium labelled pyridoxine in the rat. J. Physiol. 164, 282-294.
BOYETT, J. D., and SULLIVAN, J. F. 1970. Distribution of protein-bound zinc in normal and cirrhotic serum. Metabolism 19, 148-157.
BRAIN, M. C., and BOOTH, C. C. 1964. The absorption of tritium-labelled pyridoxine. HCl in control subjects and in patients with malabsorption. Gut 5, 241-247.
BRISE, H., and HALLBERG, L. 1962. Absorbability of different iron compounds. Acta Med. Scand. 171, (Suppl. 376) 23-51.
BROCKLEHURST, J. C. et al. 1968. The clinical features of chronic vitamin deficiency. A therapeutic trial in geriatric hospital patients. Geront. Clin. 10, 309-320.
BROWN, J. P. et al. 1973. Ingestion and absorption of naturally occurring pteroylmonoglutamates in man. Gastroenterology 64, 223-232.

60   DRUG-INDUCED NUTRITIONAL DEFICIENCIES

BUCHANAN, J. M. 1964. The function of vitamin B_{12} and folic acid co-enzymes in mammalian cells. Medicine *43*, 697-709.
BURNS, J. J. 1965. Ascorbic acid (vitamin C) in the pharmacological basis of therapeutics. *In* Water Soluble Vitamins, 3rd Edition, L. S. Goodman, and A. Gilman (Editors). Macmillan Co., New York.
BURNSTEIN, L. H., GUTSTEIN, S. and WEINER, S. V. 1970. Gamma-glutamyl carboxypeptidase (conjugase), the folic acid-releasing enzyme of intestinal mucosa. Am. J. Clin. Nutr. *23*, 919-925.
CALABRESI, P., and WELCH, A. D. 1965. Cytotoxic drugs, hormones, and radioactive isotopes. *In* The Pharmacological Basis of Therapeutics, L. S. Goodman, and A. Gilman (Editors). Macmillan Co., New York.
CALLENDER, S. T. 1973. Fortification of food with iron—is it necessary or effective? *In* Nutritional Problems in a Changing World, D. Hollingsworth, and M. Russell (Editors). Applied Sci. Publishers, London.
CAMPBELL, J. A., and MORRISON, A. B. 1963. Some factors affecting the absorption of vitamins. Am. J. Clin. Nutr. *12*, 162-169.
CARTEI, G. *et al.* 1970. Current concepts on transferrin. Factors affecting serum transferrin including pregnancy and hormonal therapy. Folia Endocrinol. (Roma) *23*, 579-592.
CAUGHEY, J. E. 1973. Zinc deficiency in man. Lancet *2*, 376-377.
CAWTHORNE, J. M., and SMITH, R. M. 1973. The synthesis of pteroylpoly-glutamates in sheep liver enzymes *in vitro*. Biochem. J. *136*, 295-301.
CHANARIN, I. 1969A. The Megaloblastic Anaemias. Blackwell Scientific Publishers, Oxford and Edinburgh.
CHATTERJEE, A. K., and GHOSH, B. B. 1970. Effect of cortisone and of adrenalectomy on plasma total ascorbic acid level in riboflavin deficiency. Endokrinologie *56*, 218-222.
CHEN, T. C., and DeLUCA, H. F. 1973. Receptors of 1,25-dihydroxychole-calciferol in rat intestines. J. Biol. Chem. *248*, 4890-4895.
CHRISTENSEN, S. 1969. Studies on riboflavin metabolism in the rat. 1. Urinary and faecal excretion after oral administration of riboflavin-5'-phosphate. Acta Pharmacol. (Kobenhavn) *27*, 27-33.
CHRISTIANSEN, C., RØDBRO, P., and LUND, M. 1973. Effect of vitamin D on bone mineral mass in normal subjects and in epileptic subjects on anticonvulsants: A controlled therapeutic trial. Brit. Med. J. *2*, 208-209.
COFFEY, G., and WILSON, C. W. M. 1975. Ascorbic acid deficiency and aspirin induced haematemesis. Brit. Med. J. *1*, 208.
COHN, E. J. *et al.* 1949. The state in nature of the active principle in pernicious anemia of catalase, and of other components of liver. Science *109*, 443 (abst.).
COHN, V. H., and MANDEL, H. G. 1965. Fat soluble vitamins. II. Vitamin K and vitamin E. *In* The Pharmacological Basis of Therapeutics, 3rd ed., L. S. Goodman, and A. Gilman (Editors). Macmillan Co., New York.
COLE, M. *et al.* 1969. Extraoccular palsy and thiamine therapy in Wernicke's encephalopathy. Am. J. Clin. Nutr. *22*, 44-51.
COLLIGAN, J. J., and MARCUS, F. I. 1974. Coagulopathy associated with vitamin E ingestion. J. Am. Med. Assoc. *230*, 1300-1301.
CONNEY, A. H. 1969. Drug metabolism and therapeutics. New Eng. J. Med. *280*, 653-660.
CONNEY, A. H., and BURNS, J. J. 1962. Factors influencing drug metabolism. Adv. Pharmacol. *1*, 31-58.
CONNEY, A. H. *et al.* 1961. Metabolic interactions between L-ascorbic acid and drugs. Vitamin C. Ann. N.Y. Acad. Sci. *92*, 115-127.
CONRAD, M. 1970. Factors Affecting Iron Absorption in Iron Deficiency. L. Hallberg, H. G. Harwerth, and A. Vannotti (Editors). Academic Press, London and New York.
DAVIS, R. K., and ROSE, M. E. 1973. Ascorbic acid status of the drug addict patient. Am. J. Clin. Nutr. *26*, 1042.

DEUS, B., and BLUM, H. 1970. Subcellular distribution of thiamin pyrophosphokinase activity in rat liver and erythrocytes. Biochem. Biophys. Acta *219*, 489-492.
DIETRICH, L. S. 1971. Regulation of nicotinamide metabolism. Am. J. Clin. Nutr. *24*, 800-804.
DiLORENZO, P. A. 1967. Pellagra-like syndrome associated with isoniazid therapy. Acta Dermat. Dermato-Venereol. *47*, 318-322.
ELSBORG, L. 1972. Binding of folic acid to human plasma proteins. Acta Haemat. *48*, 207-212.
EVANS, G. W., and GRACE, C. I. 1973. Homeostatic regulation of zinc absorption. Fed. Proc. *32*, 3804.
FALOON, W. W. 1970. Drug production of intestinal malabsorption. N.Y. State J. Med. *70*, 2189-2192.
FANKUSHEN, D. *et al.* 1964. The significance of hypermagnesemia in alcoholic patients. Am. J. Med. *37*, 802-812.
FAUSA, O. 1970. Salicylate-induced hypoprothrombinemia. Acta Med. Scand. *188*, 403-408.
FELL, G. S. *et al.* 1973. Urinary zinc levels as an indicator of muscle catabolism. Lancet *1*, 280-282.
FELL, H. B. 1965. The effect of vitamin A on the breakdown and synthesis of intercellular material in skeletal tissue in organ culture. Proc. Nutr. Soc. *24*, 166-169.
FENNELLY, J., FRANK, O., BAKER, H., and LEEVY, C. M. 1967. Red blood cell transketolase activity in malnourished alcoholics with cirrhosis. Am. J. Clin. Nutr. *20*, 946-949.
FIDGE, N. H., REESE-SMITH, F. and GOODMAN, D. S. 1969. Vitamin A and carotenes. The enzymatic conversion of β-carotene into retinal in hog intestinal mucosa. Biochem. J. *114*, 689-694.
FINCH, C. A. 1969. Iron deficiency anemia. Am. J. Clin. Nutr. *22*, 512-517.
FLYNN, A. *et al.* 1973. Zinc deficiency with altered adrenocortical function and its relation to delayed healing. Lancet *1*, 789-791.
FOY, H., KONDI, A., and MacDOUGALL, L. 1961. Pure red cell aplasia in marasmus and kwashiorkor—treated with riboflavin. Brit. Med. J. *1*, 937-941.
FOY, H., KONDI, A., and VERJEE, Z. H. M. 1972. Relation of riboflavin deficiency to cortisteroid metabolism and red cell hypoplasia in baboons. J. Nutr. *102*, 571-582.
FRIEDEMANN, T. E., KMIECIAK, T. C., KEEGAN, T. K., and SHEFT, B. B. 1948. Absorption, destruction and excretion of orally administered thiamin by human subjects. Gastroenterology *11*, 100-114.
FRIEDEN, E. 1973. The ferrous to ferric cycles in iron metabolism. Nutr. Rev. *31*, 41-44.
GALLO-TORRES, H. E. 1970. Obligatory role of bile for the intestinal absorption of vitamin E. Lipids *5*, 379-384.
GARABEDIAN, M. *et al.* 1972. Control of 25-hydroxycholecalciferol metabolism by parathyroid glands. Proc. Nat. Acad. Sci. U.S.A. *69*, 1673-1676.
GAURTH HANSEN, R. 1973. An index of food quality. Nutr. Rev. *31*, 1-7.
GAYLOR, J. L. 1962. Cutaneous vitamin D. N.Y. State J. Med. *62*, 251-253.
GEORGE, W. K. *et al.* 1962. Vitamin D and magnesium. Lancet *1*, 1300.
GHITIS, J. 1967. The folate binding in milk. Am. J. Clin. Nutr. *20*, 1-4.
GILLETTE, J. R., BRODIE, B. B., and LaDU, B. N. 1957. The oxidation of drugs by liver microsomes: On the role of TPNH and oxygen. J. Pharmacol. Exp. Therap. *119*, 532-540.
GIRDWOOD, R. H. 1971. Problems in the assessment of vitamin deficiency. Proc. Nutr. Soc. *30*, 66-73.
GIROUD, E. L., and HENKIN, R. I. 1972. Competition for zinc among serum albumin and amino acids. Biochem. Biophys. Acta *273*, 64-72.
GOLDMAN, H. I., and AMADIO, P. 1969. Vitamin K deficiency after the newborn period. Pediatrics *44*, 745-749.

GOLDSMITH, G. A.   1964.   The B vitamins: thiamin, riboflavin, niacin. *In* Nutrition: A Comprehensive Treatise, Vol. 2., G. H. Beaton, and E. W. McHenry (Editors). Academic Press, New York.

GOLDSTEIN, A., ARONOW, L., and KALMAN, S. M.   1968.   Principles of Drug Action. The Basis of Pharmacology. Hoeber Med. Div., Harper and Row Publishers, Evanston, London.

GOMPERTZ, D., and HOFFBRAND, A. V.   1970.   Methylmalonic aciduria. Brit. J. Haemat. *18*, 377–381.

GOODWIN, T. W.   1963.   The Biosynthesis of Vitamins and Related Compounds. Academic Press, London and New York.

GRAHAM, W. D.   1951.   *In vitro* inhibition of liver aldehyde dehydrogenase by tetraethylthiuram disulfide. J. Pharmacol. *3*, 160–168.

GREENBERGER, N. J.   1973.   Effects of antibiotics and other agents on the intestinal transport of iron. Am. J. Clin. Nutr. *26*, 104–112.

GROSS, S., and MELHORN, D. K.   1972.   Vitamin E, red cell lipids and red cell stability in prematurity. Ann. N.Y. Acad. Sci. *203*, 141–162.

GUENTER, W., and SNELL, J. L.   1971.   Magnesium absorption and secretion along the gastrointestinal tract of the chicken. Fed. Proc. *30*, 346.

GURNANI, S., MISTRY, S. P., and JOHNSON, B. C.   1960.   Function of vitamin B_{12} in methylmalonate metabolism. 1. Effect of a cofactor form of B_{12} on the activity of methylmalonyl-CoA isomerase. Biochem. Biophys. Acta *38*, 187–188.

HAHN, T. J. *et al.*   1972.   Phenobarbital-induced alterations in vitamin D metabolism. J. Clin. Invest. *51*, 741–748.

HALSTED, J. A., CECIL SMITH, J., JR., and IRWIN, M. I.   1974.   A conspectus of research on zinc requirements of man. J. Nutr. *104*, 345–378.

HALSTED, J. A., HACKLEY, B. M., and SMITH, J. C. JR.   1968.   Plasma, zinc and copper in pregnancy and after oral contraceptives. Lancet *2*, 278.

HANSEN, R. G.   1973.   An index of food quality. Nutr. Rev. *31*, 1–7.

HARRIS, A. B., HARTLEY, J., and MOOR, A.   1973.   Reduced ascorbic acid excretion and oral contraceptives. Lancet *2*, 201–202.

HASTINGS-WILSON, T.   1962.   Intestinal Absorption. W. B. Saunders Co., Philadelphia and London.

HAUSSLER, M. R.   1974.   Vitamin D: Mode of action and biomedical applications. Nutr. Rev. *32*, 257–266.

HAUTVAST, J. G. A. J., and BARNES, M. J.   1974.   Collagen metabolism in folic acid deficiency. Brit. J. Nutr. *43*, 457–469.

HEGSTED, D. M., FINCH, C. A., and KINNEY, T. D.   1949.   The influence of diet on iron absorption. II. The interrelationship of iron and phosphorus. J. Exp. Med. *90*, 147–156.

HELLMAN, E. S., TSCHUDY, D. T., and BARTTER, F. C.   1962.   Abnormal electrolyte and water metabolism in acute intermittent porphyria; transient inappropriate secretion of antidiuretic hormone. Am. J. Med. *32*, 734–746.

HENKIN, R. I. *et al.*   1971.   Idiopathic hypogeusia with dysgeusia, hyposmia and dysosmia. J. Am. Med. Assoc. *217*, 434–440.

HERBERT, V.   1963.   Megaloblastic anaemia. New Eng. J. Med. *268*, 201–203 and 368–371.

HERBERT, V.   1964.   Studies of folate deficiency in man. Proc. Roy. Soc. Med. *57*, 377–384.

HERBERT, V., and JACOB, E.   1974.   Destruction of vitamin B_{12} by ascorbic acid. J. Am. Med. Assoc. *230*, 241–242.

HERBERT, V., and ZALUSKY, R.   1961.   Selective concentration of folic acid activity in cerebrospinal fluid. Fed. Proc. *20*, 453.

HERBERT, V., and ZALUSKY, R.   1962.   Interrelationships of vitamin B_{12} and folic acid metabolism. Folic acid clearance studies. J. Clin. Invest. *41*, 1263–1276.

HERNDON, J. G., *et al.*   1958.   Iron absorption and metabolism. III. The enhancement of iron absorption in rats by D-sorbitol. J. Nutr. *64*, 615–623.

HODGES, R. E. *et al.* 1969. Experimental scurvy in man. Amer. J. Clin. Nutr. 22, 535-548.

HODGKIN, P. *et al.* 1973. Vitamin-D deficiency in Asians at home and in Britain. Lancet 2, 167-172.

HOFFBRAND, A. V. *et al.* 1974. Thymidylate concentrations in megaloblastic anemia. Nature 248, 602-604.

HOLLANDER, D. 1973. Vitamin K_1 absorption by everted intestinal sacs of the rat. Am. J. Physiol. 225, 360-364.

HOLLANDER, D., and TRUSCOTT, T. C. 1974. Mechanism and site of vitamin K_3 small intestinal transport. Am. J. Physiol. 226, 1516-1522.

HORNE, C. W. *et al.* 1970. Effect of combined oestrogen-progestagen oral contraceptives on serum levels of α_2-macroglobulin, transferrin, albumin, and lgG. Lancet 1, 49-51.

HOROWITZ, M. D. *et al.* 1972. Relationship between tocopherol and serum lipid levels for determination of nutritional adequacy of vitamin E and its role in cellular metabolism. Ann. N.Y. Acad. Sci. 203, 223-236.

HORWITT, M. K., and WITTING, L. A. 1972. Biochemical systems, riboflavin. *In* The Vitamins, Chemistry, Physiology, Pathology, Methods. 2nd Edition, Vol. 5., W. H. Sebrell, and R. S. Harris (Editors). Academic Press, New York and London.

HSU, J. M., ANTHONY, W. L., and BUCHANON, P. J. 1969. Zinc deficiency and incorporation of ^{14}C-labeled methionine into tissue proteins in rats. J. Nutr. 99, 425-432.

HURANI, F. I. 1973. Vitamin B_{12} and the megaloblastic development. Science 182, 78-79.

JACOBS, A. and MILES, P. M. 1969. Intraluminal transport of iron from stomach to small intestinal mucosa. Brit. Med. J. 4, 778-781.

JOHNS, D. G., SPERTI, S., and BERGEN, A. S. V. 1965. The metabolism of tritiated folic acid in man. J. Clin. Invest. 40, 1684-1695.

JUSKO, W. J., and LEVY, G. 1967. Absorption, metabolism and excretion of riboflavin-5'-phosphate in man. J. Pharm. Sci. 56, 58-62.

JUSKO, W. J., and LEVY, G. 1969. Plasma protein binding of riboflavin and riboflavin-5'-phosphate in man. J. Pharm. Sci. 58, 58-62.

JUSKO, W. J. *et al.* 1971. Riboflavin absorption in children with biliary obstruction. Am. J. Dis. Child 121, 48-52.

KAHN, S. B., and BRODSKY, I. 1966. Vitamin B_{12}, ascorbic acid and iron metabolism in scurvy. Am. J. Med. 40, 119-126.

KAMIN, H. 1969. Microsomes and Drug Oxidations, J. R. Gillette, *et al.* (Editors). Academic Press, New York.

KATUNUMA, N. *et al.* 1972. Mode of action of specific inactivating enzymes for pyridoxal enzymes and NAD-dependent enzymes and their biological significance. *In* Advances in Enzyme Regulation 10, G. Weber (Editor). Pergamon Press, Oxford, New York.

KOMAI, T., KAWAI, K., and SHINDO, H. 1974. Active transport of thiamine from rat small intestine. J. Nutr. Sci. Vitaminol. 20, 163-177.

KOMAI, T., and SHINDO, H. 1974. Structural specificities for the active transport system of thiamine in rat small intestine. J. Nutr. Sci. Vitaminol. 20, 179-187.

KONDI, A. *et al.* 1963. Anaemias of marasmus and kwashiorkor in Kenya. Arch. Dis. Child. 38, 267-275.

KROE, B. *et al.* 1963. The influence of amino acids on iron absorption. Blood 21, 546-552.

KROGER, A., and KLINGENBERG, M. 1970. Quinones and nicotinamide nucleotides associated with electron transfer. *In* Vitamins and Hormones 28, R. S. Harris, P. L. Munson, and E. Diczfalusy (Editors). Academic Press, New York and London.

KRUSE, H. D. *et al.* 1940. Ocular manifestations of ariboflavinosis. Public Health Rep. 55, 157-169.

KUTSKY, R. J. 1973. Handbook of Vitamins and Hormones. Van Nostrand Reinhold Co., New York.
LANE, M., and ALFREY, C. P. 1965. The anemia of human riboflavin deficiency. Blood 25, 432–442.
LARNER, J. 1971. Intermediary Metabolism and its Regulation. Prentice-Hall, Englewood Cliffs, N.J.
LEEVY, C. M. et al. 1965. Incidence and significance of hypovitaminemia in a randomly selected municipal hospital population. Am. J. Clin. Nutr. 17, 259–271.
LEVINE, R. R. 1971. Intestinal absorption. In Topics in Medicinal Chemistry 4, J. L. Rabinowitz, and R. M. Myerson (Editors). John Wiley & Sons, New York and London.
LEVINE, P. H., LEVINE, A. J., and WEINTRAUB, L. R. 1972. The role of transferrin in the control of iron absorption: studies on a cellular level. J. Lab. Clin. Med. 80, 333–341.
LEVY, G., and JUSKO, W. J. 1966A. Apparent renal tubular secretion of riboflavin in man. J. Pharm. Sci. 55, 1322.
LEVY, G., and JUSKO, W. J. 1966B. Factors affecting the absorption of riboflavin in man. J. Pharm. Sci. 55, 285–289.
LEVY, G., MacGILLIVRAY, M. N., and PROCKNAL, J. A. 1972. Riboflavin absorption in children with thyroid disorders. Pediatrics 50, 896–900.
LEVY, L., and HEWITT, R. R. 1971. Evidence in man for different specialized intestinal transport mechanisms for riboflavin and thiamin. Am. J. Clin. Nutr. 24, 401–404.
LIM, P., and JACOB, E. 1972A. Magnesium status of alcoholic patients. Metabolism 21, 1045–1051.
LINK, K. P. et al. 1943. Studies on the hemorrhagic sweet clover disease. IX. Hypoprothrombinemia in the rat induced by salicylic acid. J. Biol. Chem. 147, 463–474.
LOSOWSKY, M. S. et al. 1972. Intake and absorption of tocopherol. Vitamin E and its role in cellular metabolism. Ann. N.Y. Acad. Sci. 203, 212–222.
LUMENG, L., CLEARY, R. E., and LI, T.-K. 1974. Effect of oral contraceptives on the plasma concentration of pyridoxal phosphate. Am. J. Clin. Nutr. 27, 326–333.
MACFARLANE, M. D. 1974. Penicillamine and zinc. Lancet 2, 962.
MANIS, J., and SCHACHTER, D. 1966. Active transport of iron by intestine: Effect of erythropoiesis stimulated by phenylhydrazine. Nature 209, 1356.
MARKKANEN, T., VIRTANEN, S., PAJULA, R. L., and HIMANEN, P. 1974. Hormonal dependence of folic acid protein binding in human serum. Internat. J. Vit. Nutr. Res. 44, 81–94.
MATSCHINER, J. T. 1969. Occurrence and biopotency of various forms of vitamin K. In The Fat Soluble Vitamins, H. F. DeLuca, and J. W. Suttie (Editors). Univ. Wisconsin Press, Madison, Milwaukee and London.
MATSCHINER, J. T. et al. 1970. Isolation and characterization of a new metabolite of phylloquinone in the rat. Biochem. Biophys. Acta 201, 309–315.
MAWER, E. B., and SCHAEFER, K. 1969. The distribution of vitamin D_3 metabolites in human serum and tissues. Biochem. J. 114, 74P–75P.
MAYFIELD, H. L., and ROEHM, R. R. 1956. The influence of ascorbic acid and the source of B vitamins on the utilization of carotene. J. Nutr. 58, 203–217.
McBEAN, L. D., SMITH, J. C., JR., and HALSTED, J. A. 1971. Effect of oral contraceptive hormones on zinc metabolism in the rat. Proc. Soc. Exp. Biol. Med. 137, 543–547.
McCORMICK, D. B., GREGORY, M. E., and SNELL, E. E. 1961. Pyridoxal phosphokinases. I. Assay, distribution, purification and properties. J. Biol. Chem. 236, 2076–2084.

McLEAN, A., and CHANARIN, I. 1966. Urinary excretion of 5-methyl-tetrahydrofolate in man. Blood 27, 386-388.

McLEROY, V. J., and SCHENDEL, H. E. 1973. Influence of oral contraceptives on ascorbic acid concentrations in healthy, sexually mature women. Am. J. Clin. Nutr. 26, 191-196.

MELIKIAN, V. et al. 1971. Site of reduction and methylation of folic acid in man. Lancet 2, 955-957.

MELLETTE, S. J., and LEONE, L. A. 1960. Influence of age, sex, strain of rat and fat soluble vitamins in hemorrhagic syndromes in rats fed irradiated beef. Fed. Proc. 19, 1045-1049.

METHSESSEL, A. H., and SPENCER, H. 1973. Zinc metabolism in the rat. I. Intestinal absorption of zinc. J. Appl. Physiol. 34, 58-62.

METZ, J., ZALUSKY, R., and HERBERT, V. 1968. Folic acid binding by serum and milk. Am. J. Clin. Nutr. 21, 289-297.

MEZEY, E., and HOLT, P. R. 1971. The inhibitory effect of ethanol on retinol oxidation by human liver and cattle retina. Exp. Molec. Pathol. 15, 148-156.

MIALE, J. B., and KENT, J. W. 1974. The effects of oral contraceptives on the results of laboratory tests. Am. J. Obstet. Gynecol. 120, 264-272.

MIKAC-DEVIC, D. 1970. Methodology of zinc determinations and the role of zinc in biochemical processes. Adv. Clin. Chem. 13, 271-333.

MILLER, W. J. et al. 1965. Effect of zinc deficiency and restricted feeding on wound healing in bovine. Proc. Soc. Exp. Biol. Med. 118, 427-430.

MONSEN, E. R., COOK, J. D., and FINCH, C. A. 1974. The effect of meat vs. non-meat animal protein on the absorption of non-heme iron by human subjects. Fed. Proc. 33, 667.

MURPHY, F. J., and ZELMAN, S. 1965. Ascorbic acid as a urinary acidifying agent: I. Comparison with the ketogenic effect of fasting. J. Urol. 94, 297-299.

NAKAGAWA, I. et al. 1969. Effect in man of the addition of tryptophan or niacin to the diet on the excretion of their metabolites. J. Nutr. 99, 325-330.

NATHANI, M. G., and NATH, M. C. 1972. Effect of corticosteroids on ascorbic acid metabolism in rats. Metabolism 21, 779-786.

NELSESTUEN, G. L., and SUTTIE, J. W. 1973. The mode of action of vitamin K. Isolation of a peptide containing the vitamin K-dependent portion of prothrombin. Proc. Nat. Acad. Sci. 70, 3366-3370.

NELSESTUEN, G. L., ZYTKOVICZ, T. H., and HOWARD, J. B. 1974. The mode of action of vitamin K. Identification of γ-carboxyglutamic acid as a component of prothrombin. J. Biol. Chem. 249, 6347-6350.

NEUVONEN, T. J., GOTHONI, G., and HACKMAN, R. 1970. Interference of iron with the absorption of tetracyclines in man. Brit. Med. J. 4, 532-534.

NIES, A. S. 1974. Drug interaction. Med. Clin. North Am. 58, 965-975.

NORDIN, B. E. C. 1973. Nutritional aspects of calcium and vitamin D. In Nutritional Deficiencies in Modern Society, A. N. Howard, and I. McLean Baird (Editors). Newman Books, London.

NORRBY, A., RYBO, G., and SORVELL, L. 1972. The influence of a combined oral contraceptive on the absorption of iron. Scand. J. Haemat. 9, 43-51.

OLSON, R. E. 1970. The mode of action of vitamin K. Nutr. Rev. 28, 171-176.

OLSON, E. B. JR., and DeLUCA, H. F. 1973. Vitamin D metabolism and mechanism of action. In World Review of Dietetics 17. Karger, Basel, Switzerland.

OSAKI, S., JOHNSON, D. A., and FRIEDEN, E. 1971. The motilization of iron from the perfused mammalian liver by a serum copper enzyme, ferroxidase I. J. Biol. Chem. 246, 3018-3023.

OSIS, D. et al. 1972. Dietary zinc intake in man. Am. J. Clin. Nutr. 25, 582-588.

PARISI, A. F., and VALLEE, B. L. 1969. Zinc metalloenzymes: Characteristics and significance in biology and medicine. Am. J. Clin. Nutr. 22, 1222-1239.

PARISI, A. F., and VALLEE, B. L. 1970. Isolation of a zinc α_2-macro-globulin from human serum. Biochem. 9, 2421-2426.

PATEL, J. M., and PAWRR, S. S. 1974. Riboflavin and drug metabolism in adult male and female rats. Biochem. Pharmacol. 23, 1467-1477.

PATRICK, G. 1973. The regulation of intestinal calcium transport by vitamin D. Nature 243, 89-90.

PAULING, L. 1970. Vitamin C and the Common Cold. W. H. Freeman and Co., San Francisco.

PETERS, T., APT, L., and ROSS, J. F. 1971. Effect of phosphates upon iron absorption studied in normal human subjects and an experimental model using dialysis. Gastroenterology 61, 315-322.

PETERSON, P. A. 1971. Isolation and partial characterization of a human vitamin D binding plasma protein. J. Biol. Chem. 246, 7748-7754.

PIRANI, C. L. 1952. Review: Relation of vitamin C to adrenocortical function and stress phenomena. Metabolism 1, 197-222.

PIRZIO-BIROLI, G., and FINCH, C. A. 1960. Iron Absorption. III. Influence of iron stores on iron absorption in the normal subject. J. Lab. Clin. Med. 55, 216-220.

PLACK, P. A. 1965. Occurrence, absorption and distribution of vitamin A. Proc. Nutr. Soc. 24, 146-152.

POLIN, D., WYNOSKY, E. R., and PORTER, C. C. 1963. In vivo absorption of amprolium and its competition with thiamine. Proc. Soc. Exp. Biol. Med. 114, 273-277.

POLLACK, S., KAUFMAN, R. M., and CROSBY, W. H. 1964. Iron absorption: Effects of sugars and reducing agents. Blood 24, 577-581.

PRASAD, A. S., and OBERLEAS, D. 1970. Binding of zinc to amino acids and serum proteins in vitro. J. Lab. Clin. Med. 76, 416-425.

PRESCOTT, L. F. 1974. Gastrointestinal absorption of drugs. Med. Clin. North Am. 58, 907-916.

QUICK, A. J., and CLESCERI, L. 1960. Influence of acetylsalicylic acid and salicylamide on coagulation of blood. J. Pharmacol. Exp. Therap. 128, 95-98.

RAISZ, L. J. et al. 1972. 1,25-Dihydroxycholecalciferol: A potent stimulator of bone resorption in tissue culture. Science 175, 768-769.

RAUSCHKOLB, E. W. et al. 1969. Identification of vitamin D_3 in human skin. J. Invest. Dermat. 53, 289-294.

REIDENBERG, M. M. 1974. Effect of disease states on plasma protein binding of drugs. Med. Clin. North Am. 58, 1103-1109.

REINHOLD, J. G. et al. 1973. Effects of purified phytate and phytate-rich bread upon metabolism of zinc, calcium, phosphorus, and nitrogen in man. Lancet 1, 283-288.

RINDI, G., PERRI, V., VENTURA, U., and BRECCIA, A. 1962. Phosphoryl-ation of thiamin labeled with sulfur-35 in the liver of the rat. Nature 193, 581-582.

RITCHIE, J. H. et al. 1968. Edema and hemolytic anemia in premature infants: A vitamin E deficiency syndrome. New Eng. J. Med. 279, 1185-1190.

RIVERS, J. M., and DEVINE, M. M. 1970. Plasma ascorbic acid concentrations and oral contraceptives. Fed. Proc. 29, 295.

RIVLIN, R. S. 1970A. Regulation of flavoprotein enzymes in hypothyroidism and in riboflavin deficiency. Adv. Enzyme Regula. 8, 239-245.

RIVLIN, R. S. 1970B. Riboflavin metabolism. New Eng. J. Med. 283, 463-472.

RIVLIN, R. S., and LANGDEN, R. G. 1969. Effects of thyroxine upon biosyn-thesis of flavin mononucleotide and flavine adenine dinucleotide. Endo-crinology 84, 584-588.

RIVLIN, R. S., MENENDEZ, C., and LANGDON, R. G. 1968. Biochemical similarities between hypothyroidism and riboflavin deficiency. Endocrinology 83, 461-469.

ROE, D. A. 1973. A Plague of Corn: The Social History of Pellagra. Cornell Univ. Press, Ithaca and London.

ROE, D. A. 1974. Effects of drugs on nutrition. Life Sciences 15, 1219-1234.

ROE, D. A., McCORMICK, D. B. and LIN, R.-T. 1972. Effects of riboflavin on boric acid toxicity. J. Pharm. Sci. 61, 1081-1085.

ROELS, O. A. 1970. Vitamin A physiology. J. Am. Med. Assoc. 214, 1097-1102.

ROSENBERG, I. H. et al. 1969. Absorption of polyglutamic folate; participation of D-conjugating enzymes of the intestinal mucosa. New Eng. J. Med. 280, 985-988.

ROSENSTREICH, S. J., RICH, C., and VOLWILER, W. 1971. Deposition in and release of vitamin D_3 from body fat: evidence for a storage site in the rat. J. Clin. Invest. 50, 679-687.

ROSENTHAL, W. S. et al. 1973. Riboflavin deficiency in complicated chronic alcoholism. Am. J. Clin. Nutr. 26, 858-860.

SAKAMI, W., and UKSTIN, S. I. 1961. Enzymatic methylation of homocysteine by a synthetic tetrahydrofolate derivative. J. Biol. Chem. 236, PC 50.

SANDSTEAD, H. H., and SHEPHARD, G. H. 1968. Effect of zinc deficiency on the tensile strength of healing surgical incisions in the integument of the rat. Proc. Soc. Exp. Biol. Med. 128, 687-689.

SANDSTEAD, H. H. et al. 1970. Zinc and wound healing. Effects of zinc deficiency and zinc supplementation. Am. J. Clin. Nutr. 23, 514-519.

SAUBERLICH, H. E. 1967. Biochemical alterations in thiamin deficiency—their interpretation. Am. J. Clin. Nutr. 20, 528-542.

SAUBERLICH, H. E., SKALA, J. H., and DOWDY, R. P. 1974. Laboratory Tests for the Assessment of Nutritional Status. CRC Press, Cleveland.

SEEGERS, W. H., McCOY, L., and MARCINIAK, F. 1968. Blood-clotting enzymology. Clin. Chem. 14, 97-115.

SHARMA, S. K., and QUASTEL, J. H. 1965. Transport and metabolism of thiamin in rat brain cortex in vitro. Biochem. J. 94, 790-800.

SHELDON, W. 1943. Diseases of Infancy and Childhood, 5th ed. J. & A. Churchill Ltd. London.

SILBER, R., and MOLDOW, C. F. 1970. Biochemistry of vitamin B_{12} mediated reactions in man. Am. J. Med. 48, 549-554.

SIMPSON, E., and ESTABROOK, R. W. 1969. The "malate shuttle" and control of steroid hydroxylation in the adrenal cortex. In Advances in Enzyme Regulation 7, G. Weber (Editor). Pergamon Press, Oxford, London, New York.

SMITH, J. C. et al. 1973. Zinc: a trace element essential in vitamin A metabolism. Science 181, 954-955.

SMITH, J. E., and GOODMAN, D. S. 1971. The turnover and transport of vitamin D and of a polar metabolite with the properties of 25-hydroxycholecalciferol in human plasma. J. Clin. Invest. 50, 2159-2167.

SMITH, W. O., KYRIAKOPOULOS, A. A., and HAMMARSTEN, J. F. 1962. Magnesium depletion induced by various diuretics. J. Oklahoma Med. Assoc. 55, 248-250.

SPEIDEL, B. D. 1973. Folic acid deficiency and congenital malformation. Develop. Med. Child Neurol. 15, 81-83.

STEVENSON, J. W., and EARLE, I. P. 1956. Studies on parakeratosis in swine. J. Anim. Sci. 15, 1036-1045.

STRIPP, B. 1965. Intestinal absorption of riboflavin in man. Acta Pharmacol. Toxicol. 22, 353-362.

SUDA, T., DeLUCA, H. F., and TANAKA, Y. 1970. Biological activity of 25-hydroxyergocalciferol in rats. J. Nutr. 100, 1049-1052.

SULLIVAN, L. W. 1970. Differential diagnosis and management of the patient with megaloblastic anemia. Am. J. Med. 48, 609-617.

SUTHERLAND, J. F. 1962. Effect of alcohol on urinary zinc excretion. Quart. J. Stud. Alc. 23, 216.

SYDENSTRICKER, V. P. 1941. Clinical manifestations of ariboflavinosis. Am. J. Pub. Health *31*, 344–350.
TANAKA, M., and BOTTOMLY, S. S. 1974. Bone marrow delta-aminolevulinic acid synthetase activity in experimental sideroblastic anemia. J. Lab. Clin. Med. *84*, 92–98.
TANDLER, B., ERLANDSON, R. A., and WYNDER, E. L. 1968. Riboflavin and mouse hepatic cell structure and function. I. Ultrastructural alterations in simple deficiency. Am. J. Path. *52*, 69–78.
TAPPEL, A. L. 1974. Selenium-glutathione peroxidase and vitamin E. Am. J. Clin. Nutr. *27*, 960–965.
THOMPSON, G. R., OCKNER, R. K., and ISSELBACHER, K. J. 1969. Effect of mixed micellar lipid on the absorption of cholesterol and vitamin D_3 into lymph. J. Clin. Invest. *48*, 87–95.
THOMPSON, J. N. 1965. Some aspects of the metabolism and biochemistry of vitamin A. Proc. Nutr. Soc. *24*, 160–165.
THOMPSON, S. Y. 1965. Occurrence, distribution and absorption of provitamins A. Proc. Nutr. Soc. *24*, 136–146.
TISMAN, G. and HERBERT, V. 1973. B_{12} dependence of some uptake of serum folate: An explanation for high serum folate and cell folate depletion in B_{12} deficiency. Blood *41*, 465–469.
TOOHEY, J. I., and BARKER, H. A. 1961. Isolation of coenzyme B_{12} from liver. J. Biol. Chem. *236*, 560–563.
TOSKES, P. P., and DEREN, J. J. 1973. Vitamin B_{12} absorption and malabsorption. Gastroenterology *65*, 662–683.
TSAI, H. C., and NORMAN, A. W. 1973. Studies on calciferol metabolism. VIII. Evidence for a cytoplasmic receptor for 1,25-dihydroxy-vitamin D_3 in the intestinal mucosa. J. Biol. Chem. *248*, 5967–5975.
URBAN, E., and SCHEDL, H. P. 1969. Mucosal growth effect of vitamin D on the duodenum. Experientia *25*, 1270.
VALLEE, B. L. *et al.* 1959. Zinc metabolism in hepatic dysfunction. Ann. Int. Med. *50*, 1077.
VAN CAMPEN, D. 1974. Regulation of iron absorption. Fed. Proc. *33*, 100–105.
VAN THIEL, G. J., and LESTER, R. 1974. Ethanol inhibition of vitamin A metabolism in the testes: Possible mechanism for sterility in alcoholics. Science *186*, 941–942.
VICTOR, M. 1973. The role of hypomagnesemia and respiratory alkalosis in the genesis of alcohol-withdrawal symptoms. *In* Alcoholism and the Central Nervous System. Ann. N.Y. Acad. Sci. *215*, 235–248.
VIKBLADH, I. 1951. Studies on zinc in Blood. II. Scand. J. Clin. Lab. Invest. *3*, Suppl. 2, 5–73.
VILTER, R. W., MUELLER, J. F., and BEAN, W. B. 1949. The therapeutic effect of tryptophane in human pellagra. J. Lab. Clin. Med. *34*, 409–413.
VILTER, R. W. *et al.* 1953. The effect of vitamin B_6 deficiency induced by desoxypyridoxine in human beings. J. Lab. Clin. Med. *42*, 335–357.
VILTER, R. W. *et al.* 1963. Interrelationships of vitamin B_{12}, folic acid, and ascorbic acid in the megaloblastic anemias. Am. J. Clin. Nutr. *12*, 130–144.
VON WARTBERG, J. P. 1971. The metabolism of alcohol in normals and alcoholics: enzymes. *In* The Biology of Alcoholism 1: Biochemistry, B. Kissin, and M. Begleiter (Editors). Plenum Press, New York, London.
WACKER, W. E. C., and PARISI, A. F. 1968. Magnesium metabolism. New Eng. J. Med. *278*, 712–717, 772–776.
WADA, H., and SNELL, E. E. 1961. The enzymatic oxidation of pyridoxine and pyridoxamine phosphates. J. Biol. Chem. *236*, 2089–2095.
WALD, G. and Hubbard, R. 1960. The Enzymes 3. P. D. Boyer, and K. Myrback (Editors). Academic Press, New York.
WALKER, B. E. *et al.* 1973. Plasma and urinary zinc in patients with malabsorption syndromes or hepatic cirrhosis. Gut *14*, 943–948.

WALLACH, J. 1974. Interpretation of Diagnostic Tests, 2nd Edition. Little, Brown and Co., Boston.

WASSERMAN, R. H. 1969. The Vitamin D-Dependent Calcium-Binding Protein in the Fat-Soluble Vitamins. H. F. DeLuca, and J. W. Suttie (Editors). Univ. Wisconsin Press, Madison, Milwaukee, London.

WEISS, H. J. 1974. Aspirin—a dangerous drug? J. Am. Med. Assoc. *229*, 1221-1222.

WEISS, P., and BIANCHINE, J. R. 1969. The effect on serum tocopherol levels of drug-induced decreased in serum lipids. Am. J. Med. Sci. *258*, 275-281.

WHEATLEY, V. R., and REINERTSON, R. P. 1958. The presence of vitamin D precursors in human epidermis. J. Invest. Dermat. *31*, 51-54.

WHITEHEAD, V. M. 1973. Polyglutamyl metabolites of folic acid in human liver. Lancet *1*, 743-745.

WILLINGHAM, A. K., and MATSCHINER, J. T. 1974. Changes in phylloquinone epoxidase activity related to prothrombin synthesis and microsomal clotting activity in the rat. Biochem. J. *140*, 435-441.

WINDAUS, A., and BOCK, F. 1937. Provitamin from the sterol of pigskin. Hoppe Seyler's Ztschr. *245*, 168-170.

WOLF, H. *et al.* 1970. Studies of tryptophan metabolism in male subjects treated with progestational agents. Scand. J. Clin. and Lab. Invest. *25*, 237-249.

WOOLLEY, D. W. 1963. Antimetabolites of the water-soluble vitamins. *In* Metabolic Inhibitors. A Comprehensive Treatise. Vol. 1. R. M. Hochster, and J. H. Quastel (Editors). Academic Press, New York, London.

YENDT, E. R. *et al.* 1969. Clinical aspects of vitamin D. *In* The Fat Soluble Vitamins. H. F. DeLuca, and J. W. Suttie (Editors). Univ. Wisconsin Press, Madison, Milwaukee, London.

ZBINDEN, G. 1962. Therapeutic use of vitamin B_1 in diseases other than beri-beri. Ann. N. Y. Acad. Sci. *98*, 550-561.

CHAPTER 2

Factors Affecting Nutritional Requirements

While it is true that all people are somewhat equal with respect to their nutrient requirements, there is a growing awareness that genetic variation as well as acquired differences, both physiological and pathological, determine the level of nutrient intake which is required for normal tissue maintenance and growth. Williams (1963) has pointed out that individual differences in nutritional needs may have many basic causes, which may be inborn or determined by the physiological or chemical environment. He noted that the augmented need which an individual has for a particular nutrient may involve not only his own internal metabolism, but also that of the bacteria which are contained within him. If two individuals are deprived of a nutrient to the same extent, their symptoms of deficiency will vary with their genetic makeup as well as with their ages, their physiological status, their health differences, and the drugs they take.

GENETIC DIFFERENCES

A wide spectrum of inherited metabolic disorders have been shown to impose an unusual requirement either for a specific vitamin or for such nutrients as glucose or available carbohydrate. Specific enzymatic defects in the anabolic or catabolic pathways for individual amino acids, pyrroles, and sterols have been shown to alter nutrient requirements in man. Since there is evidence that in microorganisms, as also in avian and mammalian species, strain differences determine variability in nutrient needs, the same may be true in man, though this subject has, as yet, not been extensively investigated. Since population studies relative to genetic variability in nutrient requirements remain to be carried out by future investigators, discussion must be confined to inherited metabolic disturbances in which it is known that control of the abnormality is dependent on moderate or massive nutrient supplementation. Clarification of the mechanisms underlying nutrient-dependent genetic disease has laid the groundwork for interpretation of drug-induced nutritional deficiencies, since biochemical blocks or impairment of nutrient utilization may be similar in the two circumstances. Vitamins causally implicated in genetic disease are the same as those involved in drug-induced hypovitaminoses. Further, vitamin-dependent genetic disease may determine vulnerability to deficiency states caused by drugs.

With the single exception of vitamin D-dependent rickets, the recognition that certain inherited metabolic disorders demonstrate vitamin dependency is the outcome of research conducted during the last 20 years. While in each of these disorders there is a specific enzymatic defect, none of them are due to vitamin deficiency per se. Although inter-individual variation exists with respect to vitamin and other nutrient requirements, in general the intake of the recommended daily allowance of specific nutrients is sufficient to maintain nutritional status. If people or populations are subjected to progressive dietary deficiency pertaining to a vitamin, then eventually the deficiency affects all functions that are dependent on the presence of the active form of that vitamin. Diet-induced vitamin deficiencies in most cases respond to moderate intakes of the vitamin that is low in the previous diet. However, in the case of vitamin-dependent genetic disease, specific biochemical abnormalities occur affecting single reactions catalyzed by a vitamin, and these abnormalities respond only to pharmacologic amounts of that particular vitamin. Rosenberg (1969) has pointed out that reaction specificity, genetic etiology, and quantitative responsiveness constitute the essential differences between vitamin deficiency and vitamin dependency.

Several mechanisms have been proposed to explain vitamin-dependent disease, and some of these mechanisms have been proven to exist in man. In a review of this subject, Scriver (1971) summarized some of the possible conditions which may occur: (1) there may be a partial or leaky impairment of coenzyme biosynthesis; (2) a reversible disorder in the binding of coenzyme at its site of action may be present; (3) the reduced turnover of an abnormal apoenzyme may be compensated by binding to sufficient coenzyme; or (4) coenzyme may stimulate alternate pathways of biosynthesis when one is blocked.

In a review of vitamin-responsive metabolic errors, Scriver (1973) again divides these forms of genetic disease into several categories: (1) those due to defective transport and biosynthesis of the coenzyme; (2) those due to defective association of the coenzyme with the apoenzyme; (3) alterations in the cellular concentration of the mutant apoenzyme; and (4) those in which there is stimulation of an alternate metabolic pathway. In Scriver's first category are the hereditary defects of vitamin transport, both in terms of intestinal uptake and in transport of the vitamin from one compartment of the body to another or into cells. Such transport defects impair coenzyme biosynthesis because of non-availability of the necessary vitamin at the sites of their further metabolism.

Malabsorption

Folate.—Malabsorption of folate may occur as a congenital isolated defect, though it is a rare condition. Lanzkowsky (1970) described a twenty-year-old mentally retarded girl who had repeated episodes of megaloblastic anemia which responded to pharmacologic doses of folic acid in the order of 40 mg/day. Whenever this daily intake of folic acid was discontinued, not only did she show a reduction of folate levels in plasma and erythrocytes, but also her cerebrospinal fluid folate fell to 0 ng/ml. Intramuscular injection of 250 μg folic acid led to reticulocytosis, and continued administration of folate by the intramuscular route caused a rise in plasma and erythrocyte folate levels, though the cerebrospinal fluid folate could not be detected. Her defect in the absorption of folic acid included the vitamin as pteroylpolyglutamic acid, as well as pteroylmonoglutamic, pteroyldiglutamic, pteroyltriglutamic acid and 5-formyl and 5-methyltetrahydrofolic acid. It is also obvious from the data that she was unable to transport folic acid from the blood into the cerebrospinal fluid. The patient was subject to epileptiform convulsions which worsened when folic acid was given, and decreased in intensity during periods when she was folate deficient due to discontinuation of folate administration.

It is of interest that in this case, as with patients who are folate deficient due to chronic administration of anticonvulsant drugs, administration of high doses of folic acid may increase the severity and frequency of fits. While congenital malabsorption of folate of this severity is extremely rare, there is evidence to suggest that a milder folate malabsorption on a presumed congenital basis may be much more frequent. There is evidence that subclinical isolated folate malabsorption may contribute to folate deficiency with megaloblastic anemia occurring among some women receiving oral contraceptives (Shojania and Hornady 1973).

Vitamin B_{12}.—Several different transport defects selective for vitamin B_{12} have been described. The congenital forms of vitamin B_{12} deficiency can be divided into those types which are due to a defective or absent intrinsic factor production, and those which affect the ileal phase of vitamin B_{12} absorption. Patients described as having juvenile forms of pernicious anemia were cited Mollin et al. (1955) and also by Spurling et al. (1964). In these patients there was a congenital absence of intrinsic factor, and hence an inability to absorb vitamin B_{12}.

Katz et al. (1972) described a thirteen-year-old boy with megaloblastic anemia due to vitamin B_{12} deficiency who could not absorb free vitamin B_{12} given orally, but could absorb normal amounts of the vitamin given bound to gastric juice obtained from a normal patient. Studies suggested that in this patient intrinsic factor was produced but that this intrinsic factor was abnormal, and inert with respect to vitamin B_{12} binding capacity.

McKenzie et al. (1972) described a form of familial vitamin B_{12} malabsorption in which the defect appeared to be between the site where the intrinsic factor-vitamin B_{12} complex is bound to the ileal site and where vitamin B_{12} is subsequently bound to the transport protein, transcobalamin II. In this report, the patient described received 1 mg B_{12} monthly to maintain a normal hematologic status. Still another form of congenital vitamin B_{12} malabsorption was described by Hakami et al. (1971) in which there was complete absence of transcobalamin II, the globulin transport protein for newly-absorbed vitamin B_{12}. In the patient described in this report, 1 mg vitamin B_{12} was required intramuscularly twice a week or one-half mg 3–4 times/week.

Utilization

Folate.—In addition to the congenital selective defects of folate and vitamin B_{12} absorption, there exist congenital defects in the utilization of these vitamins. Arakawa (1970) divides the defects in folate utilization into several types according to the particular enzyme deficiency that exists. In one form, clinically presenting in young children with mental and physical retardation, high serum folate levels, and sometimes megaloblastic and sideroblastic anemia, a deficiency of formiminotransferase can be found using liver samples for enzyme studies. In another type of impairment in folate utilization the clinical features are those of mental retardation, megaloblastic anemia, marked dilatation of the cerebral ventricles, as shown in pneumoencephalograms, and high serum folate levels. In this type, liver enzyme studies have shown a markedly decreased activity of N 5-methyltetrahydrofolate transferase. No therapeutic approach is described with respect to these cases.

Walters (1967) described a case of congenital megaloblastic anemia which did respond to the administration of N^5-formyltetrahydrofolic acid administration. In this case, folate reductase activity in the liver was found to be defective. When 100 μg folic acid were given either orally or parenterally, there was no effect on the hematologic picture.

Vitamin B_{12}.—Several defects in vitamin B_{12} metabolism exist, but the only one which is of considerable interest in the present context is the vitamin B_{12}-responsive methylmalonic aciduria. The disease is characterized by repeated episodes of severe ketoacidosis in very early life, physical growth retardation, and the hyperexcretion of methylmalonic acid in the urine. It has been suggested in the vitamin B_{12}-responsive methylmalonic aciduria, that maintenance therapy should consist in the administration of 1 mg cobalamin (vitamin B_{12}) intramuscularly twice per week (Mahoney and Rosenberg 1970). This vitamin B_{12}-responsive disease is a clear example of one of Scriver's types of vitamin-dependent diseases; that is, where there is a partial or leaky impairment of coenzyme biosynthesis.

Vitamin B_6.—Five genetic errors of metabolism have been identified which are vitamin B_6-dependent. These include those in which there appears to be an abnormal apoenzyme, such as in the case of pyridoxine-responsive infantile convulsions, pyridoxine-responsive anemia, and pyridoxine-responsive homocystinuria, as well possibly as xanthurenic aciduria. In the case of pyridoxine-responsive cystathionuria, there is evidence that the disorder may arise because of an abnormal binding of the coenzyme to the apoenzyme. The current state of knowledge concerning pyridoxine-responsive diseases has been discussed by Rosenberg (1969). Collectively these vitamin B_6-responsive diseases result from apoenzyme defects, and it can be generalized that wherever the defect exists, it results in a deficiency of the functioning enzyme at a particular pyridoxine-dependent site. This has relevance to our understanding of drugs that have been identified as vitamin B_6 antagonists, which may also impair the binding of the coenzyme to apoenzyme or actually alter the structural configuration of the apoenzyme. However, there is no example currently known of a drug which interferes with pyridoxine metabolism that does not affect more than one and probably all vitamin B_6-dependent enzymatic pathways. In order to illustrate the complexity of the pyridoxine-responsive diseases, the example of pyridoxine-responsive anemia may best be cited. There is evidence from the work of Vogler and Mingioli (1965) that in pyridoxine-responsive anemia, the rate-limiting enzyme in heme synthesis, delta-aminolevulinic acid synthetase (ALA-synthetase), may be abnormal.

In a further study by Vogler and Mingioli (1968) of a patient with pyridoxine-responsive anemia, findings suggested that heme synthetase activity was also reduced. Since both ALA-synthetase and heme synthetase are mitochondrial enzymes, the authors speculate that there may be a mitochondrial abnormality in this disease. While in pyridoxine-responsive anemia hematological remissions are dependent on the continued administration of high levels of the vitamin, there is no evidence of a general vitamin B_6 deficiency pertaining to other functional systems of the body. Variable pyridoxine-responsiveness in this anemia has been attributed either to the fact there may be more than one primary biochemical abnormality, that the patients may differ in their pyridoxine requirements other than by virtue of their genetic disease, or that they may have an extremely high pyridoxine requirement occasioned by the intake of drugs which are pyridoxine antagonists (Horrigan and Harris 1968). Levels of pyridoxine intake required by patients with the pyridoxine-responsive diseases vary from 10 to 500 mg/day (Scriver 1973).

Vitamin D.—In the disease termed hereditary vitamin D-dependent rickets, remission until recently has been dependent upon administration of very high doses of vitamin D (Scriver 1970). Recently Frazier *et al.* (1973) produced evidence that in vitamin D-dependent rickets, a block is present in the conversion of 25-hydroxycholecalciferol to 1,25-dihydroxycholecalciferol.   These authors have postulated a genetic defect in 25-hydroxycholecalciferol-1-hydroxylase, the enzyme responsible for the production of the 1,25-dihydroxy vitamin derivative.

ACQUIRED FACTORS

Physiological Determinants

Nutrient requirements are increased by such physiological factors as active growth, pregnancy and lactation. At whatever stage of life nutrients have to be built into new tissue, over and above the physiological process of repair and replacement, nutrient requirements are increased. Growth, meaning the accretion of new tissue, begins at conception and will continue at different rates into adolescence. If growth is arrested through malnutrition, disease, or the effects of drugs, catch-up growth may follow arrest of the growth-retarding process. Adult growth and development includes the adaptations of the body to pregnancy and lactation. Increased and specific nutrient requirements for growth depend on the particular tissue being formed.

Nutrient requirements of the fetus vary with the phase of development.   Fetal drain on maternal nutrient pools is different in the period of embryogenesis from that during maturation. While it is generally believed that the fetus receives nutrients at the expense of the mother, maternal nutrient depletion can affect fetal development and growth adversely. Moreover, if a situation is created whereby a nutrient ingested by the mother cannot be utilized, then the fetal demand will not be satisfied. Arrest or aberrations of early fetal growth, occasioned by the non-availability of critical nutrients may result in malformations.   For example, the critical nutrient for nucleic acid synthesis essential to cell division is folic acid. Thus the maternal requirement for folic acid is increased during the first trimester of pregnancy to permit normal development of fetal tissues. Drugs may intervene to decrease the availability of folate to the mother and hence to the fetus, and in these circumstances the maternal requirement for folate may be heightened above those imposed by early pregnancy. Similarly in late pregnancy when the fetus is undergoing maturation and laying down nutrient stores, the maternal nutrient requirements are increased with respect to macronutrients. Drugs that cause anorexia or decrease the rate or extent of transference of nutrients via the placenta to the fetus will decrease fetal growth or retard skeletal or possibly brain maturation.

In postnatal life, genetic, endocrine, nutritional and environmental factors interact to determine growth. In considering nutritional requirements for the infant or child, the objective is to build up stores of specific nutrients to promote soft tissue development, skeletal growth and normal maturation. For the pregnant woman, nutritional needs are related not only to her requirements, but also those of the fetus, and for the lactating woman recommended nutrient intake is set at a level to support efficient milk production without causing maternal depletion. While optimal nutrient intake through periods of physiological stress allows a margin of safety to offset variable losses, it is assumed that no intervening factors, such as drug intake, exist which could further elevate nutritional requirements.

Disease Variables

Among disease categories which markedly increase nutritional requirements, the following are most significant: (1) conditions of impaired nutrient absorption, such as the celiac-sprue syndrome, (2) hemolytic anemias, such as sickle cell disease, (3) chronic infections associated with pyrexia, such as tuberculosis, (4) inflammatory bowel disease, such as ulcerative colitis, and (5) collagen diseases, such as rheumatoid arthritis.

Maldigestion and Malabsorption

These disorders are inevitably associated with nutrient depletion with or without clinical evidence of malnutrition. Multiple deficiency syndromes are common; their variety and severity depending upon the disease process, the area of the small intestine that is involved, and the extent of the disease. Weser *et al.* (1966) have divided the diseases associated with malabsorption into nine categories, including those due to inadequate digestion, those in which there is a biochemical abnormality, conditions in which the gastrointestinal mucosa is abnormal or atrophic, conditions associated with an altered intestinal bacterial flora, lymphatic obstruction, inadequate absorptive surface, conditions in which the intestinal motility is disturbed, endocrine disease, and vascular abnormalities. Malabsorption syndromes and their several etiologies are listed in Table 2.1.

Syndromes of malnutrition associated with malabsorption can be divided into four major categories, i.e. those extensive lesions of the gastrointestinal tract in which there is a predominant fecal loss of macronutrients, including fat and proteins; those in which the disease process primarily affects the upper portion of the small intestines, resulting in steatorrhea, folate deficiency, malabsorption of fat-soluble vitamins, and malabsorption of iron; those in which the malabsorption affects the lower portion of the small intestine, more especially the ileum, resulting in vitamin B_{12} deficiency; and selective forms of malabsorption in which a nutrient cannot be absorbed due to loss of a transport mechanism. Specific malabsorption syndromes within these categories are listed in Table 2.2, together with the characteristic nutritional deficiencies with which they are associated.

It should be emphasized that malnutrition resulting from disease-induced malabsorption can frequently be exacerbated by administration of drugs which also impair absorptive capacity. This is true whether the drugs act primarily on gastrointestinal enzymatic function, whether they damage the intestinal mucosa, or whether their effects are exerted after absorption. There is no definitive evidence, in primary diseases associated with malabsorption of nutrients, that impaired absorption of drugs is such that adverse effects of the pharmacologic agents on the absorptive process are decreased.

In the presence of malabsorption, the rate at which nutrient depletion occurs varies not only with the site and extent of the absorptive impairment, but also as to whether the nutrient is stored in the body. Slowly developing avitaminoses in the presence of malabsorption can be explained both as occurring because of partial loss of intestinal absorptive capacity, and also because of the gradual depletion of body stores of such vitamins as vitamin B_{12}, folate, and vitamin D. Whereas there are patients with relatively moderate degrees of malabsorption in whom it is possible to correct nutrient depletion by oral nutrient supplementation, this approach is by no means always successful. Even when correction or control of the primary disease process is possible, it is usually necessary to treat nutritional deficiencies by giving nutrients such as vitamins and iron by the parenteral route. When it is necessary to give drugs that can cause malnutrition or nutrient-depletion to patients with any one of the malabsorption syndromes, it should be realized that their nutri-

TABLE 2.1

MALABSORPTION SYNDROMES AND THEIR ETIOLOGIES

Etiology	Disease
1. Maldigestion	Chronic pancreatitis Gastric resection Hepatobiliary disease Cystic fibrosis Corticosteroids causing pancreatic necrosis Disaccharidase deficiency Cholestyramine
2. Defective transport mechanisms	Cystinuria Hartnup's disease Congenital folate malabsorption Congenital B_{12} malabsorption PAS induced B_{12} malabsorption Alcohol Biguanides Mineral oil
3. Gastrointestinal mucosal defects	Pernicious anemia Gluten-sensitive enteropathy Regional ileitis Amyloidosis Radiation injury Whipple's disease Lymphoma Kwashiorkor Pellagra Neomycin Colchicine Acute enteritis Dermatitis herpetiformis Alcohol
4. Abnormal bacterial flora	Blind loops. Fistulae Strictures Tropical sprue Scleroderma
5. Insufficient absorptive surface	Intestinal resection or bypass
6. Luminal parasites	Dibothriocephalus latus Hookworm Strongyloides Giardia lamblia
7. Vascular disease	Congestive heart failure Superior mesenteric arterial occlusion
8. Lymphatic abnormalities or obstruction	Intestinal lymphangietasia Hodgkins disease
9. Endocrine abnormalities	Diabetes mellitus Zollinger-Ellison syndrome Carcinoid syndrome Addison's disease Hypoparathyroidism

TABLE 2.2

NUTRIENT LOSSES IN COMMON MALABSORPTION SYNDROMES

Type of Defect	Diseases or Drugs	Nutrient Loss
Selective	Pernicious anemia Alcohol	Vitamin B_{12} Folate - thiamin

Proximal	Gastric, duodenal or
	  jejunal resection
	Gluten-sensitive
	  enteropathy
	Cholestyramine
		Folate, iron
		  Vitamins A, D,
		K
		Fat, calcium

Distal	Blind loop syndromes Ileal resection Regional ileitis PAS	Fat Vitamin B_{12}

Extensive	Tropical sprue
	Pancreatic insufficiency
	Neomycin
	Colchicine
		Fat, nitrogen,
		  folate, iron,
		  Vitamins A, D,
		K, B_{12}

ent stores may be severely depleted and that evidences of clinical deficiency may rapidly supervene after the drug treatment is initiated.

INCREASED CELL TURNOVER

Episodic or slowly progressive avitaminoses may develop in patients with diseases that are characterized by increased cell turnover. In hemolytic anemias associated with increased erythropoiesis, nutrient requirements for heme synthesis and red blood cell maturation may be elevated to an extent that they cannot be met by dietary intake. Megaloblastosis has been described in patients with congenital or acquired hemolytic anemias. In these conditions, folic acid deficiency is usually responsible for the megaloblastic state, though deficiency of vitamin B_{12} may be a contributory factor. A number of authors have described progressive folic acid deficiency in children and in adults with sickle cell disease (Jonsson *et al.* 1959; Oliner and Heller 1959; MacIver and Went 1960; Shaldon 1961; Lindenbaum and Klippstein 1963).

Lopez *et al.* (1973) studied a ten year old child with sickle cell anemia who had four episodes of folic acid deficiency in a period of two and a half years. The first two episodes were characterized by megaloblastic changes in the erythrocytes. Neither impaired intestinal absorption of folate, nor excessive urinary excretion of the vitamin, were apparently involved in the process. The child could only be maintained free of folic acid deficiency when he received a daily supplement of folic acid, in spite of the fact that he apparently consumed a diet that would prevent folate deficiency in a normal child of his age. Pierce and Rath (1962) described a twenty-one-year old patient with sickle cell disease who had two episodes of folic acid deficiency despite a normal food intake. Willoughby *et al.* (1961) described a woman with acquired autoimmune hemolytic anemia who developed megaloblastic erythropoiesis. On separate occasions she showed a hemolytic response to parenteral vitamin B_{12} and folic acid. However, it is difficult to interpret the relationship of vitamin administration to changes in the blood picture, because at the time she received the vitamin B_{12} she also had a blood transfusion.

In a number of reports of megaloblastic anemia developing in patients with hemolytic disease, there have been contributory factors which may predispose the patient to folic acid- or vitamin B_{12}-deficiency. These have included pregnancy or poor nutrient intake (Goldberg and Schwartz 1954; Drury and Geoghegan 1957; Jonsson 1958). It is significant in the present context that Jonsson reported that pyrimethamine, which is a folic acid antagonist, produces a megaloblastic change more rapidly in the marrow of patients with hemolytic anemia than in normal subjects.

Folate-deficiency is often present in patients with leukemia but appears to be multifactorial, and not only related to the overproduction of abnormal leukocytes. In chronic myelofibrosis, there is an increase in folate requirements because of ineffective hemopoiesis and, in certain instances, because of shortened red cell survival time (Chanarin 1970).

Increased nutrient requirements not only occur in diseases in which there is a rapid cell turnover within the hemopoietic system, but also in circumstances where there is increased epidermal cell turnover. Increased epidermal cell turnover has been found within and between the lesions of psoriasis and pityriasis rubra pilaris (Porter and Shuster 1968). While it is known that folate-deficiency occurring in patients with exfoliative psoriasis or other forms of erythroderma may be due to malabsorption, Shuster and Marks (1970) believe that the epidermal requirements for folate may contribute to the deficiency found in these diseases. The folate antagonist, methotrexate, has been extensively used in the treatment of psoriasis, but the risk of this medication has to be evaluated in face of the reports of folate-deficiency existing in the untreated disease. According to Shuster, the psoriatic lesions do not spread when supplementary or therapeutic doses of folic acid are administered.

Gough and his co-workers (1964) studied six patients with rheumatoid arthritis who also had megaloblastic anemia. In each of these cases it was established that the megaloblastic anemia was due to folate-deficiency, although the intestinal absorption of vitamin B_{12} was also depressed in three of the patients. In an extension of this study by these authors to include 46 patients with rheumatoid arthritis, it was found that there was a significant increase in the incidence of folate-deficiency as compared with the incidence in 57 control subjects. Attempting to explain the association of folate deficiency with rheumatoid arthritis, the authors offer the suggestion that the cellular proliferation in the joints of patients with rheumatoid arthritis may cause an increased demand for folic acid. While this is an interesting idea, it must be remarked that Gough's patients were, except in three cases, taking drug combinations including aspirin, which has since been documented as a pharmacological agent capable of inducing folate depletion (Alter et al. 1971).

INCREASED NUTRIENT LOSSES

Whenever the nutrient losses from the body exceed the normal range, nutrient requirements are increased. Thus, protein requirements are increased in patients with extensive burns or those with bullous dermatoses, in those with protein-losing enteropathy or nephrosis. Similarly, iron requirements are increased in the presence of hemorrhage, whether this is due to physiological causes, trauma, or disease.

Except in the circumstance of malabsorption, little is known about excess losses of vitamins via the urine or the skin. In an editorial on the nutritional status of patients with chronic renal disease before and after hemodialysis, it is pointed out that hypovitaminoses occurring in these patients are more likely to be due to inadequate intake rather than to increased loss (Nutrition Reviews 1969). Hampers et al. (1967) studied a group of uremic patients who had megaloblastic changes in the blood associated with low serum folate levels, and they suggested that the folate deficiency in their patients was due to removal of folate from the blood during hemodialysis. Serum folate is dialyzable, and Whitehead et al. (1968) have shown that a rapid fall in serum folate follows hemodialysis. Values return to predialysis values within about four days. In the 1969 editorial mentioned above, the writer comments that in anuric patients normal renal folate losses are obviated, and the losses from the body are limited to those occurring into the bile and those due to hemodialysis. Reports from Poland by Czarnecki et al. (1960) have indicated that hemodialysis may result in decreased blood levels of riboflavin, and Hasik, (1961) suggested that hemodialysis also results in decreased serum levels of ascorbic acid.

HYPERMETABOLIC STATES

Werner (1955), in his standard text on the thyroid gland states that in thyrotoxicosis there is an increased requirement for vitamin A, thiamin, pyridoxine, vitamin B_{12} and ascorbic acid, as well as increased demands for macronutrients. Rivlin (1971), in contributing to the Third Edition of this text, makes certain more up-to-date statements about the effects of thyrotoxicosis on vitamin requirements. His discussion is based on a number of investigations, including his own. The increased requirement for thiamin in this disease is substantiated, and it is pointed out that thiamin has an action which in some ways resembles that of propylthiouracil. Supplementary vitamin C appears to diminish weight loss. The pyridoxine status of hyperthyroid patients is depressed, owing apparently to an accelerated degradation of pyridoxal phosphate. Vitamin B_{12} levels in the plasma may or may not be decreased, and there is evidence that when vitamin B_{12} levels are reduced, there may be a coincidental pernicious anemia. Erythrocyte and serum folate levels as well as hepatic folate concentrations are reduced, and there is an increased FIGLU excretion following histidine load, but the reasons for folate depletion are unexplained. Since riboflavin has been found to stimulate the formation of flavin mononucleotide (FMN) and flavin adenine dinucleotide (FAD) from riboflavin, it would appear that thyrotoxicosis promotes formation of the active and storage forms of riboflavin. However, if the riboflavin status of the patient is deficient, then there might be a lessened conversion of the vitamin to FMN and FAD.

In hypermetabolic conditions associated with pyrexial disease, there is evidence that mineral and vitamin depletion develops rapidly. It is difficult to evaluate to what extent these nutritional changes are due primarily to hypermetabolism and to what extent they are associated either with depressed nutrient intake, absorption or utilization, occurring independently or together with increased metabolic rate associated with the fever.

Pekarek and Beisel (1972) found that with a number of bacterial and viral infections, serum iron and zinc concentrations were depressed from the beginning of the symptomatic illness. These authors also found that magnesium balance became negative following onset of symptoms associated with certain infectious diseases. They have suggested that changes in mineral metabolism occurring during fevers are mediated by an endogenous factor which is released into the serum by leukocytes, or that the effects may possibly be due to endotoxin production by bacteria. Increased requirements for vitamin A, thiamin, folate, riboflavin, and ascorbic acid have been recommended as necessary in pyrexial disease, though again here it is difficult to say that these are justified on the basis of increased metabolic rate (Nutrition: A Comprehensive Treatise 1964).

DECREASED NUTRIENT UTILIZATION

In acute, or more particularly, chronic diseases in which the structural integrity of organs is impaired, nutritional requirements may be increased because of inefficient nutrient utilization. For example, in hepatocellular disease such as occurs in cirrhosis, the requirement for vitamin D is increased because of impaired formation of the 25-hydroxycholecalciferol metabolite within the hepatocytes. Patients with liver disease show a slow plasma disappearance of vitamin D and also a decreased formation of vitamin D-glucuronide conjugate (Scott *et al.* 1965; Avioli *et al.* 1967). In biliary cirrhosis, the impairment in the metabolism of vitamin D in the liver is complicated by a coexistence malabsorption of vitamin D (Thompson *et al.* 1966). Evidences of folate-deficiency occurring in patients with liver disease are common, and it is believed that several factors may be responsible including impaired formation of the active form of the vitamin and impaired hepatic storage. This matter is discussed in connection with the nutritional effects of alcoholism. Herbert (1965), in discussing various hemopoietic effects of liver disease, mentions that the liver is unable to store pyridoxine or folate efficiently in these conditions. Cherrick *et al.* (1965) found that in cirrhosis, liver folate levels are affected relatively more than serum folate levels. It is suggested that relatively high serum folate levels in these patients may be related to displacement of liver folate into the serum.

According to Lear *et al.* (1954), serum vitamin B_{12} levels may be either normal or elevated in liver disease. Similarly Jones and Mills (1955) found that serum vitamin B_{12} levels were elevated in cirrhosis and these findings were confirmed by Rachmilewitz *et al.* (1956). The reduced capacity of the liver to store vitamin B_{12} in liver disease results in an increased urinary excretion of vitamin B_{12}, as shown in the Schilling test, according to Maslow *et al.* (1957). Chanarin (1969) has discussed various aspects of the liver's failure to retain folate and vitamin B_{12} in liver disease, as well as the reversal or partial reversal of changes during a period when the liver is regenerating.

An inability to utilize a specific nutrient is also evident in chronic renal disease. With chronic renal insufficiency there is impaired calcium absorption and secondary parathyroid hyperactivity. In uremia, and probably in lesser degrees of the renal insufficiency, the kidney is unable to form 1,25-dihydroxycholecalciferol from 25-

hydroxycholecalciferol, and since the former metabolite is necessary to the absorption of calcium from the intestine, this is apparently the major reason for reduced calcium absorption (Avioli *et al.* 1968). Avioli and Haddad (1973) have suggested that, in some uremic patients, alteration in the metabolism of vitamin D or its metabolites can lead to the accumulation of abnormal metabolites which then compete with 1,25-dihydroxycholecalciferol at receptor sites in various organs, including not only the intestine, but also in bones. Failure of utilization of nutrients required for synthesis of heme and maturation of erythrocytes may be secondary to lack of erythropoietin production.

VARIABLES ASSOCIATED WITH DISEASE INTERVENTION

In addition to the alterations in nutritional requirements imposed by disease or drugs, it is necessary to consider special needs of those who will undergo treatment involving physical stress and tissue trauma.

Nutritional management of the surgical patient is aimed not only towards repletion of the nutritionally depleted, but also to offset demand for nutrients in the postoperative period. Malnutrition, in a broad sense, may decrease an anesthetic tolerance, decrease a patient's ability to withstand surgical trauma, and delay wound healing (Dudrick *et al.* 1964; Gillette 1967).

Nutrient losses after surgery vary with the age of the patient, the disease condition for which surgical intervention is required, as well as with the site and magnitude of surgical trauma. In the days immediately after major surgical injury, not only is there considerable nitrogen loss, but also urinary loss of potassium, magnesium and zinc (Walker 1974; Walker *et al.* 1968; and Fell *et al.* 1973). The extent to which such nutrient depletion prejudices recovery is variable, risk being greatest if the patient has been nutritionally exhausted before the operation. Because of differences in nutrient losses, occasioned by different surgical procedures, one should be cautious about making too many generalizations concerning the nutritional requirements of surgical patients. For example, calcium requirements of the surgical patient may be related to the degree of hypercalciuria induced by the operative trauma. Hypercalciuria has been found frequently following skeletal trauma, whether produced by operation or by accident; it also may occur with immobilization or with soft tissue surgical injury (Walker 1974).

The rate of wound healing is slowed and the risk of wound dehiscence increased if nutrient gain is inadequate in the pre- or post-surgery period. Protein malnutrition, with associated hypoproteinemia, not only impairs the efficiency of tissue repair, but also may lead to edema of the wound area and cause wound edges including gastrointestinal suture lines to separate. Key nutrients in wound healing, other than protein, include ascorbic acid required for normal collagen formation, vitamin K needed to promote clot formation, and several micronutrients, including niacin, riboflavin, folate, vitamin A and zinc, to achieve optimal epithelialization of denuded surfaces. There is no evidence, however, that preoperative megadoses of these nutrients offer any protection against the complications of surgery (Williams and Zollinger 1955; Murray 1955; and Flynn et al. 1973).

Long term nutrient requirements of patients who have undergone surgery to the gastrointestinal tract may be greatly altered. This is particularly true of the post-gastrectomy patients, who can not only become malnourished due to diminished food intake, but also due to malabsorption of iron, vitamin B_{12}, folate, calcium, vitamin D and fats (McLean Baird 1973). Deliberate use of the jejuno-ileal bypass procedure to treat gross obesity by creating a state of malabsorption has been advocated by some physicians in spite of the risks involved. Not only may this procedure be quite frequently complicated by hepatic dysfunction, but also hypokalemia, hypomagnesemia and hypocalcemia may occur unless these nutrients are replenished by dietary means or by supplements (Nutrition Reviews 1974).

Nutritional status may be compromised as a result of radiation sickness or radiation injury to the gastrointestinal tract. While nausea, vomiting, anorexia and weight loss are commonly associated with any extensive therapeutic exposure to ionizing radiation, radiation damage to the small intestine results in a post-irradiation malabsorption syndrome (Jacobson 1963; Duncan and Leonard 1965; and Greenburger and Isselbacher 1964). Steatorrhea, disaccharidase deficiency and protein-losing enteropathy are associated with villous atrophy, and lymphangiectasia may follow abdominal radiation (Reeves et al. 1965; Tarpila 1971; and Tarpila and Jussila 1969).

Malnutrition following radiation enteritis may be complicated by administration of cancer chemotherapeutic agents, such as actinomycin D, which inhibits protein synthesis (D'Angio et al. 1959). However, Donaldson et al. (1975) have shown that, at least in children, recovery from radiation enteritis is promoted by dietary management aimed to reverse nutrient depletion and to circumvent food intolerance due to effects of radiation. They recommend temporary use of a gluten- and lactose-free diet in the treatment of children with malignant disease undergoing or having undergone radiation therapy with or without addition of chemotherapeutic agents.

NUTRITION AND CANCER

Whether or not nutrient intake can be manipulated to inhibit carcinogenesis of the spread of cancer in man cannot yet receive a definitive answer. While anorexia, inanition and cachexia are common features of advanced or widespread malignant disease, nutrient supplementation has little effect in sparing host tissues. Though parenteral alimentation with carbohydrates and purified amino acids may have a temporary beneficial effect on the nutrition of cancer patients, there is no evidence that a positive nitrogen balance can be maintained by this means (Waterhouse 1974; Dudrick *et al.* 1968). Nutritional rehabilitation of the cancer patient implies control of tumor growth, except in those instances where the malnutrition is primarily due to malignant disease of the gastrointestinal tract which can be relieved by surgery.

On the basis that tumors require specific nutrients for growth, numerous attempts have been made to inhibit tumor development by producing specific avitaminoses, or deliberate under-nutrition. Whereas tumor growth in experimental animals may be inhibited by giving vitamin-deficient diets, the use of vitamin-deficient diets alone in the management of human cancer has been singularly unsuccessful. Combination of a vitamin-deficient diet with the administration of a synthetic antivitamin may produce a significant antitumor effect. For example, induction of dietary riboflavin deficiency together with administration of galactoflavin, a riboflavin antagonist, has induced partial remission in isolated cases of Hodgkin's disease and lymphosarcoma (Rivlin 1973).

The possibility that nutrient requirements are peculiarly increased in malignant disease has been recently advanced. In tumor-bearing rats it has been shown by Heilman and Swarm (1975) that the cis isomer of vitamin A acid can inhibit the growth and development of chondrosarcomata. Under certain experimental conditions, chemical carcinogenesis may also be inhibited by vitamin A (Sporn and Wendell 1975). However, the relationship between vitamin A and tumor suppression is not uniform and large doses of the vitamin can potentiate lung tumor growth in laboratory animals (Smith *et al.* 1975).

Whereas the statement that nutritional requirements are altered by the development of malignant disease is a gross oversimplification of a very complex problem, it may have practical significance. Cancer chemotherapeutic drugs frequently have adverse effects on nutritional status. The patient's ability to withstand these cytotoxic drugs depends in part on appropriate nutritional rehabilitation during and immediately after the period of treatment.

DRUG METABOLISM AND NUTRIENT REQUIREMENTS

Numerous animal experiments have indicated that in induced nutritional deficiency states drug metabolism may be altered. Conversely, in certain instances, nutrient supplementation may increase the efficiency of drug biotransformation. Effects of dietary manipulation on drug metabolism are complex. For example, whereas a reduction in either the quantity or quality of dietary protein decreases the activity of the hepatic microsomal mixed function oxidase system, this may have a beneficial effect if the drug intermediate is more toxic than the parent drug, and an adverse effect if the parent drug is more toxic than the metabolites. It has been identified that not only protein but also carbohydrate, lipids, riboflavin, ascorbic acid, magnesium and zinc deficiencies have marked effects on mixed function oxidase activity (Campbell and Hayes 1974).

Despite the large number of animal studies indicating the relationship between nutritional status and drug metabolism, very little is known as to whether the data can be extrapolated to man. Poskitt (1974) has commented that "considering the extensive use of drugs in malnutrition, it is perhaps unfortunate that there are so few studies of drug metabolism." Investigations are indeed needed to show whether drug metabolism is markedly altered in people with nutritional deficiency diseases, whether the malnutrition is due to an inadequate diet or the presence of disease. Nutritional rehabilitation in malnourished people receiving drugs should take into account the special requirements for drug biotransformation.

The emphasis given to the various pathological conditions which increase nutrient requirements is justified, because these may determine the depleted nutritional status of any patient who may be receiving medications which in themselves further increase nutritional requirements, and hence increase the likelihood of clinical nutritional deficiency disease. Herbert (1973) has suggested that it should be possible to define the minimal daily requirements for a nutrient, knowing the utilizable body stores of that nutrient, and the days over which that nutrient would be depleted. This means that if the state of nutrient depletion due to disease were known at the time that a drug therapy is initiated, and the rate of nutrient depletion due to the drug is known, it might be possible to overcome the defect by appropriate administration of nutrient supplements. Practical difficulties in estimating body stores of nutrients do not detract from the need to measure the nutritional status of patients with conditions that increase nutrient requirements and cause nutrient depletion before drug therapy is initiated, so that an attempt can be made to overcome resultant nutrient depletion.

BIBLIOGRAPHY

ALTER, H. J., ZVAIFLER, N. J., and RATH, C. E. 1971. Interrelationship of rheumatoid arthritis, folic acid and aspirin. Blood 38, 405-416.

ANON. 1969. Dialysis, renal failure, and vitamin homeostasis. Nutr. Rev. 27, 75-78.

ANON. 1974. Current status of jejuno-ileal bypass for obesity. Nutr. Rev. 32, 333-336.

ARAKAWA, T. 1970. Congenital defects in folate utilization. Am. J. Med. 48, 594-598.

AVIOLI, L. V., BURGET, S., LEE, S. W., and SLATOPOLSKY, E. 1968. The metabolic fate of vitamin D_3-^{3}H in chronic renal failure. J. Clin. Invest. 47, 2239-2252.

AVIOLI, L. V., and HADDAD, J. G. 1973. Vitamin D current concepts. Progress in endocrinology and metabolism. Metabolism 22, 507-531.

AVIOLI, L. V., et al. 1967. Metabolism of vitamin D_3-^{3}H in human subjects: distribution in blood, bile, feces and urine. J. Clin. Invest. 46, 983-992.

BEATON, G. H., and McHENRY, E. W. 1964. Nutrition: A Comprehensive Treatise, Vol. 2. Academic Press, New York and London.

CAMPBELL, T. C., and HAYES, J. R. 1974. Role of nutrition in the drug-metabolizing enzyme system. Pharmacol. Rev. 26, 171-197.

CHANARIN, I. 1969. The Megaloblastic Anaemias. Blackwell Scientific Publ., Oxford and Edinburgh.

CHANARIN, I. 1970. Folate deficiency in myeloproliferative disorders. Am. J. Clin. Nutr. 23, 855-860.

CHERRICK, G. R., BAKER, H., FRANK, O. and LEEVY, C. M. 1965. Observations on hepatic avidity for folate in Laennec's cirrhosis. J. Lab. Clin. Med. 66, 446-451.

CZARNECKI, R., BIALECKI, M., BACZYK, K., and KOPCZYK, T. 1960. Effect of therapeutic use of hemodialysis on riboflavin concentration in blood. Pol. Tyg. Lek. 15, 1691-1693.

D'ANGIO, G. J., FARBER, S., and MADDOCK, C. L. 1959. Potentiation of x-ray effects by actinomycin D. Radiology 73, 175-177.

DONALDSON, S. S. et al. 1975. Radiation enteritis in children—a retrospective review. Chemico pathologic correlation, and dietary management. Cancer 35, 1167-1178.

DRURY, M. I., and GEOGHEGAN, F. 1957. Congenital haemolytic anemia complicated by megaloblastic anaemia of pregnancy. Brit. Med. J. 2, 393-394.

DUDRICK, S. J. et al. 1964. Nutritional care of the surgical patient. Med. Clin. N. Am. 48, 1253-1269.

DUDRICK, S. J. et al. 1968. Long-term total parenteral nutrition with growth development and positive nitrogen balance. Surgery 64, 134-142.

DUNCAN, W., and LEONARD, J. C. 1965. The malabsorption syndrome following radiotherapy. Quart. J. Med. 34, 319-329.

FELL, G. S. et al. 1973. Urinary zinc levels as an indication of muscle catabolism. Lancet 1, 280-282.

FLYNN, A. et al. 1973. Zinc deficiency with altered adrenocortical function and its relation to delayed healing. Lancet 1, 789-791.

FRAZIER, D. et al. 1973. Pathogenesis of hereditary vitamin-D-dependent rickets. An inborn error of vitamin D metabolism involving defective conversion of 25-hydroxy-vitamin D to 1,25-dihydroxyvitamin D. New Eng. J. Med. 289, 817-822.

GILLETTE, J. R. 1967. Individually different responses to drugs according to age, sex and functional or pathological state. In Drug Responses in Man. CIBA Foundation. G. Wolstenholme, and R. Porter (Editors). J. & A. Churchill Ltd., London.

GOLDBERG, M. A., and SCHWARTZ, S. O. 1954. Mediterranean anaemia in a Negro complicated by pernicious anemia of pregnancy. Blood 9, 648-654.
GOUGH, E. R. et al. 1964. Folic acid deficiency in rheumatoid arthritis. Brit. Med. J. 1, 212-217.
GREENBURGER, N. J., and ISSELBACHER, K. J. 1964. Malabsorption following radiation injury to the gastrointestinal tract. Am. J. Med. 36, 450-456.
HAKAMI, N., NEIMAN, P. E., CANELLOS, G. P., and LAZERSON, J. 1971. Neonatal megaloblastic anemia due to inherited transcobalamin II deficiency in two siblings. New Eng. J. Med. 285, 1163-1170.
HAMPERS, C. L. et al. 1967. Megaloblastic hematopoiesis in uremia and in patients on long term hemodialysis. New Eng. J. Med. 276, 551-554.
HASIK, J. 1961. Ascorbic acid during the course of extracorporial dialysis. Poznan. Towarz. Przyjaciol Navk Wydzial Lekar. 21, 161-166 (Polish).
HEILMAN, T. C., and SWARM, R. L. 1975. Effects of 13 cis vitamin A acid on chondrosarcoma. Fed. Proc. 34, 822 (Abs.).
HERBERT, V. 1965. Hemopoietic factors in liver disease. In Progress in Liver Disease, H. Popper, and F. Schaffner (Editors). Grune and Stratton, New York and London.
HERBERT, V. 1973. The five possible causes of all nutrient deficiency, illustrated by deficiencies of vitamin B$_{12}$ and folic acid. Am. J. Clin. Nutr. 26, 77-88.
HORRIGAN, D. L., and HARRIS, J. W. 1968. Pyridoxine-responsive anemias in man. In Vitamins and Hormones, Vol. 26, R. S. Harris, I. G. Wohl, and J. A. Loraine (Editors). Academic Press, New York and London.
JACOBSON, L. O. 1963. Radiation injury. In Cecil-Loeb Textbook of Medicine, P. B. Beeson, and W. McDermott (Editors). W. B. Saunders Co., Philadelphia, London.
JONES, P. N., and MILLS, E. H. 1955. Serum vitamin B$_{12}$ concentrations in liver disease. (Abst.) J. Lab. Clin. Med. 46, 927.
JONSSON, U. 1958. Nutritional megaloblastic anaemia in sickle cell states and the relation of folic acid to blastic crises in hemolytic anaemias. Internat. Soc. Hematol. 7th Proc. Inter. Congr., Vol. 2. Intercontinental Med. New York, 1960.
JONSSON, U., ROATH, O. S., and KIRKPATRICK, C. I. F. 1959. Nutritional megaloblastic anemia associated with sickle cell states. Blood 14, 535-547.
KATZ, M., LEE, S. K., and COOPER, B. A. 1972. Vitamin B$_{12}$ malabsorption due to a biologically inert intrinsic factor. New Eng. J. Med. 287, 425-429.
LANZKOWSKY, P. 1970. Congenital malabsorption of folate. Am. J. Med. 48, 580-583.
LEAR, A. A., HARRIS, J. W., CASTLE, W. B., and FLEMING, E. M. 1954. The serum vitamin B$_{12}$ concentration in pernicious anemia. J. Lab. Clin. Med. 44, 715-722.
LINDENBAUM, J., and KLIPPSTEIN, F. A. 1963. Folic acid deficiency in sickle cell anemia. New Eng. J. Med. 269, 875-882.
LOPEZ, R., SHIMIZU, N., and COOPERMAN, J. M. 1973. Recurrent folic acid deficiency in sickle cell disease. Am. J. Dis. Child 125, 544-548.
MacIVER, J. E., and WENT, L. N. 1960. Sickle cell anaemia complicated by megaloblastic anaemia of infancy. Brit. Med. J. 1, 775-779.
MAHONEY, M. J., and ROSENBERG, L. E. 1970. Inherited defects of B$_{12}$ metabolism. Am. J. Med. 48, 584-593.
MASLOW, W. C., DONNELLY, W. J., KOPPEL, D. M., and SCHWARTZ, S. O. 1957. Observations on the use of CO^{60}-labeled vitamin B$_{12}$ in the urinary excretion test: clinical implications of the radioisotope technique. Acta Hemat. 18, 137-147.
McKENZIE, I. L., DONALDSON, R. M. JR., TRIER, J. S., and MATHAN, V. I. 1972. Ileal mucosa in familial selective vitamin B$_{12}$ malabsorption. New Eng. J. Med. 286, 1021-1025.

McLEAN BAIRD, I. 1973. Malnutrition due to malabsorption. *In* Nutritional Deficiencies in Modern Society, A. N. Howard, and I. McLean Baird (Editors). Newman Books, London.

MOLLIN, D. L., BAKER, S. J., and DONIACH, I. 1955. Addisonian pernicious anaemia without gastric atrophy in a young man. Brit. J. Haemat. *1*, 278-290.

MURRAY, P. JR. 1955. Nutrition and wound healing. Am. J. Clin. Nutr. *3*, 461-465.

OLINER, H. L., and HELLER, P. 1959. Megaloblastic erythropoiesis and acquired hemolysis in sickle cell anemia. New Eng. J. Med. *261*, 19-26.

PEKAREK, R. S., and BEISEL, W. R. 1972. Metabolic losses of zinc and other trace elements during acute infection. *In* Proc. Western Hemisphere Nutrition Congress III. Future Publishing Co.

PIERCE, L. E., and RATH, C. E. 1962. Evidence of folic acid deficiency in the genesis of anemic sickle cell crisis. Blood *20*, 19-32.

PORTER, D. I., and SHUSTER, S. 1968. Epidermal renewal and amino acids in psoriasis and pityriasis rubra pilaris. Arch. Dermat. *98*, 339-343.

POSKITT, E. M. E. 1974. Clinical problems related to the use of drugs in malnutrition. Proc. Nutr. Soc. *33*, 203-207.

RACHMILEWITZ, M., ARONOVITCH, J., and GROSSOWICZ, N. 1956. Serum concentrations of vitamin B_{12} in acute and chronic liver disease. J. Lab. Clin. Med. *48*, 339-344.

REEVES, R. J. *et al.* 1965. Fat absorption studies and small bowel x-ray studies in patients undergoing CO^{60} teletherapy and/or radium application. Am. J. Roentgenol. *94*, 848-851.

RIVLIN, R. S. 1971. Vitamin metabolism. *In* The Thyroid. A Fundamental and Clinical Text, 3rd Edition, S. C. Werner, and S. H. Ingbar (Editors). Harper and Rowe, New York and London.

RIVLIN, R. S. 1973. Riboflavin and cancer: A review. Cancer Res. *33*, 1977-1986.

ROSENBERG, L. E. 1969. Inherited amino acidopathies demonstrating vitamin dependency. New Eng. J. Med. *281*, 145-153.

SCOTT, K. G. *et al.* 1965. Measurements of the plasma levels of tritiated labeled vitamin D_3 in control and rachitic, cirrhotic and osteoporotic patients. Strahlentherapie (Suppl.) *60*, 317.

SCRIVER, C. R. 1970. Vitamin D dependency. Pediatrics *45*, 361-363.

SCRIVER, C. R. 1971. Mutant consumers with special needs. Nutr. Rev. *29*, 155-158.

SCRIVER, C. R. 1973. Vitamin responsive inborn errors of metabolism. Metabolism *22*, 1319-1343.

SHALDON, S. 1961. Megaloblastic erythropoiesis associated with sickle-cell anaemia. Brit. Med. J. *1*, 640-641.

SHOJANIA, A. M., and HORNADY, G. J. 1973. Oral contraceptives and folate absorption. J. Lab. Clin. Med. *82*, 869-875.

SHUSTER, S., and MARKS, J. 1970. Systemic Effects of Skin Disease. William Heinemann Med. Books, London.

SMITH, D. M. *et al.* 1975. Vitamin A (retinyl acetate) and benzo(a) pyrene-induced respiratory tract carcinogenesis in hamsters fed a commercial diet. Cancer Res. *35*, 11-16.

SPORN, M. B., and WENDELL, H. 1975. Griffith Memorial Symp., FASEB 59th Annual Meeting, April 13-18, Atlantic City, N.J.

SPURLING, C. L., SACKS, M. S., and JIJI, R. M. 1964. Juvenile pernicious anemia. New Eng. J. Med. *271*, 995-1003.

TARPILA, S. 1971. Morphological and functional response of human small intestine to ionizing irradiation. Scand. J. Gastroenterol. Suppl. *6*, 9-48.

TARPILA, S., and JUSSILA, J. 1969. The effect of radiation on the disaccharidase activities of human small intestinal mucosa. Scand. J. Clin. Lab. Invest. Suppl. *23*, Abs. 44.

THOMPSON, G. R., LEWIS, B., and BOOTH, C. C. 1966. Absorption of vitamin D_3-^{3}H in control subjects and patients with intestinal malabsorption. J. Clin. Invest. 45, 94-102.
VOGLER, W. R., and MINGIOLI, E. S. 1965. Heme synthesis in pyridoxine-responsive anemia. New Eng. J. Med. 273, 347-352.
VOGLER, W. R., and MINGIOLI, E. S. 1968. Porphyrin synthesis and heme synthetase activity in pyridoxine-responsive anemia. Blood 32, 979-988.
WALKER, W. F. 1974. Nutrition after injury. In World Rev. Nutr. and Dietetics 19, 173-204.
WALKER, W. F., FLEMING, L. W., and STEWART, W. K. 1968. Urinary magnesium excretion in surgical patients. Brit. J. Surg. 55, 466-469.
WALTERS, T. R. 1967. Congenital megaloblastic anemia responsive to N^5-formyltetrahydrofolic acid administration. J. Pediat. 70, 686.
WATERHOUSE, C. 1974. How tumors affect host metabolism. Ann. N.Y. Acad. Sci. 230, 86-93.
WESER, E., JEFFRIES, G. H., and SLEISENGER, M. H. 1966. Malabsorption. Gastroenterology 50, 811-828.
WERNER, S. C. 1955. The Thyroid. Hoeber-Harper, New York.
WHITEHEAD, V. M., COMTY, C. H., POSEN, G. A., and KAYE, M. 1968. Homeostasis of folic acid in patients undergoing maintenance hemodialysis. New Eng. J. Med. 279, 970-974.
WILLIAMS, R. J. 1963. Biochemical Individuality. John Wiley & Sons., New York (Science Editions, 1963).
WILLIAMS, R. D., and ZOLLINGER, R. M. 1955. Principles of surgical nutrition. Am. J. Clin. Nutr. 3, 449-455.
WILLOUGHBY, M. L. N., PEARS, M. A., SHARP, A. A., and SHIELDS, M. J. 1961. Megaloblastic erythropoiesis in acquired hemolytic anemia. Blood 17, 351-356.

CHAPTER 3

Variables Determining Incidence and Risk

While it can now be accepted that drugs of widely differing chemistry and pharmacologic action have the potential to cause nutritional deficiency, the actual incidence of drug-induced malnutrition in persons and populations receiving such drugs varies widely. Except in circumstances when the nutritional effect of drugs is inseparable from desired therapeutic effects, nutrient depletion by drugs is preventable, provided that the hazard is recognized. Unwarranted nutritional reactions from drugs are observed and reported more frequently today than in the past, and in part this change has been brought about by the same factors which have determined the increasing incidence of other forms of iatrogenic disease. According to Melmon (1971), major factors contributing to the upsurge of drug reactions are the greater availability of prescription and nonprescription drugs, as well as the physicians' lack of knowledge of pharmacology and the factors which predispose the drug reactions. Whereas escalating drug use is an important determinant of the numbers of people at risk for nutritional side effects, the major occurrence of nutritional deficiency in drug users is among those whose intake of drugs is prolonged, and in those whose dietary intake of the nutrients depleted by the drug is marginal.

NUTRIENT GAIN VERSUS REQUIREMENTS

Drug-induced nutritional deficiency is determined not only on a pharmacologic basis, i.e., on the characteristics of the drugs taken and their uses, but also by coexisting variables which singly or collectively impose nutrient requirements exceeding nutrient gain. Nutrient gain comprises intake and limited endogenous synthesis of nutrients, as well as their absorption and utilization, such that nutrient stores are sufficient for continued maintenance despite increasing nutrient requirements. In most circumstances, nutrient gain is quantitatively related to intake over time. Bearing this in mind, the risk of nutritional depletion and deficiency from drug intake can be conceptualized by following the models depicted in Fig. 3.1. It can be seen that if nutrient intake exceeds nutrient requirement both before and after a drug or drugs are taken, then depletion will not occur. When the drug regimen causes a major loss of nutrients, then maintenance of the original nutrient intake may be insufficient to prevent deficiency.

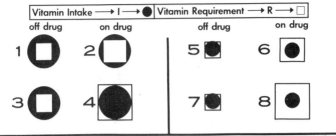

Increased vitamin requirements imposed by drug intake may be innocuous if
vitamin intake is ample (2).
Marginal vitamin intake (6) and/or major increase in requirements during period
of drug intake condition the degree of vitamin depletion (4,8).

FIG. 3.1. VITAMIN INTAKE AND REQUIREMENT AS INDICATORS OF
DRUG-INDUCED DEPLETION OR DEFICIENCY

On the other hand, if the subject has a nutrient intake prior to drug
usage which is equal to or less than requirements, then a moderate
nutrient loss caused by a drug will induce deficiency, that deficiency
being increased by the level and rate of drug-determined nutrient
losses.

Since requirements for individual nutrients exhibit genetic, physiological and pathological variability, as well as changes due to intake
of medication, it is necessary to consider all of these factors to use
the model in Fig. 3.1 realistically to decide whether an individual is
likely to become nutritionally depleted from the medications that he
or she is receiving.

GENETIC VARIABILITY IN DRUG METABOLISM

Pharmacogenetics

Among the factors identified as influencing the incidence of drug-
induced nutrient depletion, genetically determined differences in the
rate of drug metabolism may be considered as a relatively unexplored
field. However, from presently available evidence, it is clear that, if
the inactivation of a drug known to cause nutrient depletion is slow,
then the risk of such side effects is enhanced (Devadatta *et al.* 1960).

Slow Acetylation

Isonicotinic acid hydrazide (INH) is inactivated by acetylation.
Slow acetylation, which is an autosomal recessive trait, has been
demonstrated by Peters *et al.* (1965) to be due to lowered synthesis
of hepatic N-acetyl transferase. Hughes *et al.* (1955) first recognized,
and Devadatta *et al.* (1960) confirmed, that among those people who
are slow acetylators of INH, commonly prescribed doses of the drug

can result in persistently high blood levels and an unusually frequent incidence of peripheral neuritis, due to pyridoxine deficiency. According to LaDu (1972), other hydrazide drugs such as hydralazine are inactivated by the INH, N-acetyl transferase, and it is therefore suspected that pyridoxine deficiency due to this antihypertensive drug would tend to arise more commonly in those who have low activity of this enzyme.

A rare inborn error of drug metabolism is associated with inefficient hydroxylation of diphenylhydantoin (DPH). The inability of these persons to hydroxylate DPH is relative, but Kutt et al. (1964) described a family who demonstrated DPH toxicity while receiving a moderate dosage of this drug. Genetic incapacity to hydroxylate DPH appears to be confined to this drug, and such persons are able, according to Price Evans (1969), to hydroxylate phenobarbital and phenylalanine as well as normal people. As yet there is no convincing evidence that those who are slow hydroxylators of DPH are more likely to develop nutritional side effects from this drug than others receiving it, though this requires further investigation.

ACQUIRED FACTORS AFFECTING DRUG METABOLISM

Important acquired factors which influence drug metabolism include the rate of intestinal absorption and delivery of the drug to the liver, liver function, the presence of other disease including malnutrition, and the concomitant administration of other drugs which can either increase or inhibit the metabolism of the initial drug. There are numerous factors which are known to stimulate or damp down microsomal drug-metabolism, but our discussion here will be limited to examples where stimulation or inhibition of drug-metabolism has an effect on nutrient requirements.

Conney and Burns (1972) cite examples of drugs which are stimulators of hepatic microsomal enzyme systems and cause nutrient depletion in rats and in man. Whereas they cite examples where drugs such as the anticonvulsants, which are microsomal enzyme-inducers, increase the metabolism and breakdown of nutrients such as vitamin D, in a multiple drug regimen, one drug may stimulate or inhibit the metabolism of another. Whether or not an enzyme-inducer causes nutrient depletion may indeed depend in part upon the rate of breakdown of that drug, or conversely, on its persistence in the body.

When a patient has been taking a single drug with impunity and then other drugs are added to the regimen which inhibit the metabolism of the first drug, then side effects may occur and these may have nutritional implications. Kutt et al. (1966) studied the inhibition of parahydroxylation of DPH by antituberculous drugs. They observed the development of DPH intoxication in epileptic patients who developed tuberculosis and were given INH, PAS, and cycloserine. Blood levels of DPH rose after the antituberculous drug therapy was initiated. In an earlier study, they had found that pyridoxine and folic acid increased the urinary output of the metabolite of DPH, 5-phenyl-5'-parahydroxyphenylhydantoin in a patient whose DPH metabolism was depressed because of hepatic disease. In another patient who had developed high blood levels of DPH due to the co-administration of INH and PAS, they gave pyridoxine which, however, did not change the blood level of DPH. Subsequently, they gave this patient folic acid and the DPH blood level fell and then stabilized, and the urinary output of the DPH metabolites increased. They suggest that the folic acid may have promoted parahydroxylation of the DPH, though this theory is unproven.

Conney et al. (1972) have drawn our attention to the fact that certain environmental and industrial chemicals are capable of inhibiting drug metabolism. It is possible that this might cause an inhibition of microsomal enzyme-inducing-drugs which cause nutrient depletion.

DRUG DOSAGE AND DURATION OF DRUG USE

It has earlier been shown that whether a person is on a diet which is inadequate with respect to one or more nutrients, or whether he has a disease which causes increased nutrient requirements which are not covered by dietary intake, nutrient depletion is gradual, and evidences of malnutrition do not make their appearance until nutrient stores are exhausted. The same situation pertains to drug-induced malnutrition, and it is important, therefore, to remember that the patients most likely to develop drug-induced malnutrition are those who are on drugs for a long period of time. In general, those most at risk are persons or populations who receive drugs for the control of chronic disease, such as epileptics who may take anticonvulsant therapy for many years. Drug dosage has a less clear-cut effect upon the incidence of drug-induced malnutrition, except that a high dose of drug given for a prolonged period is more likely to cause nutritional side effects than when a low dose is given for a short time. Excessive self-medication with laxatives or antacids may cause nutrient depletion either through induction of malabsorption or by increased urinary loss of nutrients, or both.

DRUG-BINDING

Drugs which produce adverse effects on nutrient utilization have been grouped according to their mode of actions, but within these groups, drugs vary in their interaction with or binding to vitamins or to enzymes required in vitamin metabolism. Thus, a vitamin B_6-deficiency from hydrazide drugs varies not only with the degree of inhibition of metabolism of this vitamin by any one of these drugs, but also on the stability of the Schiff base between the drug and pyridoxal phosphate. If the Schiff base is stable, as in the case of the INH-pyridoxal phosphate complex, it is more likely that urinary excretion of the vitamin, as this complex, will be enhanced.

All folate inhibitors produce a similar pattern of derangement of DNA synthesis and all are capable of partial or complete blockade of the dihydrofolate reductase enzyme. The relative potency of the antifolates in causing interference with folate metabolism in human subjects is related to their differential affinity for this enzyme.

Methotrexate has a greater affinity for the human dihydrofolate reductase than pyrimethamine, and both these drugs have a greater power of enzyme-binding than either triamterene or pentamidine isethionate. Whereas folic acid has no value in overcoming the antifolate effects of excess methotrexate, it may be used to combat the effects of certain other "weaker" folate antagonists. There is evidence that, when folate is given to patients who have received methotrexate, there is hyperexcretion of nonutilizable folate in the urine. While it has also been shown that bound methotrexate can be displaced from tissue-binding sites by folic acid, folic acid has no practical therapeutic effect, as previously mentioned, in reversing the acute toxicity of methotrexate, because its efficiency in removing methotrexate from the receptor site on the reductase enzyme is inadequate. Another contributory factor is that, in acute or subacute methotrexate poisoning, free methotrexate will preferentially displace bound methotrexate from binding sites, thus preventing entry of folic acid.

Folinic acid (5-formyltetrahydrofolate), which is readily converted to active tetrahydrofolic compounds of the body, is not bound to the dihydrofolate reductase enzyme and does not displace methotrexate from this enzyme. It is used as the antidote to acute methotrexate intoxication or acute toxicity from other antifolates (Hryniuk and Bertino 1969). Studies by Nixon and Bertino (1972) suggest that it is effective when given by the oral as well as by parenteral routes. Folic acid deficiency with megaloblastic anemia due to prolonged low dosage methotrexate therapy can be treated with folic acid only provided that no further methotrexate is being administered.

DIET

In populations or individuals receiving drugs which interact with nutrients, diet is a critical factor in the estimation of the risks of nutritional side effects. Maintenance of vitamin stores in the tissues is dependent primarily on dietary intake and also, on a more limited basis, on endogenous synthesis. The lower the tissue stores of a vitamin before the drug is taken, the less drug will be required to induce nutrient depletion to a point of deficiency. Whereas vitamin antagonists can so reduce the availability of vitamins by metabolic inhibitions so that deficiency states are created in spite of adequate dietary intake, hypovitaminoses from most of the drugs under consideration result from a gradual depletion. Eventually, any nutrient-depleting-drug will adversely affect nutritional balance, unless the diet is modified to overcome the increased nutrient requirements or dietary supplements taken.

Factors which affect food availability, such as income and seasonal availability, may determine intake of a vitamin such as folic acid. Drug-induced deficiency may be discernible only during the periods of the year when intake of the required vitamin is lowest. In a study of the folate status of pregnant women who had taken oral contraceptives within six months of becoming pregnant, decreased plasma and erythrocyte folate levels were found in the previous OCA users during the first trimester. A subgroup of these women studied during the summer had erythrocyte folate levels which, though reduced over the control population, were within the normal range, whereas in the winter group, average erythrocyte folate levels in ex-OCA users were in the depletion range. These differences could be explained by seasonal changes in folate intake from fresh vegetables (Martinez and Roe 1974).

Florid rickets has been found in a minority of children receiving anticonvulsants, but with greater frequency in those whose vitamin D intake is marginal, or in those who through custom or disability are house-bound (Lifshitz and MacLaren 1973). When the requirement for vitamin D is increased by intake of anticonvulsants, the increased need must be met, either by giving supplementary vitamin D by mouth, or by increasing ultraviolet light exposure so that more cholecalciferol is synthesized in the skin. It has recently been pointed out that the incidence of vitamin D deficiency found in a vulnerable population increases during the winter and decreases during the summer months when sunlight exposure is increased (Gupta et al. 1974).

In the literature on drug-induced malnutrition, adequacy of diet has often been assumed; in fact, variability in the reported incidence of drug-induced hypovitaminosis may be explained largely by group or individual differences in food intake.

PHYSIOLOGICAL STRESS

Symptomatic drug-induced malnutrition is more likely to develop in those whose nutrient requirements are suddenly or repeatedly increased, as, for example, in periods of rapid or catch-up growth, or with multiple pregnancies. There is evidence that the epileptic child on anticonvulsant drugs is more likely to develop rickets than an adult on similar drugs to develop osteomalacia, this difference being due to differing vitamin D requirements in the two age groups. Women on anticonvulsant drugs during a single pregnancy may develop biochemical evidence of folate depletion, but if they have successive pregnancies and continue intake of these drugs they are at high risk for the development of megaloblastic anemia. In this situation, the high folate requirements of pregnancy, both for the fetus and the mother, must be considered.

PRE-EXISTENT DISEASE

Earlier, the factors which increase nutritional requirements have been discussed. It has been explained that in pathological conditions associated with malabsorption, with increased loss of nutrients other than via the gastrointestinal tract, with increased cell turnover, or with decreased utilization, requirements for particular nutrients may be substantially elevated. When drugs causing nutrient depletion are prescribed to treat one or more of these conditions, the effects of the drug and the disease are additive, and, therefore, overt malnutrition is more likely to supervene.

PROBLEMS OF AGING

It is postulated that the elderly are more likely to develop drug-induced malnutrition, not only because they are prominent drug users, but also because they may consume marginal diets and suffer chronic diseases leading to nutritional impairment. Exton-Smith (1973) has emphasized the multifactorial origin of nutritional deficiency in the aged. He cites, as primary causes of malnutrition in old age, ignorance, social isolation, physical disability, mental disturbance, iatrogenic causes, and poverty. As secondary causes he mentions impaired appetite, masticatory inefficiency, malabsorption, alcoholism, drugs and increased requirements. Balacki and Dobbins (1974) have emphasized that malabsorption syndromes in the elderly are directly or indirectly related to chronic diseases found in this population group, or to the treatment of these diseases. As causes of malabsorption and consequent malnutrition in the elderly, these authors cite sequelae of surgical resections, pancreatic insufficiency from chronic pancreatitis or carcinoma, hepatobiliary disease including cirrhosis, "blind loop" syndrome, and drug-induced changes. Among the drugs considered as causative of malabsorption in geriatric patients the following are included: alcohol, cathartics, cholestyramine, clofibrate, colchicine, certain diuretics, neomycin, para-amino salicylic acid, phenindione, mannitol, and certain antimetabolites.

Haghshenass and Rao (1973) studied serum folate levels in 27 elderly patients receiving anticonvulsant therapy with diphenylhydantoin. Although none of their patients showed overt evidence of megaloblastic anemia, the serum folate levels were extremely low in their patient group as contrasted with the values from 25 control subjects. Dietary intakes of folic acid were considered to be adequate. The authors commented that the lowest serum folate levels found were those from persons on DPH who were over sixty years of age.

There is excellent documentation in the U.S. that the elderly are the chief users of drugs. In a listing of long-term maintenance drugs for persons aged sixty-five and over, prepared for the U.S. Department of Health, Education and Welfare in 1968, the following drug categories appear prominently: antiarthritics, anticoagulants, anticonvulsants, cardiovascular preparations, hypotensives, drugs for the treatment of diabetes, diuretics, hormones, and isoniazid for the treatment of senile tuberculosis. As previously indicated, many drugs in these categories are known to be capable of inducing vitamin or mineral deficiencies.

ENVIRONMENTAL FACTORS

In addition to dietary physiological disease and drug factors, nutritional status may be affected by either the physical or the chemical environment. It has long been known that children who are housebound are subject to rickets if they do not consume adequate amounts of vitamin D in their diets or receive supplements of vitamin D. Similarly, osteomalacia has frequently been recognized in Indian women living in purdah. The rate of cutaneous synthesis of cholecalciferol depends on the availability of ultraviolet light from solar or artificial sources. Far back, Hess and Unger (1922) related the seasonal incidence of rickets to variability in available sunlight. McLaughlin *et al.* (1974) studied serum 25-hydroxycholecalciferol concentrations among a group of healthy Caucasians living in the U.K. Blood samples were obtained throughout various seasons of the year, and it was found that there were marked seasonal variations in the levels of this vitamin D metabolite. Prevalence of rickets among immigrant populations in Great Britain has been variously attributed to lack of sunlight exposure, together with deeper skin pigmentation and low dietary intake of vitamin D (Cooke *et al.* 1974).

Hahn *et al.* (1972) who studied 25-cholecholesterol levels in epileptics on anticonvulsants and in control subjects found significantly lower levels of this vitamin D metabolite in the patient group. However, the lowest levels were found in patients with low vitamin D intake and "the least" exposure to sunlight.

Industrial chemicals related to drugs in therapeutic use may be capable of interfering with nutritional status. The toxicological properties of missile fuels and propellants was reviewed by Bach (1970). This author discusses the relative toxicity of monomethylhydrazine (MMH) and unsymmetrical-dimethylhydrazine (UDMH). Both of these chemicals are vitamin B_6-inhibitors or antimetabolites. Toxicity can be aborted or prevented by administration either of pyridoxine or pyridoxamine. Concurrent use of drugs and exposure to environmental chemicals should be considered in establishing the relative hazards of drug-induced malnutrition.

BIBLIOGRAPHY

BACH, K. C. 1970. Aerospace toxicology. I. Propellant toxicology. Fed. Proc. *29*, 2000–2005.
BALACKI, J. A., and DOBBINS, W. O. 1974. Maldigestion and malabsorption: making up for lost nutrients. Geriatrics *29*, 157–166.
CONNEY, A. H., and BURNS, J. J. 1972. Metabolic interactions among environmental chemical and drugs. Science *178*, 576–586.
COOKE, W. T. *et al.* 1974. Rickets, growth, and alkaline phosphatase in urban adolescents. Brit. Med. J. *2*, 293–297.
DEVADATTA, S. *et al.* 1960. Peripheral neuritis due to isoniazid. Bull. World Health Organ. *23*, 587–598.
EXTON-SMITH, A. N. 1973. Nutritional deficiencies in the elderly. *In* Nutritional Deficiencies in Modern Society, A. N. Howard, and I. McLean (Editors). Baird-Newman Books, London.
GUPTA, M. M., ROUND, J. M., and STAMP, T. C. B. 1974. Spontaneous cure of vitamin-D deficiency in Asians during summer in Britain. Lancet *1*, 586–588.
HAGHSHENASS, M., and RAO, D. B. 1973. Serum folate levels during anticonvulsant therapy with diphenylhydantoin. J. Am. Geriatric Soc. *21*, 275–277.
HAHN, T. J., HENDIN, B. A., SCHARP, C. R., and HADDAD, J. G. 1972. Effect of chronic anticonvulsant therapy on serum 25-hydroxycalciferol levels in adults. New Eng. J. Med. *287*, 900–909.

HESS, A. F., and UNGER, L. J. 1922. Infantile rickets: The significance of clinical, radiographic and chemical examinations in its diagnosis and incidence. Am. J. Dis. Child 24, 327-338.

HRYNIUK, W. B., and BERTINO, J. R. 1969. Treatment of leukemia with large doses of methotrexate and folinic acid: Clinical-biochemical correlates. J. Clin. Invest. 48, 2140-2155.

HUGHES, H. G., SCHMIDT, L. H., and BIEHL, J. P. 1955. The metabolism of isoniazid; its implications in therapeutic use. Trans. Conf. Chemotherap. Tuberc. 14, 217.

KUTT, H., WINTERS, W., and MacDOWELL, F. H. 1966. Depression of parahydroxylation of diphenylhydantoin by antituberculous chemotherapy. Neurology 16, 594-602.

KUTT, H., WOLK, M., SCHERMAN, R., and MADELL, F. 1964. Insufficient parahydroxylation as a cause of diphenylhydantoin toxicity. Neurology 14, 542.

LaDu, B. N. 1972. Isoniazid and pseudocholinesterase polymorphisms. Fed. Proc. 3, 1276-1285.

LIFSHITZ, F., and MacLAREN, N. K. 1973. Vitamin D-dependent rickets in institutionalized, mentally retarded children receiving longterm anticonvulsant therapy. I. A survey of 288 patients. J. Pediatrics 83, 612-620.

MARTINEZ, O., and ROE, D. A. 1974. Diet and contraceptive steroids (OCA) as determinants of folate status in pregnancy. Fed. Proc. 33, 715. (Abst.)

McLAUGHLIN, M. et al. 1974. Seasonal variations in serum 25-hydroxycholecalciferol in healthy people. Lancet 1, 536-538.

MELMON, K. L. 1971. Preventable drug reactions—causes and cures. New Eng. J. Med. 284, 1361-1368.

NIXON, P. F., and BERTINO, J. R. 1972. Effective absorption and utilization of oral formyltetrahydrofolate in man. New Eng. J. Med. 286, 175-179.

PETERS, J. H., MILLER, K. S., and BROWN, P. 1965. Studies on the metabolic basis for the genetically determined capacities for isoniazid inactivation in man. J. Pharmacol. Exp. Therap. 150, 298.

PRICE EVANS, D. A. 1969. Recent advances in knowledge of genetically controlled idiosyncratic reaction to drugs. In Proc. European Soc. for Study of Drug Toxicity 10, Sensitization to drugs. Excerpta Med. 11-18.

U.S. DEPT. HEALTH, EDUCATION AND WELFARE. 1968. The Drug Users. U.S. Task Force on Prescription Drugs. USDA/HEW, Washington, D.C.

CHAPTER 4

Diagnosis of Drug-Induced Malnutrition

GENERAL CRITERIA

In considering the diagnosis of drug-induced nutritional deficiency, several facts must be kept in mind. There are three groups of cases: 1) those in which there is nutrient depletion which can be recognized by biochemical evaluation of nutritional status; 2) cases of nutritional deficiency which are manifested by biochemical and/or hematologic or radiographic changes, characteristic of one or more deficiency diseases; and 3) those cases of overt clinical deficiency in which signs and symptoms are present which can be confirmed as being nutritional in origin by laboratory and/or radiological investigation.

Nutrient depletion cannot be considered as being drug-induced unless there is an immediately antecedent or current history of drug intake. In the instance of prenatal malnutrition, causing fetal malformation, growth failure, immaturity or nutritional deficiency in the neonate, the mother must have received one or more drugs during a part or the whole of the period of gestation.

Drugs may produce nutritional deficiencies which are rarely due to dietary inadequacy. For example, a number of drugs induce pyridoxine deficiency which is rarely due to poor intake of this vitamin. Drugs can also produce deficiencies such as vitamin D deficiency, which, though prevalent in certain social or ethnic groups, may be uncommon in the general population.

These nutritional deficiencies usually develop slowly after the initiation of drug intake. Slow evolution of the deficiency reflects a gradual nutrient store depletion, because increased nutrient requirements, imposed by the drug, are not met by increased nutrient intake or parenteral supplementation.

Drugs may produce unusual and complex nutritional syndromes, such as combined vitamin D and folate deficiency in epileptics on anticonvulsant drugs, or combined folate, pyridoxine and niacin deficiency in patients on drugs used for the control of tuberculosis.

Drug-induced nutritional deficiencies are likely to be single or multiple hypovitaminoses, because drugs impair the absorption or utilization of vitamins more than of other nutrients. As indicated in a previous publication by the author (Roe 1971), deficiencies of B vitamins are produced by more drugs and with greater frequency than deficiencies of other water-soluble or fat-soluble vitamins.

Vitamin or other nutritional deficiencies that ensue from drug intake are likely to be multifactorial in origin. The interacting causes are: marginal nutrient intake or synthesis, physiological stress, or diseases in which nutrient requirements are increased.

Proof of the causal relationship between drug intake and nutritional deficiency may require withdrawal of the drug under suspicion as an etiological agent. Since this approach may be indefensible from a clinical standpoint, proof may be sought from studies of animal models and/or from previous experience, and/or from statistical techniques showing a constant relationship between intake of a particular drug and the development of nutritional depletion or deficiency. If specific nutrient supplementation overcomes the deficiency state, then it may be assumed that a drug received has produced the condition only if no other causes of malnutrition can be found in the patient's diet or nutritional demands or disease.

Pitfalls explaining the misdiagnosis of nutrient depletion or deficiency due to drugs include: 1) absence of an awareness from the literature of drug-nutrient interactions; 2) absence of prior experience of such cases; 3) attribution of the symptoms to the primary disease under drug treatment; 4) confidence in the drug's safety derived from short-term usage; 5) lack of appreciation of high risk groups. This would include those, who by virtue of diet, alcoholism, disease or disability, are in a state of suboptimal nutrition at the onset of drug therapy, or at some point thereafter, which would make them more prone to develop malnutrition due to the added effects of the drug or drugs; and 6) multiple drug regimens in which one or more long-term drugs taken by the patient are unknown. This particularly applies to the situation of laxative abuse or other forms of excessive self-medication. When several drugs are taken, it might be difficult to associate a particular drug with the impaired nutritional status.

Diagnosis requires the following knowledge and investigations: 1) an index of suspicion derived from previous published reports and/or experience of drug-induced malnutrition; 2) understanding the potential causes of nutrient depletion in the patient; 3) a complete drug history; 4) knowledge of the patient's diet from food frequency data, food diaries, recall, or by actual measurement of food intake; 5) complete evaluation of the patient's medical history and physical examination; 6) biochemical, radiologic and/or hematologic evaluations of nutritional status; 7) assessment of evidence of nutritional depletion with respect to specific macro- or micronutrients; 8) determination of the relative importance of drugs, diet and disease as determinants of the nutritional impairment; 9) identification of the specific drug or drug groups which are contributing to the impairment of the nutritional status, and an understanding of how this impairment developed; and 10) trial withdrawal of drugs as medically feasible, and observation and evaluation of nutritional status thereafter.

CLINICAL HISTORY

Certain generalizations can be made about the points in a medical history which may lead a physician to consider the possibility of drug-induced malnutrition. Any patient who is taking a drug and has symptoms, which cannot be explained by the primary disease or in relation to drug hypersensitivity or intoxication, should be investigated with respect to nutritional status. This applies not only to the situation in which the patient is taking a drug known to increase nutrient requirements, but also when he or she is on a drug which has not yet been reported to have this potential. Cases presenting with symptoms of a nutritional deficiency which is rare in the general population should be questioned about drug intake. Since patients with chronic diseases on multiple drug regimens are prime candidates for drug-induced malnutrition, they, or if they are children, their families, should be questioned particularly about symptoms suggestive of deficiency disease.

Whereas the clinical history alone yields insufficient information on which to make a diagnosis of drug-induced malnutrition, it is a necessary step in the investigations for the following reasons: 1) it will allow identification of genetic or acquired disease for which the patient may have been receiving long term medication, e.g. epilepsy, tuberculosis; 2) it will give information on those factors which may predispose the patient to drug-induced malnutrition; i.e., a disease in which the nutrient requirements are increased and at the same time medication has been given with drugs known to impair nutritional status; and 3) it may reveal a change of symptomatology which cannot be explained as due to the primary disease and which may lead to a suspicion of the development of malnutrition. A listing of symptoms commonly associated with nutritional deficiency is given in Table 4.1.

Identification of people with drug-induced malnutrition depends on recognition of a characteristic story of antecedent events. Drugs known to increase nutrient requirements rarely cause clinical deficiency except with prolonged intake, and then only when the diet has been marginal with respect to those nutrients which are depleted by the drug or drugs in question. The number of cases found varies with the physician's awareness of the risk. Provided that this risk is

TABLE 4.1

SYMPTOMS ASSOCIATED WITH
DRUG-INDUCED MALNUTRITION

Symptom	Deficit or Condition
Weight loss	Protein-caloric
Growth retardation (children)	deficit
Diarrhea	Malabsorption
Dermatitis of face and scalp, "burning" feet and depression	Vitamin B_6
Sore tongue, weakness, breathlessness	Folate
Dermatitis (light exposed areas), diarrhea and confusion	Niacin
Bone pain, difficulty in walking; muscle (adults) weakness / Thickening of wrists, progressive limb deformity, muscle weakness (children)	Vitamin D
Bleeding gums, bruising, rectal bleeding, bleeding after injury or surgery	Vitamin K

acknowledged, then the next step is to obtain an accurate account of drug and diet intake.

DRUG INTAKE

The drug history must include a listing of medications taken, by generic or proprietary names. Information must be obtained as to the reason why each medication is used, whether for the cure or control of disease, for alleviation of complaints, or for purposes of contraception. Records must be obtained, not only of prescription drugs, but also of those obtained across the counter without prescription, and of those obtained from other persons including members of the family. The interviewer obtaining a drug history should always use a structured questionnaire and appropriate record forms in order that there will be a complete coverage of all medications taken (Tables 4.2 and 4.3). Frequently, dose and duration of drug intake should be established. Prior history of adverse drug reactions in the patient or in relatives of the patient should also be recorded. When the patient is unclear about the indication for his or her medication, is confused or ignorant of the preparations ingested, or has only a vague idea about the dose, the family physician may be able to supply the missing information. This approach is helpful if the patient has a family doctor, and if he knows what the patient has been given by other doctors that have been consulted. A striking fact about drug-induced vitamin deficiencies is the long duration of

TABLE 4.2

DRUG HISTORY (ADULT)

1a. Do you have any health problems for which you are taking prescription medications at the present time? Yes _____ No _____

If yes:

Health Problems	Drug		Duration of Intake	Frequency	Dose
	Proprietary Name	Generic Name			
_____	_____	_____	_____	_____	_____
_____	_____	_____	_____	_____	_____
_____	_____	_____	_____	_____	_____
_____	_____	_____	_____	_____	_____

1b. Are you taking any other medication which a doctor has prescribed (name or reason unknown)? Yes _____ No _____

If yes:

Description	Duration of Intake	Frequency	Dose	Identity
_____	_____	_____	_____	_____
_____	_____	_____	_____	_____
_____	_____	_____	_____	_____
_____	_____	_____	_____	_____

2a. Have you taken prescription medication for any of the following health problems within the past 3 months? Yes _____ No _____

If yes:

Health Problem	Drug Name	Duration of Intake	When Discontinued	Reason for Stopping	Still Taking*
Asthma					
Arthritis					
High blood pressure					
Fluid retention					
Infection (specify)					
Tuberculosis					
Malaria					
Psoriasis					
Colitis					
High cholesterol					
Parkinson's disease					

TABLE 4.2 (*Continued*)

Health Problem	Drug Name	Duration of Intake	When Discontinued	Reason for Stopping	Still Taking*
Liver disease					
Kidney disease					
Blood disease					
Bone disease					
Gout					
Blood clots					
Diabetes					
Other (specify)					

*Check (√)

2b. Have you taken any other medication within the past 3 months which a doctor has prescribed (name or reason unknown)? Yes _____ No _____

If yes:

Description	Duration of Intake	Frequency	Dose	Identity

3a. Do you take medications, self-prescribed, for any of the following complaints?

Complaint	Yes	No	Constantly	Frequently	Occasionally
Constipation					
Indigestion					
Headache					
Nervousness					
Insomnia					
Pain					
Menstrual cramps					
Colds & sinus trouble					
Other (state)					

If response to 3a is positive in 1 or more categories:

3b. What medication do you take to relieve these complaints, and how much do you need to gain relief?

Complaint	Drug	Duration	Frequency	Dose
Constipation				
Indigestion				
Headache				

TABLE 4.2 (*Continued*)

Complaint	Drug	Duration	Frequency	Dose
Nervousness				
Insomnia				
Pain				
Menstrual cramps				
Colds & sinus trouble				
Other (state)				

4. Are you taking birth control pills now? Yes _____ No _____
    If yes, name:
    Duration of intake:

    Have you taken birth control pills within the past 6 months?
    Yes _____ No _____
    If yes, name:
    Duration of intake:
    Date discontinued:
    Reason for stopping the Pill:

TABLE 4.3

DRUG HISTORY (INFANT OR CHILD)—MOTHER AS RESPONDENT

1. Did you have any health problems, treated by medication, during your pregnancy with this child? Yes _____ No _____

    If yes:

Health Problem	Drug	Duration of Intake Trimester		
		1st	2nd	3rd
_____	____	____	____	____
_____	____	____	____	____

2. Has this child been breastfed? Yes _____ No _____

    If yes, have you (did you) take medications during the period of breastfeeding? Yes _____ No _____

    If yes, specify

3a. Does your child take any medications prescribed by the doctor for known health problems? Yes _____ No _____

    If yes:

TABLE 4.3 *(Continued)*

Drug Name	Duration of Intake	Frequency	Dose	Reason

3b. Does your child take any other medications prescribed by the doctor?
Yes _____ No _____
(Name or reason unknown)

If yes:

Drug Name	Duration of Intake	Frequency	Dose	Reason

4a. Has your child taken prescription medication for any of the following health problems within the past 3 months? Yes _____ No _____

If yes:

Health Problem	Drug Name	Duration of Intake	When discontinued	Reason stopping
Asthma				
Eczema (dermatitis)				
Infection (specify)				
Tuberculosis				
Convulsions (seizures)				
Liver disease				
Kidney disease				
Blood disease				
Bone disease				
Behavior problem				
Other (specify)				

4b. Has your child taken any other prescription medications during the past 3 months? Yes _____ No _____ (name or reasons unknown)

If yes:

Description	Duration of Intake	Frequency	Dose	Identity

TABLE 4.3 (Continued)

5a. Do you give your child (baby) medications for any of the following complaints?

	Yes	No	Constantly	Frequently	Occasionally
Teething					
Constipation					
Colds					
Growing pains					
Colic					
Headache					
Nervousness					
Behavior problems					
Other (specify)					

5b. If response to 5a is positive in 1 or more categories, what medications do you give him (her) to relieve complaints?

Complaint	Drug	Duration	Frequency	Dose
_____	____	_____	_____	____
_____	____	_____	_____	____

drug intake prior to the appearance of symptoms. However, when a patient is asked how long a drug has been taken, the period stated may be inaccurate. Nor can this time always be reliably obtained from the family doctor or from other physicians seen only recently, because none of them may have been the original prescriber. Thus, communication with past physicians may be necessary in order to find out exactly how long the drug has been taken. Pharmacy records may be used to check prescription renewals when this information is not obtainable from physicians. Identification of unlabeled drugs may be available through use of the "Physician's Desk Reference" (1976) or through consultation with pharmacists. In cases where identification is not possible through these means, drug analysis may be necessary using area laboratories.

DIETARY HISTORY

The least satisfactory feature of published reports of drug-induced malnutrition is the description of the patient's diet. Commonly, diets are stated to be satisfactory or unsatisfactory. This has come about because the writers have omitted to supply dietary information, or because a diet history was never obtained. If the patient is asked whether he eats well, the answer is usually in the affirmative.

The physician has several options as to how to proceed. He can obtain a 24-hr diet recall from the patient, but this is not a very accurate method for dietary assessment, because the last day's food intake may not be representative of the norm. Further, it is known that the total amount of the actual food recalled and the recall of component foods varies inversely with the educational status of the patient. Reticence or wishful thinking about food intake may also be conditioned by fear of the doctor or by a desire to have the doctor believe that a certain type of diet is consumed. An alternate and more satisfactory approach is to ask the patient to keep a food diary for five or seven days. During that time, everything that is put in the mouth is recorded. This is a good method, not only for recording food, but also for drugs and supplementary nutrient intakes. A useful food diary format is illustrated in Table 4.4. The patient brings the completed food diary back to the doctor at the end of the stipulated period. It is then used to obtain the frequency of intake of specific nutrients with which the investigator is concerned. For example, in the case of rickets or osteomalacia the major concern would be with the intake of vitamin D-fortified milk, or in a patient with megaloblastic anemia, the physician requires information on the intake or otherwise of rich sources of folic acid, including green, leafy vegetables, orange juice and fresh fruits, liver and other meats. Major sources of key nutrients, affected by drug intake (including alcohol) are listed in Table 4.5 and recommended levels of intake of such nutrients in Table 4.6.

The food diary method of obtaining dietary information can only be applied in a select group of patients who have the health, intelligence, motivation and time to provide valid information. However, often the pattern, quality and quantity of food intake has to be discovered on the basis of one interview with the patient. Under these circumstances, a dietary questionnaire based on food frequency only can be used to assess adequacy or otherwise of nutrient intake (Table 4.7).

Self-imposed and therapeutic diets should be discussed with special reference to palatability and to foods which are not allowed. The exact medical indication for any therapeutic diet should be noted. When the diet has been self-imposed, not only should the composition of the diet be described and its expected effect, but also questions should be asked as to whether the individual adheres strictly to the diet. It is important to learn whether diet imposes restriction of the total quantity of all foods, whether specific foods are left out because they are considered to be fattening, and if so, what sorts of foods are eliminated for this reason. Inquiries should be made about

TABLE 4.4

INTAKE DIARY—1 WEEK

Woman Aged 20
Day 1

Date	Time	Item	Amount
July	7:30 a.m.	Coffee—black	1 cup
	10:30 a.m.	Doughnut—sugar	1
		Coffee—black	1 cup
	Noon	Potato chips	1 package
		Carbonated beverage	1 can
	6:00 p.m.	Hamburger	$\frac{1}{4}$ lb.
		Bun	1
		French Fried Potatoes	1 frozen package
		Cookies/Choc. Chip	4
	10:00 p.m.	Candy bar/Choc.	1 (2 oz.)
		Beer	1 large glass
		1 birth control pill	

1) Compute patient's weekly food and beverage consumption: (kinds and amounts), i.e. Milk and milk products; eggs; meat and poultry, liver, fish; bread, cereal, cake; vegetables (raw) green, yellow, other; vegetables (cooked) green, yellow, other; nuts and legumes; fruits (raw and cooked), fruit juices; butter, margarine; alcoholic beverages; and nutrient supplements.

2) Average daily intake in these food groups:

3) Using Tables 5 and 6 determine whether rich sources of specific nutrients are included to combat depletion effects of drug regimen.

4) Summarize findings.

5) If assistance of dietitian is available, compute nutrient intake from dietary information per se and in relation to recommended dietary allowances.

TABLE 4.5

MAJOR SOURCES OF VITAMINS AND MINERALS
AMONG COMMON FOODS AND BEVERAGES

Ascorbic Acid*	Lemons, oranges, grapefruit, tangerines, strawberries, canteloupe Citrus fruit juices, canned fruit beverages fortified with vitamin C Sweet peppers, broccoli, brussel sprouts, cabbage, turnip greens, collards, cauliflower, spinach, collard greens, kale, tomatoes, onions
Folic Acid*	Liver (beef, calf, lamb, pork, chicken) Asparagus, spinach, lettuce, onions, brussel sprouts, cauliflower, broccoli, cabbage, peas, beans, nuts Orange juice Berries

TABLE 4.5 *(Continued)*

Vitamin B_6 (includes pyridoxine, pyridoxamine and pyridoxal)	Liver Meats, Fish Eggs Whole grain cereals Green leafy and yellow vegetables Bananas, grapes, pears
Vitamin B_{12}	Liver, other meats Clams, sardines, salmon, oysters, herring, other fish Cheeses Milk Eggs
Niacin	Liver Lean meats. Fish and shellfish Enriched breads and cereals Eggs
Riboflavin	Eggs, Liver Lean meats Enriched bread and cereals Leafy green vegetables Milk
Thiamin	Enriched bread and cereals Liver Peas and lima beans Leafy green vegetables
Vitamin A and carotenes	Milk, butter, fortified margarine Liver Eggs Leafy green and yellow vegetables (e.g. carrots)
Vitamin D	Vitamin D fortified milk and margarine Herring
Vitamin K	Spinach, cauliflower, cabbage, kale, liver
Iron	Liver, Shellfish, lean meat Eggs Spinach, peas and beans Tomato juice Nuts Enriched bread and cereals
Magnesium	Dried beans and peas Soybeans Nuts
Zinc	Liver, other animal protein foods
Calcium	Milk, Buttermilk Ice cream and Ice milk Cheese Cottage cheese

*Major losses occur due to storage or cooking.

TABLE 4.6

DAILY NUTRIENT REQUIREMENTS FOR CHILDREN AND ADULTS
ON COMMON DRUGS

	Vitamin D	Ascorbic Acid	Folacin	Vitamin B_6	Vitamin B_{12}
	IU	mg	μg	mg	μg
Anticonvulsants (Including phenobarbital, diphenylhydantoin, and primidone)	400–800[1]	45–60	400–1000[2]	1.2–2.5	2–4[3]
Oral Contraceptives	400[1]	60–100	400–1000[2]	25[2]	2–4[3]
Antituberculous Drugs (Including INH, PAS and cycloserine)	400	45–60	400–1000[2]	50[2]	2–4[3]
Antimalarials (Including pyrimethamine)	400	45–60	5000[4]	1.2–2.5	2–4[3]

[1] 1 qt. of fortified milk supplies 400 IU vitamin D.
[2] Will require intake of nutrient supplement.
[3] Supplement required for vegans.
[4] May be replaced by 5 mg folinic acid per day.
[5] Values should be compared with Recommended Dietary Allowances, 8th ed., 1974. Nat. Acad. Sci., Washington, D.C.

TABLE 4.7

FOOD FREQUENCY INTERVIEW

1. How many times per week do you consume (does your child consume):

Meat	0 1 2 3 4 5 6 7 >7 specify
Poultry	0 1 2 3 4 5 6 7 >7 specify
Fish	0 1 2 3 4 5 6 7 >7 specify
Hot dogs	0 1 2 3 4 5 6 7 >7 specify
Liver	0 1 2 3 4 5 6 7 >7 specify
Eggs	0 1 2 3 4 5 6 7 >7 specify
Cheese	0 1 2 3 4 5 6 7 >7 specify
Cottage cheese	0 1 2 3 4 5 6 7 >7 specify
Fruit juice	0 1 2 3 4 5 6 7 >7 specify
Raw fruit	0 1 2 3 4 5 6 7 >7 specify
Cooked fruit	0 1 2 3 4 5 6 7 >7 specify
Raw vegetables	0 1 2 3 4 5 6 7 >7 specify
Cooked green leafy vegetables	0 1 2 3 4 5 6 7 >7 specify
Beans and peas	0 1 2 3 4 5 6 7 >7 specify
Instant Breakfast	0 1 2 3 4 5 6 7 >7 specify
Peanut butter	0 1 2 3 4 5 6 7 >7 specify
Nuts	0 1 2 3 4 5 6 7 >7 specify
Doughnuts	0 1 2 3 4 5 6 7 >7 specify
Cereal breakfast foods	0 1 2 3 4 5 6 7 >7 specify
Crackers or pretzels	0 1 2 3 4 5 6 7 >7 specify
Macaroni, spaghetti, rice, noodles	0 1 2 3 4 5 6 7 >7 specify
Soft drinks	0 1 2 3 4 5 6 7 >7 specify

TABLE 4.7 *(Continued)*

Coffee or tea	0 1 2 3 4 5 6 7 >7 specify
Beer	0 1 2 3 4 5 6 7 >7 specify
Wine	0 1 2 3 4 5 6 7 >7 specify
Liquor	0 1 2 3 4 5 6 7 >7 specify
Ice cream	0 1 2 3 4 5 6 7 >7 specify
Cookies	0 1 2 3 4 5 6 7 >7 specify
Pie, cake	0 1 2 3 4 5 6 7 >7 specify

2. How many servings per day do you eat of the following foods:

Bread, toast, rolls, muffins   0 1 2 3 4 >4 specify
(1 slice or 1 item is a serving)

Milk—including addition to other foods   0 1 2 3 4 >4 specify
(8 ounces is a serving)

Butter or margarine   0 1 2 3 4 >4 specify
(1 tsp. is a serving)

3. Estimate frequency of food and beverage intake on the basis of food and drink groups.

Low frequency   = <7 times per week
Intermediate frequency   = 7 times per week
High frequency   = >7 times per week

Low frequency   = <4 times per day
Intermediate frequency   = 4 times per day
High frequency   = >4 times per day

Adjust frequency rating to age, sex, physiological status and activity of population group.

Ref: Nutritional Assessment in Health Programs. 1973. G. Christakis (Editor). Amer. J. Public Health. Suppl. 16–17.
Abramson J. H., Slome, C., and Kosovsky, C. 1963. Food Frequency interview as an epidemiological tool. Amer. J. Public Health *53* 1093–1101.

unusual or fad diets with respect to composition, intent, moral or spiritual justification, and anticipated results. If the patient has been on a peculiar diet, it should be found out if he or she is a devotee of health foods or an advocate of the macrobiotic principle. Whenever vegetarianism is discovered, careful questioning is required to find out if eggs and dairy products are or are not included. If it is found that the patient is a vegan (strict vegetarian), then further questions should be addressed about the intake of protein-rich foods such as legumes and vitamin-rich foods such as citrus fruits or fruit juices and leafy green vegetables.

The optimal method for determination of nutrient intake is by actual measurement of foods and beverages consumed. This method requires the services of a trained dietitian or nutritionist and can only be satisfactorily carried out when the patient is under observation, as under hospital conditions. Nutrient intake can then be assessed from food composition tables (Watt and Merrill 1963), or from food data banks available in major hospital dietetics departments. The reader may ask why, in the case of a suspected drug-induced malnutrition, so much attention should be given to the diet. Justification is based on the experience that those with deficiency states related to drug intake have often been eating badly. Nutrient requirements which are most commonly elevated by drug intake are those of folic acid, vitamin B_{12}, pyridoxine and vitamin D. It is therefore of primary importance to consider the record of the patient's diet history as it relates to the level of intake of these nutrients. Further, as the complete drug history has been obtained and reviewed prior to the diet history, it is possible to be more specific. For example, if the patient has received anticonvulsants which eventually cause the depletion of folic acid, vitamin B_{12} and vitamin D, then it is necessary to look at the diet with respect to information which would suggest low intake of one or more of these vitamins. The epileptic girl who dislikes vegetables, skips breakfast, relies mainly on snack foods from vending machines to reduce foods costs, and will not drink milk because she considers it to be fattening, is a candidate for folate deficiency. For one reason or another

TABLE 4.8

EXAMPLES OF MARGINAL DIETS FOR DRUG RECIPIENTS

Drug Group	Nutrients Depleted	Marginal Diet
Anticonvulsants	Folate	*Fruits↓
		*Vegetables↓
		*Liver↓
	Vitamin D	Milk↓
		Vegan
Antituberculosis Drugs	Folate	see above*
	Vitamin B_{12}	Vegan
	Vitamin B_6	Animal protein↓
	Niacin	Refined cereals↑
		(cornmeal)
Oral contraceptives	Folate	see above*
	Vitamin B_6	Snack foods↑
Alcohol	Folate	Fruit↓
	Thiamin	Vegetables↓
		Liver↓
	Magnesium	Animal protein↓
	Zinc	Refined cereals↑
		Alcohol↑

↓ = low frequency or omitted
↑ = high frequency or major source of calories
* = major folate (folacin) sources

she denies herself sources of folic acid, including not only such vegetables as spinach, but also orange juice, because breakfast is omitted, and meats because they are too expensive. Her deliberate omission of milk from her diet increases the hazard of vitamin D deficiency unless she makes use of opportunities to get out in the sunshine. Similar composite pictures can be built from drug and dietary information in other kinds of individuals. These are summarized in Table 4.8 in which nutritional hazards of people on specific drugs or drug groups are indicated in relation to diet.

PHYSICAL EXAMINATION AND NUTRITIONAL EVALUATION

There is a common misconception that drug-induced nutritional deficiencies are always or nearly always asymptomatic. This idea has arisen because, in many instances, drug-induced malnutrition has been discovered accidentally by the finding of abnormal biochemical parameters of nutritional status. Nevertheless, syndromes of malnutrition associated with drug intake should be recognized. These can be grouped in the following manner:

Malabsorption

Drugs capable of producing massive malabsorption induce diarrhea, usually associated with steatorrhea and weight loss. Muscle-wasting may be evident and may be severe. Flatulence, colicky abdominal pain and exacerbation of diarrhea may follow ingestion of milk due to secondary lactose intolerance, due to lactase deficiency. Ingestion of other disaccharide sugars such as sucrose may have similar effects. Symptoms referable to the development of a deficiency of fat-soluble vitamins, while rare, should be looked for, and may include bone pain associated with osteomalacia, and bleeding from the intestine or from hemorrhoids associated with vitamin K deficiency. As with other forms of drug-induced disease, the symptoms and signs of drug-induced malabsorption vary with the primary disease which is under treatment, as well as with the duration and magnitude of drug therapy.

Laboratory investigation includes the identification of malabsorption in association with drug intake, and demonstration of nutrient depletion or deficiency. The following tests are of particular value with respect to the identification of malabsorption:

(1) *The D-xylose absorption test* using a 25 gm dose of xylose (Rinaldo and Gluckman 1964). Impaired renal function causes significant retention of xylose so that the blood concentration remains elevated and the urinary excretion lowered, rendering the

test unusable in patients with renal disease such as may be present in elderly subjects. For this reason, MacLennan (1971) has suggested that the xylose absorption test should not be used as a single screening procedure for malabsorption.

(2) *Serum carotene levels* may be measured using the method of Yudkin (1941) and provides a useful index of absorption from the gastrointestinal tract. Serum carotene levels may, however, be low when there is an unusually poor intake of carotenoids as has been demonstrated by Wenger *et al.* (1957). Steatorrhea can be evaluated by extracting and determining fat in freeze-dried feces by the method of Bowens *et al.* (1964).

(3) *Fecal nitrogen determination* provides a useful measure of protein malabsorption except in instances where there is significant protein-losing enteropathy (Wilson and Dietschy 1972). Studies with ^{51}Cr-albumin will demonstrate an excessive loss of plasma proteins into the gastrointestinal tract as may occur in laxative abuse (Waldmann 1961; Waldmann and Wochner 1965).

(4) Where facilities exist, *peroral intestinal mucosal biopsy* is of value as a diagnostic test which can be repeated when the drug is withdrawn to find out whether the intestinal mucosal damage has been reversed (Rubin and Dobbins 1965).

(5) Basic studies of nutritional status in cases of drug-induced malabsorption should include estimation of total serum proteins by the biuret method, serum albumin determinations by electrophoretic separation, serum sodium and potassium, serum calcium and phosphorus, alkaline phosphatase, and prothrombin time. Serum vitamin A levels should be determined in fasting blood samples according to a fluorometric technique such as that developed by Thompson *et al.* (1971). However, it should be realized that low serum vitamin A levels may reflect low intake of this vitamin or the presence of liver disease, and therefore cannot be considered as diagnostic of malabsorption.

A reduced serum calcium $\times$ phosphorus (Ca $\times$ P) product in mg/% is indicative of insipient or overt rickets or osteomalacia, more particularly when associated with elevated alkaline phosphatase levels. Where there is indication from these biochemical parameters of vitamin D deficiency, radiological studies should be carried out in order to confirm or establish whether or not clinical rickets is present. While vitamin D deficiency is an uncommon complication of drug-induced malabsorption alone, it may occur in those whose vitamin D status is marginal prior to the occurrence of the malabsorption.

Because a number of drugs induce folate and/or vitamin B_{12} malabsorption, it is necessary to study the patients' status with respect to these two vitamins, as will be described.

Anemia

Drug-induced anemias are not uncommon, but are rarely diagnosed on the basis of symptomatology. Any severe anemia may present with pallor, weakness and dyspnea on exertion, but these signs give no indication of the etiology. If, however, these symptoms develop in a patient receiving a drug, and they cannot be explained satisfactorily as clinical features of the primary disease under treatment, it should be assumed that there is a drug-induced problem present until proven otherwise. Any persons who will be receiving or who have received chronic therapy with drugs known to induce nutritional anemia should have regular complete blood counts, preferably using an automated technique. An anemia can be said to be present if the erythrocyte count and the hemoglobin levels are reduced.

Hematologic changes indicative of nutritional deficiency may occur in the absence of anemia. Drug-induced anemias may be due to folate or vitamin B_{12} deficiency (megaloblastic), to vitamin B_6 deficiency (sideroblastic), or to iron deficiency associated with salicylate-induced gastrointestinal bleeding. By far the largest number of drug-induced anemias are megaloblastic and are due to folate depletion. Drug-induced vitamin B_{12} deficiency with anemia is extremely rare (Heinivaara and Palva 1965). Folate deficiency and vitamin B_{12} deficiency are identical with respect to hematologic changes. A reduction in the red cell count in excess of a reduction in hemoglobin level is suggestive of megaloblastic anemia. Further hematological studies should include evaluation of erythrocyte size and morphology, a leukocyte count, examination of leukocytes including neutrophils in stained films, and if possible bone marrow examinations. Particular attention should be given to the mean corpuscular volume of the erythrocytes. In megaloblastic anemia, values may be in the range of 96–164 μ^3 (normal values 76–90 μ^3). Moderate macrocytosis may be indicative of regular ingestion of alcohol, and it has been suggested that this is not due to folate deficiency, but to a direct toxic effect of the alcohol. In folate deficiency, the first hematologic change is hypersegmentation of the neutrophils, and this is followed by the appearance of macrocytes in the peripheral blood, visible in stained films. As the severity of folate deficiency increases, the anemia will be manifested particularly by reduction in the erythrocyte count. Leukopenia is exhibited in those subjects who have severe megaloblastic anemia. The bone marrow exhibits megaloblastic changes involving the red cell precursors as well, in several cases, as other cell series. Severely megaloblastic marrows show morphological abnormalities in the granulocyte precursors and in the megakaryocytes (Chanarin 1969).

Differentiation of folate from vitamin B_{12} deficiency must be made on the basis of laboratory findings. Serum and red cell folate levels are usually determined using microbiological assays (L. casei) (Waters and Mollin 1961; Hoffbrand et al. 1966). In folate deficiency both the serum and the red cell folate levels are reduced, but in vitamin B_{12} deficiency the serum folate levels are either in the normal range or elevated, and the red cell folate is lowered (Cooper and Lowenstein 1966). In acute folate deficiency, decreases in serum folate levels precede decreases in erythrocyte levels of folate. However, in chronic folate deficiency, reduction in erythrocyte folate levels is a better indicator of folate depletion than serum folate levels, because the latter may reflect recent folacin intake. An indirect method for the evaluation of folate status is by the FIGLU test, in which the urinary output of formiminoglutamic acid is measured following a histidine load. A marked increase in FIGLU excretion is indicative of folate depletion or deficiency (Hla-Pe and Aung-Than-Batu 1967). When microbiological methods are used for the assay of serum and erythrocyte folate, falsely low values may be obtained if the patient is currently taking an antibiotic. Attempts are being made to obviate these technical difficulties by substituting a radioassay technique for the more conventional microbiological methods for folate estimation (Rothenberg et al. 1972; Mincey et al. 1973).

Three major methods are available for the estimation of vitamin B_{12} depletion. The procedure that is most useful for the diagnosis of this condition is a measurement of serum vitamin B_{12} levels. Serum vitamin B_{12} levels may be determined either by a microbiological method or by the use of the radioisotope of vitamin B_{12} (Skeggs 1963; Britt et al. 1969). The urinary excretion of methylmalonic acid had been used as a measure of vitamin B_{12} deficiency (Giorgio and Luhby 1969). Sauberlich et al. (1974) have indicated that this test lacks sensitivity for the determination of vitamin B_{12} deficiency. The Schilling test has been used extensively for the evaluation of vitamin B_{12} deficiency, but in fact, it measures vitamin B_{12} absorption or malabsorption. A tracer dose of radiolabeled vitamin B_{12} is administered orally followed by a flushing dose of stable vitamin B_{12} given by the intramuscular route. The excretion of the radiolabeled vitamin B_{12} is then measured in the urine. Decreased urinary excretion of the radioisotope is indicative of vitamin B_{12} malabsorption (Schilling 1953; Corcino *et al.* 1970).

The Schilling test should also be performed after administration of a purified intrinsic factor preparation. If this has no effect on vitamin B_{12} malabsorption, it can be assumed that production of intrinsic factor is adequate.

Vitamin B_6 deficiency anemia is a rare complication of therapy with drugs acting as pyridoxine antagonists. The anemia has the following features: hypochromic erythrocytes, elevated serum iron levels, and saturation of total iron binding capacity, erythroid hypoplasia of the bone marrow, and also the presence of ringed sideroblasts in the bone marrow (Sullivan and Weintraub 1973). A characteristic feature of pyridoxine deficiency anemia is the presence of two red cell populations, one normochromic and the other hypochromic. While sideroblastic anemia may be diagnosed from evaluation of the erythrocyte count, examination of stained blood films, bone marrow examination, and determination of serum iron and iron-binding capacity, the finding of such an anemia is not necessarily indicative of pyridoxine deficiency. In order to determine whether pyridoxine deficiency is causative of the sideroblastic anemia, it is necessary to carry out tests of vitamin B_6 status, using biochemical techniques. Iron deficiency anemia associated with chronic GI blood loss and high aspirin intake produces a hypochromic microcytic anemia. Hemoglobin levels are reduced relatively more than the erythrocyte count. The mean corpuscular volume is decreased. As with simple iron deficiency of dietary origin, the serum iron is decreased and total iron-binding capacity increased.

The prothrombin time is occasionally prolonged. Feces may be dark or black due to the presence of occult blood which can be confirmed by the guiac test. A labeled chromium test should be carried out for gastrointestinal bleeding. A 10 ml sample of the patient's blood is tagged with 200 μCi of ^{51}Cr and then given intravenously. Daily stools and blood samples are collected and radioactivity measured. Radioactivity in the stool confirms blood loss and comparison of radioactivity measurements of 1 ml blood samples indicates the amount of blood loss (Wallach 1974).

Proof that a drug is the etiological agent in the development of a nutritional anemia can only be obtained by drug withdrawal. Evidence that an anemia is due to a deficiency of a particular nutrient is completed when it is shown that substitution therapy with a specific nutrient reverses the anemia. The latter procedure is not without risk, as for example in the case of vitamin B_{12} deficiency when administration of folate may cure the anemia but also, by so doing, delay the correction of the vitamin B_{12} deficiency with its attendant neuropathy.

Pharmacologic doses of vitamins may decrease the therapeutic effect of drugs. While proof of folate deficiency in epileptics on anticonvulsant therapy can be attained by administering folic acid, seizure control may thereby be decreased. Similarly, high doses of pyridoxine may obviate the therapeutic effects of L-dopa in patients with Parkinsonism.

Neuropathies

Drug-induced deficiency of vitamin B_6 or vitamin B_{12} can lead to the development of a neuropathy. From the clinical standpoint, these conditions could be confused. Common to both are the slow development of paresthesias, numbness and the development of pareses of the lower limbs. Examination of tendon reflexes in the lower limbs is not really helpful, because in either of these vitamin deficiencies associated with neuropathy, the reflexes may be either increased or decreased according to the stage of the disease. Further, in both conditions vibration sense may be impaired, though it is more likely that this would be impaired in vitamin B_{12} deficiency. Characteristic features of the vitamin B_6 neuropathy include the "burning feet" syndrome, muscle soreness in the legs, and atrophy of the peroneal muscles. Ataxia is characteristic of vitamin B_{12} deficiency, and with progression of this condition, spastic paraplegia or flaccid paralysis of the lower limbs may develop. Visual impairment as a result of retrobulbar neuritis and optic atrophy are rarer components of vitamin B_{12} deficiency. In both vitamins B_6 and B_{12} deficiencies, psychological symptoms may be prominent with depression as a common occurrence. It must be emphasized that vitamin B_{12} neuropathy has not been documented as due to drug therapy alone and could only occur in those with preexistent B_{12} depletion if treatment with drugs such as PAS were prolonged.

Several laboratory tests are in use for the diagnosis of vitamin B_6 deficiency. Where one or more drugs appear to be implicated as causes of vitamin B_6 deficiency, a combination of the following tests should be performed. The tryptophan load test can be carried out routinely, provided that it is possible to obtain a 24 hourly specimen collection of urine. Either a 2 or 5 gm L-tryptophan load is given orally and thereafter a 24 hourly collection of urine is made and this sample is analyzed for the presence of tryptophan metabolites, but most frequently this examination is limited to xanthurenic acid. Increased xanthurenic acid values in this test are indicative of vitamin

B_6 depletion (Sauberlich 1972; Linkswiler 1967). Erythrocyte transaminase activities are also used to determine vitamin B_6 status. These include erythrocyte glutamate-oxaloacetate transaminase (EGOT), and erythrocyte glutamate-pyruvate transaminase (EGPT). Activity of these enzymes declines in vitamin B_6 deficiency, but there is considerable individual variability in values obtained. A modification of the transaminase tests is through *in vitro* addition of pyridoxal phosphate, which will stimulate EGOT and EGPT activities in persons with vitamin B_6 deficiency and also to a smaller extent in normal subjects (Raica and Sauberlich 1964; Cinnamon and Beaton 1970).

There are many other tests which have been proposed as measures of vitamin B_6 status, but difficulties of performance or interpretations limit their use, particularly in patients with B_6 deficiency induced by drugs. The most promising among these tests is the determination of vitamin B_6 levels of plasma, erythrocytes and whole blood. According to Sauberlich *et al.* (1974), the method of Haskell and Snell (1972) and of Chabner and Livingston (1970) have enough sensitivity so that accurate measurements of pyridoxal phosphate in plasma and erythrocytes can be obtained. Serum pyridoxal levels appear to reflect intake of this vitamin, whereas it is assumed that values in erythrocytes are a measure of tissue levels.

It has recently been suggested by Lumeng *et al.* (1974) that in evaluating vitamin B_6 status in oral contraceptive users, the plasma level of vitamin B_6 may be a better indicator of depletion rather than the tryptophan load test. These authors mentioned that the effect of oral contraceptives on tryptophan metabolism is not only related to direct interference in pyridoxal phosphate dependent reactions, but also on direct effects of the estrogen component on tryptophan metabolism.

Measurements of the urinary excretion of vitamin B_6 are not of value in any patients receiving drugs that are pyridoxine antagonists. While low urinary levels of vitamin B_6 indicate an inadequate intake of this vitamin, it should be remembered that when drugs such as INH are administered there is a hyperexcretion of vitamin B_6 in the urine (Biehl and Vilter 1954).

When peripheral neuritis is encountered among persons who are receiving drugs known to inhibit vitamin B_6 metabolism, the chances are that biochemical evidences of vitamin B_6 deficiency are causally related to the neuropathy. However, it is also possible that these people have a vitamin B_{12} deficiency on the basis of disease, such as pernicious anemia, or that their peripheral neuritis is due to thiamin deficiency, due for example to high alcohol intake. Erythrocyte transketolase measurements have been shown to be satisfactory indicators of early thiamin deficiency, this test representing a functional evaluation of thiamin adequacy (Chong and Hou 1970).

Dermatitis

Dermatitis developing in persons receiving medications is rarely of nutritional origin, and it usually occurs either as a direct toxic manifestation of the drug or more commonly on an allergic basis. Exceptions are the seborrhoeic dermatitis which may develop in those taking such vitamin B_6 antagonists as L-dopa, and pellagra, a dermatosis of light-exposed areas which may occur also in those on B_6 antagonists who also have a marginal intake of niacin. In the author's limited experience, seborrhoeic dermatitis occurring in patients on a high dosage of L-dopa clears promptly when large doses of pyridoxine are administered, this being the diagnostic test. If a light-sensitive dermatitis develops in a patient receiving INH, or possibly another vitamin B_6 antagonist, diagnostic tests should include measurement of the 24 hourly excretion of N^1-methylnicotinamide, as well as a therapeutic trial of niacin. N^1-methylnicotinamide is one of the major urinary metabolites of niacin. In niacin deficiency, the excretion of this niacin metabolite decreases markedly (Pelletier and Campbell 1962; Frazier *et al.* 1955).

Riboflavin deficiency, under conditions of experimental depletion or dietary lack, is manifested by seborrhoeic dermatitis, dermatitis over sites of trauma, as well as glossitis, angular stomatitis and corneal vascularization (Sydenstricker 1941; Kruse *et al.* 1940).

Clinical evidence of riboflavin deficiency is rarely attributable to drug ingestion per se. In several chronic alcoholics among whom riboflavin depletion is prevalent, specific signs of riboflavin deficiency have been conspicuous by their absence (Rosenthal *et al.* 1973).

The degree of stimulation (activity coefficient) of erythrocyte glutathione reductase by flavin adenine dinucleotide is presently considered the most sensitive functional test of riboflavin nutrition (Tillotson and Baker 1972; Sauberlich *et al.* 1972).

Blood levels and urinary levels of riboflavin are generally accepted to reflect recent intake rather than tissue deficiency (Burch *et al.* 1948; Horwitt *et al.* 1950). The competitive protein-binding assay for urinary riboflavin (Fazekas *et al.* 1974) offers great promise as a means of screening population groups such as alcoholics for marginal intake of riboflavin. However, as noted elsewhere in this text, boric acid absorption causes an increased urinary excretion of riboflavin in contrast to dietary lack of the vitamin which reduces both blood and urinary levels (Roe *et al.* 1972).

Bone Disease

The only form of drug-induced malnutrition presenting as a skeletal disease is vitamin D deficiency, most commonly induced by long-term intake of anticonvulsant drugs. As already indicated, rickets and osteomalacia can both be diagnosed from the classical symptomatology, from radiological studies, from biochemical determination of serum calcium, serum phosphorus, and serum alkaline phosphatase, as well as computation of the calcium phosphorus product. A more functional test of vitamin D deficiency in those on anticonvulsants is through determination of serum 25-hydroxycholecalciferol. Serum levels of 25-hydroxycholecalciferol are decreased in a significant

TABLE 4.9

INTERPRETATION OF LABORATORY TESTS FOR THE
EVALUATION OF NUTRITIONAL STATUS (ADULTS)

Test	Deficient (high risk)	Low (medium risk)	Acceptable (low risk)	Nutrient Evaluation
Serum iron μg/100 ml	<30	30–59.9	⩾60	Iron
Serum albumin g/100 ml	<2.8	2.8–3.4	⩾3.5	Protein
Plasma carotene μg/ 100 ml	<20	20–39	⩾40	GI absorption
Plasma retinol μg/100 ml	<10	10–19	⩾20	Vitamin A
Serum folate ng/ml	<3	3.0–5.9	>6.0	Folate
Erythrocyte folate ng/ml	<140	140–159	>160	Folate
Serum vitamin B_{12} pg/ml	<150	150–200	>200	Vitamin B_{12}
Serum ascorbic acid mg/ 100 ml	<0.20	0.20–0.29	⩾0.30	Vitamin C
Erythrocyte transketo- lase % (Thiamine pyro- phosphate stim.)	>20	16–20	0–15	Thiamin
Erythrocyte glutathione reductase-activity coefficients	>1.40	1.20–1.40	<1.20	Riboflavin
Erythrocyte transami- nase indices				
EGPT	>1.25		⩽1.25	Vitamin B_6
EGOT	>2.0		⩽2.0	Vitamin B_6
Tryptophan load test— increase in excretion xanthurenic acid mg/day	>50	25–50	<25	Vitamin B_6
N^1-methyl nicotinamide excretion mg/g creatinine	<0.5	0.5–1.59	1.6–4.29	Niacin
Serum Ca $\times$ P product mg%	<40		>40	Vitamin D
Alkaline phosphatase— King-Armstrong units/ 100 ml	>40		8–14	Vitamin D

number of patients receiving phenobarbital and diphenylhydantoin (Hahn *et al.* 1972).

SCREENING TESTS

In most instances the diagnosis of drug-induced malnutrition can be made by the physician if he can obtain the cooperation of the regional or local laboratory in order that certain simple biochemical tests can be carried out. Laboratory tests for drug-induced malabsorption should include a quantitative assay of fecal fat, and serum carotene estimations. Serial blood counts should be a routine procedure for all patients on long-term drug therapy. The biochemical profile should include erythrocyte transaminases, serum calcium and phosphorus, total serum protein, serum albumin, serum and erythrocyte folate, serum alkaline phosphatase, as well as the Quick one-stage prothrombin time and/or the two stage prothrombin time procedure (Hemker *et al.* 1970). In some instances it is possible to prove drug-induced malnutrition by withdrawing the pharmacologic agent and repeating laboratory tests at intervals thereafter. Reversal of nutrient depletion effects will occur if the deficiency was drug-induced. Drug substitution may be similarly used. When neither of these methods is medically feasible, therapeutic trial using vitamin(s) known to be depleted by particular drugs can be carried out (Table 4.9).

BIBLIOGRAPHY

BAKER, JR., C. E. 1976. Physicians Desk Reference. Medical Economics Co., Oradell, N.J.

BIEHL, J. P., and VILTER, R. W. 1954. Effect of isoniazid on vitamin B_6 metabolism; its possible significance in producing isoniazid neuritis. Proc. Soc. Exp. Biol. Med. *85*, 389–392.

BOWENS, M. A., LUND, P. K., and MATHIES, J. C. 1964. A rapid, reliable procedure for the determination of total fecal lipids; with the observation on the composition of the lipids excreted by human subjects in normal and pathological states. Clin. Chim. Acta *9*, 344–347.

BRITT, R. P., BOLTON, F. G., CULL, A. C., and SPRAY, G. H. 1969. Experience with a simplified method of radio-isotopic assay of serum vitamin B_{12}. Brit. J. Haemat. *16*, 457–464.

BURCH, H. B., BESSEY, O. A., and LOWRY, O. H. 1948. Fluorometric measurements of riboflavin and its natural derivatives in small quantities of blood serum and cells. J. Biol. Chem. *175*, 457–470.

CHABNER, B. and LIVINGSTON, D. 1970. A simply enzymic assay for pyridoxal phosphate. Anal. Biochem. *34*, 413–423.

CHANARIN, I. 1969. The Megaloblastic Anemias. Blackwell Scientific Publishing Co., Oxford, Edinburgh.

CHONG, Y. H., and HOU, G. S. 1970. Erythrocyte transketolase activity. Am. J. Clin. Nutr. *23*, 261–266.

CINNAMON, A. D., and BEATON, J. R. 1970. Biochemical assessment of vitamin B_6 status in man. Am. J. Clin. Nutr. *23*, 696–702.

COOPER, B. A., and LOWENSTEIN, L. 1966. Vitamin B_{12}-folate interrelations in megaloblastic anemia. Brit. J. Haemat. 12, 283-296.
CORCINO, J. J., WAXMAN, S., and HERBERT, V. 1970. Absorption and malabsorption of vitamin B_{12}. Am. J. Med. 48, 562-569.
FAZEKAS, A. G., MENENDES, C. E., and RIVLIN, R. S. 1974. A competitive protein binding assay for urinary riboflavin. Biochem. Med. 9, 167-176.
FRAZIER, E. I., PRATHER, M. E., and HOENE, E. 1955. Nicotinic acid metabolism in humans. I. The urinary excretion of nicotinic acid and its metabolic derivatives on four levels of dietary intake. J. Nutr. 56, 501-516.
GIORGIO, A. J., and LUHBY, A. L. 1969. A rapid screening test for the detection of congenital methylmalonic aciduria in infancy. Am. J. Clin. Path. 52, 374-379.
HAHN, T. J., HENDIN, B. A., SCHARP, C. R., and HADDAD, J. D. 1972. Effect of chronic anticonvulsant therapy on serum 25-hydroxycalciferol levels in adults. New Eng. J. Med. 287, 900-909.
HASKELL, B. E., and SNELL, E. E. 1972. An improved apotryptophanase assay for pyridoxal phosphate. Anal. Biochem. 45, 567-576.
HEINIVAARA, O., and PALVA, I. P. 1965. Malabsorption and deficiency of vitamin B_{12} caused by treatment of paraaminosalicylic acid. Acta. Med. Scand. 177, 337-341.
HEMKER, H. C., MULLER, A. D., and LOELIGER, E. A. 1970. Two types of prothrombin in vitamin K deficiency. Thromb. Diath. Haemorrh. 23, 633-637.
HLA-PE, U., and AUNG-THAN-BATU. 1967. A new colorimetric method for determination of formiminoglutamic acid in urine. Anal. Biochem. 20, 432-438.
HOFFBRAND, A. V., NEWCOMBE, B. F. A., and MOLLIN, D. L. 1966. Method of assay of red cell folate activity and the value of the assay as a test for folate deficiency. J. Clin. Path. 19, 17-28.
HORWITT, M. K., HARVEY, C. C., HILLS, O. W., et al. 1950. Correlation of urinary excretion of riboflavin with dietary intake and symptoms of ariboflavinosis. J. Nutr. 41, 247-264.
KRUSE, H. D., SYDENSTRICKER, V. P., SEBRELL, W. H., and CLEEKLEY, H. M. 1940. Ocular manifestations of ariboflavinosis. Public Health Rep. 55, 157-169.
LINKSWILER, H. 1967. Biochemical and physiological changes in vitamin B_6 deficiency. Am. J. Clin. Nutr. 20, 547-557.
LUMENG, L., CLEARY, R. E., and LI, P-K. 1974. Effect of oral contraceptives on the plasma concentration of pyridoxal phosphate. Am. J. Clin. Nutr. 27, 326-333.
MacLENNAN, W. J. 1971. Xylose absorption and serum carotene levels in the elderly. Geront. Clin. 13, 370-378.
MINCEY, E. K., WILCOX, E., and MORRISON, R. T. 1973. Estimation of serum and red cell folate by a simple radiometric technique. Clin. Biochem. 6, 274-284.
PELLETIER, O., and CAMPBELL, J. A. 1962. A rapid method for the determination of N^1-methylnicotinamide in urine. Anal. Biochem. 3, 60-67.
RAICA, N., JR. and SAUBERLICH, H. E. 1964. Blood cell transaminase activity in human vitamin B_6 deficiency. Am. J. Clin. Nutr. 15, 67-72.
RINALDO, J. A., JR. and GLUCKMAN, R. F. 1964. Maximal absorption capacity for xylose in nontropical sprue. Gastroenterology 47, 248-250.
ROE, D. A. 1971. Drug induced deficiency of B vitamins. N. Y. State J. Med. 71, 2770-2777.
ROE, D. A., McCORMICK, D. B., and LIN, R-T. 1972. Effects of riboflavin on boric acid toxicity. J. Pharm. Sci. 61, 1081-1085.
ROSENTHAL, W. S., ADHAM, N. F., LOPEZ, R., and COOPERMAN, J. M. 1973. Riboflavin deficiency in complicated chronic alcoholism. Am. J. Clin. Nutr. 26, 858-860.

ROTHENBERG, S. P., DaCOSTA, M., and ROSENBERG, Z. 1972. A radio-assay for serum folate: use of a 2-phase sequential-incubation, ligand-binding system. New Eng. J. Med. *286*, 1335-1339.

RUBIN, C. E., and DOBBINS, W. O. 1965. Peroral biopsy of the small intestine. A review of its diagnostic usefulness. Gastroenterology *40*, 676-697.

SAUBERLICH, H. E., et al. 1972. Biochemical assessment of the nutritional status of vitamin B_6 in the human. Am. J. Clin. Nutr. *25*, 629-642.

SAUBERLICH, H. E., JUDD, J. H., NICHOALDS, G. E., BROQUIST, H. P. et al. 1972. Application of the erythrocyte glutathione reductase assay in evaluating riboflavin nutritional status in a high school student population. Am. J. Clin. Nutr. *25*, 756-762.

SAUBERLICH, H. E., SKALA, J. H., and DOWDY, R. P. 1974. Laboratory Tests for the Assessment of Nutritional Status. C.R.C. Press, Cleveland, Ohio.

SCHILLING, R. F. 1953. Intrinsic factor studies. II. The effect of gastric juice on the urinary excretion of radioactivity after the oral administration of radioactive vitamin B_{12}. J. Lab. Clin. Med. *42*, 860-866.

SKEGGS, H. R. 1963. Lactobacillus leichmannii assay for vitamin B_{12}. In Analytical Microbiology, E. Kavanagh (Editor). Academic Press, New York.

SULLIVAN, A. L., and WEINTRAUB, L. R. 1973. Sideroblastic anemias. An approach to diagnosis and management. Med. Clin. N. Am. *57*, 335-342.

SYDENSTRICKER, V. P. 1941. Clinical manifestations of ariboflavinosis. Am. J. Public Health *31*, 344-350.

THOMPSON, J. N., ERDODY, P., BRYAN, R., and MURRAY, T. K. 1971. Fluorometric determination of vitamin A in human blood and liver. Biochem. Med. *5*, 67-89.

TILLOTSON, J. A., and BAKER, E. M. 1972. An enzymatic measurement of the riboflavin status in man. Am. J. Clin. Nutr. *25*, 425-431.

WALDMANN, T. A. 1961. Gastrointestinal protein loss demonstrated by Cr-51 labelled albumin. Lancet *2*, 121-123.

WALDMANN, T. A., and WOCHNER, R. D. 1965. The measurement of gastrointestinal protein loss by means of Cr^{51}-albumin and Cu^{67}-caeruloplasmin. In Radioisotope Techniques in the Study of Protein Metabolism, Technical Reports, Series 45, Intern. At. Energy Agency, Vienna.

WALLACH, J. 1974. Interpretation of Diagnostic Tests. 2nd Edition, Little, Brown and Co., Boston.

WATERS, A. H., and MOLLIN, D. L. 1961. Studies on the folic acid activity of human serum. J. Clin. Pathol. *14*, 335-344.

WATT, B. K., and MERRILL, A. L. 1963. Composition of foods. Agr. Handbook No. *8*, USDA, Washington, D.C.

WENGER, J., KIRSNER, J. B., and PALMER, W. L. 1957. Blood carotene in steatorrhea and the malabsorption syndromes. Am. J. Med. *22*, 373-380.

WILSON, F. A., and DIETSCHY, J. M. 1972. Approach to the malabsorption syndromes associated with bile acid metabolism. Arch. Internal Med. *130*, 584-594.

YUDKIN, S. 1941. Estimation of vitamin A and carotene in human blood. Biochem. J. *35*, 551-556.

CHAPTER 5

Drug-Induced Malabsorption

Drugs can induce malabsorption through a number of mechanisms. These mechanisms can be divided into those which exert their effects in the intestinal lumen, and those which impair mucosal absorption of nutrients and metabolic factors, whereby nutrients which are required for an absorptive process are impaired.

LUMINAL FACTORS

Drugs can provide a solution for nutrients. Such a situation exists in the case of mineral oil which may be used for laxative purposes. The intestinal transit time may be greatly reduced by cathartics, and thereby nutrients pass through the small intestine too rapidly for optimal absorption. Other pharmacologic agents, such as neomycin and cholestyramine, bind bile acids and thus impair the absorption of fats and of fat-soluble vitamins. There is also evidence that when a drug binds bile acids, the absorption of vitamin B_{12} may be decreased. Inhibition of pancreatic enzymes, such as lipases, will result in maldigestion of nutrients, and this in turn can lead to malabsorption.

MUCOSAL FACTORS

Alterations in the histology of the small intestine with cellular damage can result from intake of certain pharmacologic agents. These may cause destruction of the villous epithelium, can obliterate microvilli, or can interfere with the mitotic activity of intestinal epithelium so that the reparative process within the small intestine is abnormal. When the microvilli, composing the brush border of the small intestinal mucosa, are destroyed, there may be a concomitant loss or inhibition of intestinal enzymes located along the brush border, including disaccharidases and peptidases.

Primary malabsorption occurs when drugs depress uptake of nutrients from the small intestine without interfering with subsequent nutrient metabolism. Drugs known to have this potential, their usage, the malabsorption they produce, and their mode of action are summarized in Table 5.1. Impairment of intestinal absorption may be limited or nutrient specific, when the drug has a particular affinity for the nutrient, when there is a blockade of a single transport system, when intestinal enzymes are inactivated, or when bile salts

TABLE 5.1

PRIMARY INTESTINAL ABSORPTIVE DEFECTS INDUCED BY DRUGS

Drug	Usage	Malabsorption or Fecal Nutrient Loss	Mechanism
Mineral oil	Laxative	Carotene, Vit. A, D, K	Physical barrier Nutrients dissolve in mineral oil and are lost Micelle formation.↓
Phenolphthalein	Laxative	Vitamin D, Ca	Intestinal hurry K depletion Loss of structural integrity
Neomycin	Antibiotic to "sterilize" gut	Fat, nitrogen, Na, K, Ca, Fe, lactose, sucrose, vit. B_{12}	Structural defect Pancreatic lipase↓ Binding of bile acids (salts)
Cholestyramine	Hypocholesterolemic agent Bile acid sequestrant	Fat, Vit. A, K, B_{12}, D, Fe	Binding of bile acids (salts) and nutrients, e.g. Fe
Potassium chloride	Potassium repletion	Vitamin B_{12}	Ileal pH↓
Colchicine	Anti-inflammatory agent in gout	Fat, carotene, Na, K, Vit. B_{12}, lactose	Mitotic arrest Structural defect Enzyme damage
Biguanides: Metformin Phenformin	Hypoglycemic agents (in diabetes)	Vitamin B_{12}	Competitive inhibition of B_{12} absorption
Para-amino salicylic acid	Anti-tuberculosis agent	Fat, folate, Vitamin B_{12}	Mucosal block in B_{12} uptake
Salicylazosulfapyridine (Azulfidine)	Anti-inflammatory agent in ulcerative colitis, and regional enteritis	Folate	Mucosal block in folate uptake

are removed from the sites of absorption of fat-soluble vitamins. Similarly, drugs can impair nutrient absorption when they are capable of adsorbing a specific nutrient. Drugs can produce one or more of these effects. Those drugs that interfere with the structural integrity of the villi, causing malabsorption syndromes, which vary according to the area and severity of mucosal damage, consist in irritants and cytotoxic agents. Effects observed depend on the physical and chemical properties of the drug, as well as on drug dosage, on the mechanism or mechanisms whereby the drug exerts its deleterious effects, and on whether there is a pre-existing intestinal disease. It cannot be assumed, because a drug causes malabsorption by acting within the intestinal lumen, that it does not exert unrelated nutritional effects after absorption.

LAXATIVES AND CATHARTICS

The first drug which was discovered to cause malabsorption was mineral oil, at one time commonly used as a laxative and also as a substitute for olive oil in low-calorie salad dressings. In a series of animal experiments and human studies dating from 1927 onwards, it was shown that mineral oil impairs the absorption of carotene, vitamins A, D, and K (Burrows and Farr 1927; Smith and Spector 1940A and 1940B; Javert and Maeri 1941). Morgan (1941) suggested that the adverse effects of mineral oil on the absorption of fat-soluble vitamins was due to the physical barrier created at the mucosal surface. If this were the situation, then it might be anticipated that a more profound and uniform effect on nutrient absorption might be produced by intake of mineral oil. Curtis and Ballmer (1939), studying human volunteers, showed that when mineral oil or mineral oil emulsions were administered in 20 ml doses 3 times/day, carotene was removed from the diet and excreted with the mineral oil. If the mineral oil was presaturated with carotene, this provitamin ingested in the diet was still in part removed from the food, but in lesser amounts. This latter experiment was first carried out with the mineral oil-carotene mixture at $22°C$. When the experiment was repeated with the mineral oil-carotene mixture at $37°C$, this prevented the removal of carotene from the food in the gastrointestinal tract. The presence of mineral oil in the upper small intestine may impair micelle formation and thus hamper absorption of vitamins A, D, and K. Alternatively, as with carotene, solubility of these vitamins in the mineral oil may potentiate excretion. Rickets and osteomalacia from excessive mineral oil intake have been documented (Meulengracht 1939; Sinclair 1967).

Abuse of cathartics, which is still a public health problem, has resulted in severe malabsorption syndromes (Cummings et al. 1974). The fact that there are only a few case reports in the literature does not necessarily mean that further cases have not occurred. Two cases of factitious diarrhea, due to excessive ingestion of phenolphthalein and bisacodyl were reported by Heizer et al. (1968). Protein-losing enteropathy as well as malabsorption syndromes were demonstrated in both of these patients. Diarrhea from overuse of cathartics has previously been reported, and in some cases hypocalcemia has been found (Staffurth and Allott 1962). Frame et al. (1971) described a woman whose massive and prolonged intakes of phenolphthalein resulted in osteomalacia. Impaired absorption of xylose suggested a malabsorption state. Discontinuation of the drug relieved the signs and symptoms of her vitamin D deficiency. Malabsorption due to phenolphthalein may be associated with loss of structural integrity of the intestinal mucosa, but this has not been established. French *et al.* (1956) have suggested that it may be due to "intestinal hurry." Heizer *et al.* (1968) consider that there may be a disturbance in the integrity of the intestinal epithelial cells due to potassium depletion. Massive diarrhea associated with intake of castor oil or saline cathartics has not been shown to be associated with enteric loss of plasma proteins (Race *et al.* 1970).

ANTIBACTERIAL AGENTS INCLUDING ANTIBIOTICS

Among normal subjects, antibiotics such as tetracycline, kanamycin, polymyxin and bacitracin produce minimal interference with intestinal absorption (Dobbins 1968; Powell *et al.* 1962; Greenberger *et al.* 1966). However, decreased nutrient absorption associated with diarrhea has been documented in patients receiving broad spectrum antibiotics. In many of these cases there is evidence for primary malabsorption independent of drug intake. That is to say, patients developing malabsorption while they are taking antibiotics, such as tetracycline, have minimal malabsorption prior to drug intake such as celiac sprue syndrome (Jones 1973). The antibacterial agent, neomycin, was first reported to cause malabsorption by Faloon *et al.* (1958). Neomycin, when administered orally to man in doses of 3-12 gm/day for 3-7 days, causes a reversible malabsorption syndrome. Increased fecal excretion of fat, nitrogen, sodium, potassium and calcium have been found. Serum cholesterol is lowered due to impaired uptake of lipids. Impaired absorption of vitamin B_{12}, iron, lactose and sucrose, have also been demonstrated. Morphological and functional changes are induced by neomycin which can explain these effects. Villi are shortened and the lamina propria of the intestinal mucosa is infiltrated with inflammatory cells and macrophages (Jacobson *et al.* 1960; Jacobson and Faloon 1961). Keusch *et al.* (1970) showed that in Thai subjects structural changes in the epithelial cells near the tips of the villi appear within six hours of the first dose of neomycin. At this same time after the initiation of drug therapy, sucrose absorption is depressed. The authors suggest, but do not prove, that sucrose malabsorption is due to damage to the brush border where sucrase is located.

In vitro studies have revealed that at the pH found within the duodenum, neomycin forms a precipitate with bile salts (Faloon 1966). Pancreatic lipase activity is also decreased by neomycin (Mehta *et al.* 1964). In studies reported by Gordon *et al.* (1968), neither administration of bile salts nor pancreatic enzymes consistently affected steatorrhea induced by neomycin. Faloon (1970), however, considered that increased fecal fat excretion with neomycin was related to the unusual ability of the drug to bind fatty and bile acids. Corcino *et al.* (1970) have concluded that vitamin B_{12} malabsorption with neomycin is due to structural defects in the small intestine, but no experimental proof is available. It is now considered that neomycin induces maldigestion and malabsorption by three mechanisms: inhibition of pancreatic lipase, precipitation of bile salts, and mucosal damage. The mucosal damage is likely to be the major factor when the drug is given in high dosages (Dobbins 1968).

Para-aminosalicylic acid (PAS) was shown by Levine (1968) to cause malabsorption of fat at high levels of intake (12 g/daily) but no significant steatorrhea when given in smaller amounts (6 g/daily). Megaloblastic anemia was described by Heinivaara and Palva (1965) in two patients treated with PAS for tuberculosis. Subsequently these authors demonstrated malabsorption of vitamin B_{12} in other patients given PAS and in PAS-fed mice (Palva and Heinivaara 1965). In the rat they showed that PAS did not interfere with the production of intrinsic factor or with its binding to vitamin B_{12} and they proposed a mucosal block in B_{12} uptake to explain the findings. Additionally, they have suggested that PAS inhibition of B_{12} absorption is due to a drug-induced block in a folate-dependent enzyme in the wall of the ileum (Palva *et al.* 1966). Vitamin B_{12} malabsorption, induced by PAS, is rapidly reversible on withdrawal of the drug (Toskes and Deren 1972).

HYPOLIPEDEMIC AGENTS

The bile acid sequestrant, cholestyramine, has been shown to induce frank steatorrhea in normal subjects receiving 30 g of this resin per day (Hashim *et al.* 1961). Decreased serum cholesterol, associated with high dose cholestyramine intake, is due not only to fecal excretion of bile acids, but also to steatorrhea (Roe 1968). Malabsorption of fat-soluble vitamins can be induced. In subjects receiving vitamin A in olive oil, peak serum levels of the vitamin are suppressed as compared to control subjects not receiving this drug (Longenecker and Basu 1965). Heaton *et al.* (1972) reported osteomalacia in a woman receiving cholestyramine therapy for postileectomy diarrhea. The authors suggest that her vitamin D deficiency may have been due to a malabsorption induced by the drug, but initial bile salt catharsis may have contributed to the condition (Heaton *et al.* 1972). Prolonged intake of cholestyramine at high dosage has been shown by Visintine *et al.* (1961) to cause vitamin K deficiency, reversible by parenteral vitamin K.

Thomas *et al.* (1971) showed in rats that cholestyramine can bind both inorganic and organic iron, causing significant malabsorption of both forms of the mineral. More recently Cook *et al.* (1974) studied the *in vitro* binding of iron by cholestyramine and the utilization of dietary iron in laboratory animals fed cholestyramine. They found that the *in vitro* binding of iron by cholestyramine was negligible. In weanling rats, neither hemoglobin nor serum iron levels were significantly affected by cholestyramine. On the basis of these studies they concluded that cholestyramine does not interfere with the utilization of dietary iron, at least in rats. In view of these conflicting papers, further studies are required to define whether cholestyramine exerts any effect on the absorption of iron both in normal and anemic patients.

Cholestyramine has been shown by Coronato and Glass (1973) to lower the absorption of radio-B_{12} in normal volunteers and in those with pernicious anemia. Results of *in vitro* studies by these same authors using guinea pig intestinal mucosa indicated that cholestyramine may decrease the uptake of vitamin B_{12} by binding a portion of the same sites on the intrinsic factor molecule which normally binds B_{12} and thus prevents the formation of the intrinsic factor-B_{12} complex. Although these authors showed that cholic and possibly deoxycholic acids decrease absorption of radio-B_{12}, they do not believe that cholestyramine induces B_{12} malabsorption due to sequestration of bile acids.

Clofibrate (Atromid S) has effects on the intestinal mucosa which may increase its hypolipidemic potential. This drug has also been reported to increase the fecal excretion of neutral sterols (Grundy *et al.* 1969). Zakim *et al.* (1969) reported that clofibrate decreases the activity of enzymes involved in the mucosal metabolism of carbohydrates. Clinical evidence of malabsorption has not been established in patients taking this drug.

ANTI-INFLAMMATORY AGENTS

Colchicine, long used in the treatment of gout, is known to induce gastrointestinal side effects in many patients (Woodbury 1965). Race *et al.* (1971) studied the effects of colchicine on intestinal function in human subjects. The drug produced consistent increases in the fecal excretion of sodium, potassium, fat and nitrogen; also, it impaired absorption of radio-B_{12}, suggesting an impairment of ileal function. Disaccharidase inhibition was demonstrated to occur rapidly after initiation of colchicine administration. These nutritional effects of colchicine were all found to be reversible. Variable changes in the histology of the jejunal mucosa were seen in sections of biopsy material from subjects receiving colchicine, but the degree of malabsorption could not be related to the severity of histological changes (Webb et al. 1968). Colchicine is known to be a spindle poison which arrests cell mitosis in metaphase (Taylor 1965). In man, as in laboratory animals, similarities exist between the effects of colchicine and x-rays on the intestinal mucosa (Dustin 1963; Hampton 1966). Lack of quantitative relationships between histological changes in the intestinal mucosa and the degree of malabsorption suggest that absorptive defects, induced by colchicine, may be due to interference with transport mechanisms. Serum cholesterol levels have been shown by Robulis et al. (1969) to be depressed by colchicine, and concomitantly there is enhanced excretion of bile acids in the stool.

The anti-inflammatory drug, salicylazosulfapyridine (Azulfidine), does not induce malabsorption in itself, but can exacerbate malabsorption of folate which occurs in those forms of inflammatory bowel disease for which the drug is prescribed (Franklin and Rosenberg 1973).

ORAL HYPOGLYCEMIC DRUGS

The biguanides used in the oral therapy of diabetes since 1957 have been shown to cause malabsorption of vitamin B_{12}. Berchtold et al. (1969) and Tomkin et al. (1971) have shown that long term metformin therapy may result in impairment of vitamin B_{12} status. The latter authors have shown that this is not due to lack of intrinsic factor. Malabsorption of vitamin B_{12} has also been demonstrated by Tomkin (1973) in patients receiving the related biguanide phenformin over prolonged periods. In both instances this selective malabsorption is reversible when the drug is discontinued. The biguanides impair glucose as well as vitamin B_{12} absorption, and it has been suggested that the action of the biguanides in lowering blood sugar is due to the former effect. Biguanide-induced malabsorption of vitamin B_{12} may either be due to competitive inhibition of vitamin absorption in the distal ileum or due to drug inactivation of vitamin B_{12}.

POTASSIUM CHLORIDE

It has been shown in vitro that the uptake of vitamin B_{12} by normal ileal homogenates is dependent on the pH of the environment. Uptake of this vitamin is maximal at pH 6.6 and above and absent below pH 5.5 (Carmel et al. 1969). Palva et al. (1972) showed that, in patients with no evidence of prior vitamin B_{12} malabsorption, administration of slow release potassium chloride led to abnormal Schilling test values, indicating impairment of B_{12} absorption by the drug. Normalization of Schilling test values occurred when the drug was withdrawn. Radiotelemetric measurements of the ileal pH were performed on patients during KCl administration, and the results indicated that patients receiving this drug have lower ileal pH values, and that those with lower ileal pH values also had depressed Schilling test values.

OTHER DRUGS

Selective vitamin malabsorption has been invoked to account for low serum and erythrocyte folate values in patients receiving oral contraceptives or anticonvulsants. Evidence is controversial and there is extensive data showing that these drugs can cause folate depletion by other mechanisms.

SECONDARY MALABSORPTION

Secondary malabsorption is caused by drugs which affect nutrient metabolism so that an active transport mechanism is inhibited. The examples of secondary malabsorption that have now been documented are mainly those relating to vitamin D (Table 5.2).

Glucocorticoids lower serum calcium by reducing its absorption. Based on studies of human volunteers who received tritiated vitamin D_3 before and after prednisone, Avioli, et al. (1968) suggested that antagonism of glucocorticoids to the action of vitamin D in man is related to the rapid turnover of the vitamin. While it is accepted that glucocorticoids impair calcium transport in a manner antagonistic to the action of vitamin D, Kimberg (1969) has pointed out that how

TABLE 5.2

DRUGS AFFECTING VITAMIN D AND CALCIUM TRANSPORT

Drugs	Usage	Malabsorption	Mechanism
Prednisone (other gluco-corticoids)	Allergic and collagen diseases	Calcium	Calcium transport↓
Phenobarbital	Anticonvulsants	Calcium	Accelerated
Diphenylhydantoin	Anticonvulsants	Calcium	catabolism of
Primidone	Anticonvulsants	Calcium	vitamin D and
Glutethimide	Sedative	Calcium	active metabolites
Diphosphonates	Paget's disease	Calcium	1,25-DHCC formation↓

and if glucocorticoids affect the production of active metabolites in the vitamin D is presently unsettled.

Rickets and osteomalacia can result from chronic intake of anticonvulsant drugs such as phenobarbital and diphenylhydantoin. Schmid (1967) described rickets in patients receiving long-term anticonvulsant therapy. Kruse (1968) reported that 15% of epileptic patients under treatment showed serum biochemical and radiological features of osteomalacia. The extent of these changes was related to the duration of treatment and to the dose of anticonvulsant drugs.

Richens and Rowe (1970) found subnormal serum calcium levels in 22.5% and an elevated alkaline phosphatase level in 29% of 160 residential patients in an institution who were receiving long-term anticonvulsant drugs. DeLuca and Masotti (1971) reported that a group of 34 severely retarded children in an institution who were receiving long-term anticonvulsant drugs showed lower serum calcium and phosphate levels and higher alkaline phosphatase values than control subjects. These patients had a higher incidence of bone rarefaction than did a similar group of children who were not on anticonvulsants.

Stamp (1974) described three epileptic patients who developed vitamin D deficiency while receiving anticonvulsant drugs. He pointed out and supported his thesis with case documentation that anticonvulsant rickets shows considerable resistance to treatment with vitamin D, but that the same type of cases show a rapid response to ultraviolet light irradiation. This same author also has shown that when the frequency of seizures increases in epileptics on anticonvulsants, this may be explained by the presence of hypocalcemia.

Juvenile and adult forms of vitamin D deficiency have been discovered in epileptic patients taking phenobarbital alone or diphenylhydantoin alone, but there is evidence that combinations of these drugs with or without primidone increases the rachitic effect (Bowden 1974). Subclinical as well as clinical osteomalacia among epileptics has been documented by Dent et al. (1970) and Christiansen et al. (1972).

In 288 institutionalized mentally retarded children studied by Lifshitz and MacLaren (1973), fasting serum values of calcium, phosphorus, and alkaline phosphatase were measured. X-rays of long bones were obtained from 75 of these patients. Of their 288 patients, 134 had received anticonvulsants for more than a year. All of them had a daily vitamin D_2 intake of 800–1200 IU. It was found that those children who had received anticonvulsants had lower values for both serum calcium and phosphorus, and higher values for serum alkaline phosphatase, than control subjects who were not receiving anticonvulsants. The observed biochemical changes were correlated with the duration of therapy but not with drug dosage. Sixty-eight of their patients who were receiving combinations of anticonvulsants had the most marked depression of calcium and phosphorus values and increases in alkaline phosphatase. Nine of these had biochemical and radiological evidence of rickets, and 20 of them had bone rarefaction.

In another study by Christiansen et al. (1973), the bone mineral content (BMC) of both forearms was measured by photon absorptiometry among a sample of 226 epileptic out-patients receiving anticonvulsant drugs. Initially the BMC values for all epileptic patients was 87% of normal. These patients were then treated with 2000 IU of vitamin D_2 daily for three months and there was an average increase in BMC of 4% among those receiving anticonvulsant drugs.

Livingston et al. (1973) are skeptical about the association of intakes of anticonvulsant drugs and vitamin D deficiency. They reported negatively concerning the incidence of rickets or osteomalacia among 15,000 clinic patients receiving treatment for epilepsy. In their paper these authors state that they were unable to find a single patient exhibiting chemical or radiological changes described for anticonvulsant rickets, and they also state that they do not recall having encountered such findings in any of the 15,000 patients who were referred to the clinic, except for some few patients seen approximately 30 years ago who had rickets associated with an inadequate intake of vitamin D. It is notable that their radiological studies were related only to X rays of the skull, and that no X rays were taken of long bones necessary to the early diagnosis of rickets. It may also be significant that their cases were seen on an out-patient basis, and perhaps had adequate exposure to sunlight which would be denied institutionalized patients.

Vitamin D deficiency in patients on anticonvulsant drugs has been attributed by Hahn et al. (1972B) to accelerated conversion of the vitamin and its active metabolite, 25-hydroxycholecalciferol (25-HCC) to inactive polar derivatives by drug induction of hepatic microsomal enzymes. Serum concentrations of 25-HCC are lower in drug-treated epileptics than in controls, and serum concentration of 25-HCC correlate well with serum calcium levels. This has suggested that hypocalcemia results from drug-induced inactivation of 25-HCC. Accelerated plasma disappearance rate and increased urinary excretion of vitamin D metabolites has been reported in people receiving phenobarbital and diphenylhydantoin (Hahn et al. 1972A; Silver et al. 1972).

In chicks, rickets, hypocalcemia, decreased duodenal calcium transport, and reduction of calcium-binding proteins have been produced by diphenylhydantoin and phenobarbital administration. Effects in the chick are dependent on drug dose and inversely related to the intakes of vitamin D_3 (Villareale et al. 1974A; 1974B). Evidence has been obtained in the rat for an inhibitory effect of diphenylhydantoin and phenobarbital on calcium absorption (Koch et al. 1973; Caspary 1972).

Osteomalacia has been reported by Greenwood et al. (1973) in a patient who was taking glutethimide over a prolonged period. Glutethimide structurally resembles phenobarbital and, like phenobarbital, is a potent inducer of hepatic microsomal enzymes. In the reported case of glutethimide-induced osteomalacia, evidence was obtained of hepatic enzyme induction and the plasma half-life of tritiated vitamin D_3 was decreased. It was suggested by the authors that, as with the anticonvulsant drugs, glutethimide increases the turnover rate of vitamin D, causing depletion of vitamin stores and impairment of vitamin D-dependent calcium absorption. It must be emphasized, however, that conclusive proof of anticonvulsants' induced impairment of calcium absorption through increased vitamin D turnover in the liver has not yet been obtained.

Diphosphonates have been shown to exert a beneficial effect on the clinical course of Paget's disease and myositis ossificans (Smith et al. 1973; Bassett et al. 1969), and calcinosis universalis (Cram et al. 1971). Hill et al. (1973) showed that in rats disodium ethane-1-hydroxy-1,1-diphosphonate for 14 days developed rickets and impaired calcium transport even when these animals were given large amounts of vitamin D_3. These vitamin D-deficient rats, treated with the diphosphonate, responded to 1,25-dihydroxycholecalciferol, and it was inferred by the authors that the drug inhibited the renal biosynthesis of 1,25-dihydroxycholecalciferol. There has been concern that the diphosphonates can cause calcium malabsorption in man leading to osteomalacia, and changes characteristic of rickets have been documented in certain children receiving these drugs (Bordier and Tun-Chat 1972; Russell et al. 1972). Jowsey et al. (1971) have shown that high dose therapy of osteoporosis with diphosphonate increases the osteoid content of bone biopsies. Smith et al. (1973) found that increased thickness of osteoid occurred in biopsies of Paget's bone in subjects on a dose of 20 mg/kg/day of diphosphonate (disodium etidronate). These histological changes were found to be reversible with discontinuance of the drug. In a six months double blind controlled study of 47 subjects with Paget's disease who were treated with disodium etidronate, Altman et al. (1973) found that the benefits to the primary disease process were dose related. No side effects suggestive of osteomalacia were encountered in this group. In another series of cases of patients with Paget's disease who received diphosphonates, Russell *et al.* (1974) demonstrated that the disease was suppressed, as evidenced by bone biopsy specimens. These authors found that increases in unmineralized osteoid suggestive of early vitamin D deficiency were only seen in bone biopsy specimens taken after the higher doses of the drug, and that these changes were minimal. It was considered that the risk of vitamin D deficiency incurred by those patients receiving diphosphonates was small in comparison with the great benefits which the drug conferred in the management of Paget's disease.

BIBLIOGRAPHY

ALTMAN, R. D. *et al.* 1973. Influence of disodium etidronate on clinical and laboratory manifestations of Paget's disease of bone (osteitis deformans). New Eng. J. Med. *289*, 1379–1384.

AVIOLI, L. V., BIRGE, S. J., and LEE, S. W. 1968. Effects of prednisone on vitamin D metabolism in man. J. Clin. Endocrinol. Metab. *28*, 1341–1346.

BASSETT, C. A. L., *et al.* 1969. Diphosphonates in the treatment of myositis ossificans. Lancet *2*, 845.

BERCHTOLD, P., BOLLI, P., ARBENZ, U., and KEISER, G. 1969. Intestinal malabsorption as a result of treatment with metformin. A question of the mode of action of the biguanide. Diabetologia *5*, 405–412.

BORDIER, P. J., and TUN-CHOT, S. 1972. Quantitative histology of metabolic bone disease. Clin. Endocrinol. Metab. *1*, 197–215.

BOWDEN, A. N. 1974. Anticonvulsants and calcium metabolism. Develop. Med. Child Neurol. *16*, 214–217.

BURROWS, M. T., and FARR, W. K. 1927. The action of mineral oil per os on the organism. Proc. Soc. Exp. Biol. Med. *24*, 719–723.

CARMEL, R. *et al.* 1969. Vitamin B_{12} uptake by human small bowel homogenate and its enhancement by intrinsic factor. Gastroenterology *56*, 548–555.

CASPARY, W. F. 1972. Inhibition of intestinal calcium transport by diphenylhydantoin in rat duodenum. Naunyn Schmiedeberg's Arch. Exp. Pathol. Pharmakol. *274*, 146–153.

CHRISTIANSEN, C., KRISTENSEN, M., and RØDBRO, P. 1972. Latent osteomalacia in epileptic patients on anticonvulsants. Brit. Med. J. *3*, 738–739.

CHRISTIANSEN, C., RØDBRO, P., and LUND, M. 1973. Incidence of anticonvulsant osteomalacia and effect of vitamin D: controlled therapeutic trial. Brit. Med. J. *4*, 695–701.

COOK, D. A., HAGERMAN, L. M., and SCHNEIDER, D. L. 1974. Utilization of dietary iron in rats fed diets containing cholestyramine resin. Fed. Proc. *33*, 716.

CORCINO, J. J., WAXMAN, S., and HERBERT, V. 1970. Absorption and malabsorption of vitamin B_{12}. Am. J. Med. *48*, 562–569.

CORONATO, A., and GLASS, G. B. J. 1973A. Depression of the intestinal uptake of radio-vitamin B_{12} by cholestyramine. Proc. Soc. Exp. Biol. Med. *142*, 1341–1344.

CORONATO, A., and GLASS, G. B. J. 1973B. The effect of deconjugated and conjugated bile salts on the intestinal uptake of radio-vitamin B_{12} *in vitro* and *in vivo*. Proc. Soc. Exp. Biol. Med. *142*, 1345–1348.

CRAM, R. L., BARMADA, R., GEHO, W. B., and RAY, R. D. 1971. Diphosphonate treatment of calcinosis universalis. New Eng. J. Med. *285*, 1012–1013.

CUMMINGS, J. H. *et al.* 1974. Laxative-induced diarrhea: A continuing clinical problem. Brit. Med. J. *1*, 537-541.

CURTIS, A. C., and BALLMER, R. S. 1939. The prevention of carotene absorption by liquid petrolatum. J. Am. Med. Assoc. *113*, 1785-1788.

DeLUCA, H. F., and MASOTTI, R. E. 1971. Hypocalcemia induced by anticonvulsant drugs. 48th Annual Meeting Canadian Pediatric Society, Kingston, Ontario, Canada.

DENT, C. E., RICHENS, A., ROWE, D. J. F., and STAMP, T. C. B. 1970. Osteomalacia with long term anticonvulsant therapy in epilepsy. Brit. Med. J. *4*, 69-72.

DOBBINS, W. O. 1968. Drug-induced steatorrhea. Gastroenterology *54*, 1193-1195.

DUSTIN, P., JR. 1963. New aspects of the pharmacology of antimitotic agents. Pharmac. Rev. *15*, 449-480.

FALOON, W. W. 1966. Effect of neomycin and kanamycin upon intestinal absorption. Ann. N. Y. Acad. Sci. *132*, 879-887.

FALOON, W. W. 1970. Drug production of intestinal malabsorption. N.Y. State J. Med. *70*, 2189-2192.

FALOON, W. W., FISHER, C. J., and DUGGAN, K. C. 1958. Occurrence of a sprue-like syndrome during neomycin therapy. Abst. J. Clin. Invest. *37*, 893.

FRAME, B., GUIANG, H. L., FROST, H. M., and REYNOLDS, W. A. 1971. Osteomalacia induced by laxative (phenolphthalein) ingestion. Arch. Intern. Med. *128*, 794-796.

FRANKLIN, J. L., and ROSENBERG, I. H. 1973. Impaired folic acid absorption in inflammatory bowel disease: effects of salicylazosulfapyridine (Azulfidine). Gastroenterology *64*, 517-525.

FRENCH, J. M., GADDIE, R., and SMITH, N. 1956. Diarrhea due to phenolphthalein. Lancet *270*, 551-553.

GORDON, S. J., HARO, E. N., PAES, I. C., and FALOON, W. W. 1968. Studies of malabsorption and calcium excretion induced by neomycin sulfate. J. Am. Med. Assoc. *204*, 129-134.

GREENBERGER, N. J., RUPPERT, R. D., and CUPPAGE, F. E. 1966. Inhibition of intestinal iron transport induced by tetracycline. Gastroenterology *53*, 590-599.

GREENWOOD, R. H., PRUNTY, F. T. G., and SILVER, J. 1973. Osteomalacia after prolonged glutethimide administration. Brit. Med. J. *1*, 643-645.

GRUNDY, S. M., AHRENS, E. M., SALEN, G., and QUINTOS, E. 1969. Mode of action of atromid-S on cholesterol metabolism in man. Abs. J. Clin. Invest. *48*, 33a.

HAHN, T. J., BIRGE, S. J., SCHARP, C. R., and AVIOLI, L. V. 1972A. Phenobarbital-induced alterations in vitamin D metabolism. J. Clin. Invest. *51*, 741-748.

HAHN, T. J., HENDIN, B. A., SCHARP, C. R., and HADDAD, J. G., JR. 1972B. Effect of chronic anticonvulsant therapy on serum 25-hydroxycalciferol levels in adults. New Eng. J. Med. *287*, 900-909.

HAMPTON, J. C. 1966. A comparison of the effects of X-radiation and colchicine on the intestinal mucosa of the mouse. Radiat. Res. *28*, 37-59.

HASHIM, S. A., BERGEN, S. S., JR., and VANITALLIE, T. B. 1961. Experimental steatorrhea induced in man by bile acid sequestrant. Proc. Soc. Exp. Biol. Med. *106*, 173-175.

HEATON, K. W., LEVER, J. V., and BARNARD, D. 1972. Osteomalacia associated with cholestyramine therapy for postileectomy diarrhea. Gastroenterology *62*, 642-646.

HEINIVAARA, O., and PALVA, I. P. 1964. Malabsorption of vitamin B_{12} during treatment with para-aminosalicylic acid. A preliminary report. Acta Med. Scand. *175*, 469-471.

HEINIVAARA, O., and PALVA, I. P. 1965. Malabsorption and deficiency of vitamin B_{12} caused by treatment with para-aminosalicylic acid. Acta Med. Scand. *177*, 337–341.

HEIZER, W. D., WARSHAW, A. L., WALDMANN, T. A., and LASTER, L. 1968. Protein-losing gastroenteropathy and malabsorption associated with factitious diarrhea. Ann. Intern. Med. *68*, 839–851.

HILL, L. F., LUMB, G. A., MAWER, E. B., and STANBURY, S. W. 1973. Indirect inhibition of the biosynthesis of 1,25-dihydroxycholecalciferol in rats treated with a diphosphonate. Clin. Sci. *44*, 335–347.

JACOBSON, E. D., CHODOS, R. B., and FALOON, W. W. 1960. Malabsorptive syndrome induced by neomycin. Am. J. Med. *28*, 524–533.

JACOBSON, E. D., and FALOON, W. W. 1961. Malabsorptive effects of neomycin in commonly used doses. J. Am. Med. Assoc. *175*, 187–190.

JAVERT, C. T., and MACRI, C. 1941. Prothrombin concentration and mineral oil. Am. J. Obstet. Gynecol. *42*, 409–414.

JONES, C. C. 1973. Megaloblastic anemia associated with long-term tetracycline therapy. Ann. Intern. Med. *78*, 910–912.

JOWSEY, J. *et al.* 1971. The treatment of osteoporosis with disodium ethane-1-hydroxy-1, 1-diphosphonate. J. Lab. Clin. Med. *78*, 574–584.

KEUSCH, G. T., TRONCALE, F. J., and PLAUT, A. G. 1970. Neomycin-induced malabsorption in a tropical population. Gastroenterology *58*, 197–202.

KIMBERG, D. V. 1969. Effects of vitamin D and steroid hormones on the active transport of calcium by the intestine. New Eng. J. Med. *280*, 1396–1405.

KOCH, H. U., KRAFT, D., VON HERRATH, D., and SCHAEFFER, K. 1973. Influence of diphenylhydantoin and phenobarbital on intestinal calcium transport in the rat. Epilepsia *13*, 829–834.

KRUSE, R. 1968. Osteopathies induced by chronic anticonvulsant drug therapy. (Current Information). Monatsschr. Kinderheilkd *116*, 378–381.

LEVINE, R. A. 1968. Steatorrhea induced by para-aminosalicylic acid. Ann. Intern. Med. *68*, 1265–1270.

LIFSCHITZ, F., and MacLAREN, N. K. 1973. Vitamin D-dependent rickets in institutionalized, mentally retarded children receiving long-term anticonvulsant therapy. I. A survey of 288 patients. J. Pediat. *83*, 612–620.

LIVINGSTON, S., BERMAN, W., and PAULI, L. L. 1973. Anticonvulsant drugs and vitamin D metabolism. J. Am. Med. Assoc. *244*, 1634–1635.

LONGENECKER, J. B., and BASU, S. G. 1965. Effect of cholestyramine on absorption of amino acids and vitamin A in man. Fed. Proc. *24*, 375 (Abs.).

MEHTA, S. K., WESSER, E., and SLEISENGER, M. A. 1964. The *in vitro* effect of bacterial metabolites and antibiotics on pancreatic lipase activity. Abs. J. Clin. Invest. *43*, 1252.

MEULENGRACHT, E. 1939. Osteomalacia of the spinal column from deficient diet or from disease of the digestive tract. III. Osteomalacia e abuse laxantium. Acta Med. Scand. *101*, 187–210.

MORGAN, J. W. 1941. The harmful effects of mineral oil (liquid petrolatum) purgatives. J. Am. Med. Assoc. *117*, 1335–1336.

PALVA, I. P., and HEINIVAARA, O. 1965. Drug induced malabsorption of vitamin B_{12}. Experimental studies with PAS-fed mice. Acta Med. Int. Fenn. *54*, 37–38.

PALVA, I. P., HEINIVAARA, O., and MITTILA, M. 1966. Drug-induced malabsorption of vitamin B_{12}. III. Interference of PAS and folic acid in the absorption of vitamin B_{12}. Scand. J. Haemat. *3*, 149–153.

PALVA, I. P., SALOKANNEL, S. J., TIMONEN, T., and PALVA, H. L. A. 1972. Drug-induced malabsorption of vitamin B_{12}. IV. Malabsorption and deficiency of B_{12} during treatment with slow-release potassium chloride. Acta Med. Scand. *191*, 355–357.

POWELL, R. C., NUNES, W. T., HAN, R. S., and VACCA, J. B. 1962. The influence of nonabsorbable antibiotics on serum lipids and the excretion of neutral sterols and bile acids. Am. J. Clin. Nutr. *11*, 156–168.

RACE, T. F., PAES, I. C., and FALOON, W. W. 1970. Intestinal malabsorption induced by oral colchicine. Comparison with neomycin and cathartic agents. Am. J. Med. Sci. *259*, 32–41.

RICHENS, A., and ROWE, D. J. F. 1970. Disturbance of calcium metabolism by anticonvulsant drugs. Brit. Med. J. *4*, 73–76.

ROBULIS, A., RUBERT, M., and FALOON, W. W. 1969. Cholesterol lowering, fecal bile acid and sterol changes during neomycin and colchicine. Abs. Fed. Proc. *28*, 268.

ROE, D. A. 1968. Essential hyperlipemia with xanthomatosis. Effects of cholestyramine and clofibrate. Arch. Derm. *97*, 436–445.

RUSSELL, R. G. G. *et al.* 1972. Treatment of myositis ossificans progressiva with a diphosphonate. Lancet *1*, 10–12.

RUSSELL, R. G. G. *et al.* 1974. Diphosphonates in Paget's disease. Lancet *1*, 894–898.

SCHMID, F. 1967. Osteopathies induced by anticonvulsants. Dauerbehandlung Fortschr. Med. *85*, 381–383.

SILVER J. *et al.* 1972. The effect of phenobarbitone-induction on vitamin D metabolism. Clin. Sci. *42*, 12P.

SINCLAIR, L. 1967. Rickets from liquid paraffin. Lancet *1*, 792.

SMITH, M. C., and SPECTOR, H. 1940A. Calcium and phosphorus metabolism in rats and dogs as influenced by the ingestion of mineral oil. J. Nutr. *20*, 19–30.

SMITH, M. C., and SPECTOR, H. 1940B. Some effects on animal nutrition of the ingestion of mineral oil. Univ. Ariz. Coll. Agric. Exper. Sta. Bull. *84*, 373–395.

SMITH, R. *et al.* 1973. Paget's disease of bone: experience with a diphosphonate (disodium etidronate) in treatment. Quart. J. Med. *42*, 235–256.

STAFFURTH, J. S., and ALLOTT, E. N. 1962. Paralysis and tetany due to simultaneous hypokalemia and hypocalcemia, with other metabolic changes. Am. J. Med. *33*, 800–806.

STAMP, T. C. B. 1974. Effects of long-term anticonvulsant therapy on calcium and vitamin D metabolism. Proc. Roy. Soc. Med. *67*, 64–68.

TAYLOR, E. W. 1965. The mechanism of colchicine inhibition of mitosis. I. Kinetics of inhibition and the binding of H^3-colchicine. J. Cell Biol. *25*, 145–160.

THOMAS, F. B., McCULLOUGH, F. S., and GREENBERGER, N. J. 1971. Inhibition of the intestinal absorption of inorganic and hemoglobin iron by cholestyramine. J. Lab. Clin. Med. *78*, 70–80.

TOMKIN, G. H. 1973. Malabsorption of vitamin B_{12} in diabetic patients treated with phenformin: a comparison with metformin. Brit. Med. J. *3*, 673–675.

TOMKIN, G. H., HADDEN, D. R., WEAVER, J. A., and MONTGOMERY, D. A. D. 1971. Vitamin-B_{12} status of patients on long-term metformin therapy. Brit. Med. J. *2*, 685–687.

TOSKES, P. P., and DEREN, J. J. 1972. Selective inhibition of vitamin B_{12} absorption by para-aminosalicylic acid. Gastroenterology *62*, 1232–1237.

VILLAREALE, M. *et al.* 1974A. Diphenylhydantoin: effects on calcium metabolism in the chick. Science *183*, 671–673.

VILLAREALE, M. *et al.* 1974B. Effects of anticonvulsants on calcium metabolism in the chick. Pediat. Res. Abs. *8*, 165.

VISINTINE, R. E. *et al.* 1961. Xanthomatous biliary cirrhosis treated with cholestyramine, a bile-acid-absorbing resin. Lancet *2*, 341–343.

WEBB, D. I., CHODOS, R. B., MAHAR, C. Q., and FALOON, W. W. 1968. Mechanism of vitamin B_{12} malabsorption in patients receiving colchicine. New Eng. J. Med. *279*, 845–850.

WOODBURY, D. M. 1965. Analgesics and antipyretics. Colchicine. *In* The Pharmacological Basis of Therapeutics, 3rd Edition. L. S. Goodman, and A. Gilman (Editors). Macmillan Co., New York.

ZAKIM, D., HERMAN, R. H., ROSENSWEIG, N. S., and STIFEL, F. B. 1969. Clofibrate-induced changes in the activity of human intestinal enzymes. Gastroenterology *56*, 496–499.

CHAPTER 6

Iatrogenic Hyperexcretion and Tissue Depletion of Minerals and Vitamins

MINERALS

Mineral depletion can result from drug-induced malabsorption or can be associated with excessive urinary losses of minerals.

ANTACIDS

According to Quigley *et al.* (1939) aluminum hydroxide, one of the commonest antacids, can be taken in high and chronic dosage without causing adverse effects. Harvey (1965), in Goodman and Gilman's standard text on therapeutic drugs, emphasizes that aluminum hydroxide combines with phosphates in the intestine and that the aluminum phosphates are then excreted in the feces. Abuse of aluminum hydroxide can result in phosphate depletion. These effects of phosphate depletion vary with the severity of the process. Bone demineralization may occur preceding the development of osteomalacia or rickets. Bloom and Flinchum (1960) described a fifty-year-old woman who developed osteomalacia after taking aluminum hydroxide for many years as treatment for a spastic colon. When she was first seen her serum calcium level was 10.4 mg%, but the serum inorganic phosphorus level was 2.9 mg% fasting, and 2.0 mg% in the afternoon while she was taking the aluminum hydroxide tablets. When this woman stopped taking her "stomach medicine" in the form of aluminum hydroxide and was given small doses of calcium and vitamin D, her osteomalacia resolved and she became symptom-free. Lotz *et al.* (1968) have also described a phosphorus depletion syndrome occurring in patients on prolonged antacids consisting of magnesium-aluminum hydroxides. In their cases there were clinical symptoms of malaise and bone pain associated with hypophosphatemia and hypercalciuria.

Dent and Winter (1974) made an exhaustive study of another woman who developed osteomalacia due to phosphate depletion from taking aluminum hydroxide in various forms. Their patient was a forty-nine-year-old housewife who complained of pain in the left hip, and weakness and difficulty in walking. These symptoms had been present for about five months, and more recently had become severe. She had also noticed considerable weakness. Her other relevant history was that she complained of severe heartburn which apparently was associated with esophagitis and hiatus hernia. In order to relieve the heartburn she had taken approximately 4.7 gm/day of aluminum hydroxide for nine months and thereafter about 20 gm/day of this antacid for about fifteen months. Clinical signs in this woman, suggestive of osteomalacia, included her waddling gait, weakness of the hip and knee flexor muscles, and tenderness of both humeri and the left hip. She showed a low plasma phosphorus and a high renal excretion of calcium with a low urinary phosphorus content. Her serum alkaline phosphatase level was not markedly elevated. She had an extremely high fecal excretion of phosphorus. Her symptoms and signs of drug-induced phosphate depletion and osteomalacia gradually came back towards normality when the dose of aluminum hydroxide was reduced. It is interesting that in this patient osteomalacia could not be diagnosed radiologically, but a bone biopsy taken at the time when the patient was first seen confirmed the diagnosis.

Baker *et al.* (1974) described a twenty-six-year-old woman with congenital renal dysplasia associated with uremia, who was treated by hemodialysis. When she was first seen she had no evidence of osteomalacia or of myopathy associated with vitamin D deficiency. Her serum calcium was 9.6 mg/100 ml and serum phosphate 7.0 mg/100 ml and the alkaline phosphatase level in the serum was 48 IU. In view of the presence of hyperphosphatemia, she was treated with aluminum hydroxide at a dose of 2.25 gm/day. After a period of about 22 months on this regimen she developed painful feet, and soon afterwards pain in the legs, arms and shoulders. She also had difficulty in climbing stairs because of weakness in her legs. Later she became so weak that she was unable to rise unaided to a sitting position. Although at the time that she first developed pain in her feet, x-ray examination had been normal, by the time she developed extreme weakness, which was about seven months later, she showed Looser's zones in her pubis and an iliac crest biopsy showed evidence of osteomalacia. Hypophosphatemia and raised alkaline phosphatase developed while she was on treatment with aluminum hydroxide. Aluminum hydroxide treatment was then stopped and she was given a neutral phosphate mixture. Thereafter, her plasma phosphate rose and it was possible to stop the phosphate supplementation after three weeks when phosphate levels were within normal limits. Six weeks after stopping aluminum hydroxide, x-rays of the pelvis showed healing of the Looser's zones. Alkaline phosphatase values fell gradually after aluminum hydroxide was discontinued. She subsequently had a successful renal transplant. It is suggested by the authors of this report that because the patient had a poor renal metabolism of vitamin D, she may have been particularly sensitive to the effects of hypophosphatemia induced by the drug intake.

LAXATIVES

Chronic usage of drugs containing inorganic mercury may result in osteomalacia due to phosphate depletion. Lee *et al.* (1972) described a thirty-eight-year-old woman who developed signs of the adult Fanconi syndrome after taking calomel ($Hg_2 Cl_2$) for chronic constipation. Radiological studies of this patient revealed changes of osteomalacia, and this diagnosis was confirmed by bone biopsy. She also had acidosis, hypokalemia, and elevated alkaline phosphatase, and a generalized amino aciduria. Hypocalcemia and glucosuria were present. Hypophosphatemia was found prior to treatment. When the mineral balance of this patient was corrected and the calomel discontinued, the patient recovered. The authors suggest that nutrient transport in general and that of phosphate in particular was defective in this patient as with other patients having the Fanconi syndrome not associated with drug intake. They propose that transport of phosphate across the intestinal and renal epithelium, as well as uptake into bone, is depressed in this condition. Other authors, including Wands *et al.* (1974) have described chronic inorganic mercury poisoning due to high intake of mercury-containing laxatives and have shown that this results in a renal tubular defect, severe diarrhea, and the development of renal failure. While they do not indicate that their patients had evidence of osteomalacia, this could have been present but missed due to the severity of other symptoms. It should be emphasized that there is no possible therapeutic indication for the use of mercury-containing laxatives, but that these drugs may be taken surreptitiously by those who wish to lose weight as well as with those who believe they have a special need to increase bowel function.

DIURETICS

Oral diuretics, such as furosemide, ethacrynic acid and triamterene have been shown to produce significant hypercalciuria (D'Arcy and Griffin 1972). Hanze and Seyberth (1967) showed that when either intravenous furosemide or intravenous ethacrynic acid or oral triamterene are administered to normal subjects, there is an increased clearance of calcium.

Tambyah and Lim (1969) first obtained evidence that oral furosemide decreases the renal tubular reabsorption of calcium.

Effects of furosemide, ethacrynic acid and triamterene on calcium excretion are in contrast to those induced by thiazide drugs. Hypercalcemia which is usually transient, and hypocalciuria occurs in patients receiving chlorthiazide or hydrochlorthiazide (Duarte *et al.* 1971).

Furosemide has been utilized as a temporary measure to control symptoms of hypercalcemia. Suki *et al.* (1970) administered high doses of furosemide intravenously to eight patients with advanced renal disease and secondary hyperparathyroidism whose initial serum calcium values ranged from 12.3–18.4 mg/100 ml. Diuresis occurred and serum calcium levels fell, reaching normal levels in three patients after 25.5 hours of furosemide treatment. Reductions in serum calcium were associated with hyperexcretion of calcium in the urine. Noted by the authors is the fact that the effect of furosemide is predictable because this diuretic exerts its effects maximally in the proximal convoluted tubule and the ascending loop of Henle which are sites of optimal calcium reabsorption

Magnesium deficiency has been found among patients on long-term diuretic therapy for cardiac failure. A group of such patients studied by Lim and Jacob (1972) had been on combined therapy with digoxin, and chlorthiazide, as well as furosemide. Mersalyl had been administered in some cases. The authors considered that these patients' inadequate diets associated with anorexia, as well as the administration of the diuretics, contributed to the magnesium deficiency. Ethacrynic acid has been shown to increase both calcium and magnesium excretion in the urine, the effect being proportional to the degree of natriuresis (Demartini *et al.* 1967). Cardiac glycosides, such as strophanthin and digoxin, augment the renal clearance of divalent cations including magnesium and calcium (Kupfer and Kosovsky 1965).

Increased urinary excretion of zinc has been reported during and immediately following administration of oral diuretics including the thiazides, chlorthalidone and furosemide.

Wester (1975) determined serum zinc levels in 96 healthy subjects (69 men and 27 women) and in 210 patients (95 men and 115 women) treated with diuretics for more than 6 months. Serum zinc levels tended to be higher in patients on diuretics than in the healthy individuals. The author attempts to explain this finding on the basis of the diminished blood volume produced by the diuretics. On the other hand, when the zinc content of liver tissue was determined in autopsy specimens from patients who had received diuretics as against controls, lower tissue levels of zinc were obtained in the diuretic-treated group. While it is possible that the varying causes of death between groups could possibly explain this finding, Wester feels that the differences in the zinc contents of the treated versus untreated were so great that zinc depletion due to diuretics is very likely.

CHELATING AGENTS

Since chelating agents in therapeutic use possess the common property of forming a wide range of stable but soluble metal complexes, it is predictable that they will potentiate the loss of minerals essential to physiological functions as well as combatting metal overload. D-Penicillamine used in heavy metal poisoning, in Wilson's disease, in cystinuria and more recently in rheumatoid arthritis, has been shown to potentiate the excretion of zinc. McCall *et al.* (1967) studied the effects of D-penicillamine on the urinary excretion of copper and zinc in eight patients with either Wilson's disease or cystinuria. The common dose of penicillamine was 250 mg every 8 hours. The absolute increase in excretion of zinc was greater than that of copper in six of the patients studied. Zinc excretion rose with penicillamine dosage even when levels of the drug were administered that produced no further potentiation of copper excretion. Urinary zinc excretion did not reach a maximum until at least three days after the initiation of treatment but remained elevated one week after cessation of drug administration. This was in contrast to copper excretion which peaked after 24 hours and within 24 hours of stopping D-penicillamine urinary copper fell to pretreatment levels. In order to assess the risk of zinc deficiency being induced by penicillamine, the authors carried out zinc balance studies before and during treatment. Increased absorption of zinc from the intestine offset increased urinary losses of zinc, so that a positive zinc balance was obtained in the patients studied. On the basis of these studies and of biochemical investigation of the patients' urine, the authors conclude that the effects of D-penicillamine on zinc metabolism are due to the formation of a zinc-penicillamine chelate.

Although the work of these investigators suggests that the risk of zinc deficiency from therapeutic intake of D-penicillamine is low, more recently there has been suspicion that D-penicillamine may cause symptoms indicative of zinc depletion. In the British trials of D-penicillamine in the treatment of rheumatoid arthritis in which the drug was administered to 105 patients at a dose of 1.5 g/day, two patients developed anorexia combined with loss of taste which could be explained as signs of zinc deficiency (Multicentre Trial Group 1973).

Fell *et al.* (1973) have commented that other chelating agents may cause excessive loss of zinc in the urine including intravenous EDTA and ethambutol (N,N'-diisopropylethylene diamine). The latter drug, intended for long term use as a tuberculostatic agent could induce zinc deficiency though no such side effect has been reported to date.

HYPERVITAMINURIA

An excessive urinary loss of water-soluble vitamins may be the result of several forms of drug-nutrient interaction. Hydrazide drugs, such as INH, form Schiff bases with pyridoxal phosphate, resulting in a hyperexcretion of vitamin B_6. Folate antagonists such as methotrexate can increase the urinary excretion of folate because the vitamin, displaced from its binding to the folate reductase enzyme by the drug, is non-utilizable and therefore eliminated from the body.

One situation under investigation is whether drugs that compete for vitamin-binding sites on plasma proteins can displace the vitamin in the free form so that it can be filtered by the kidney. Another similar situation would exist if a drug removed a vitamin from its plasma-protein binding site, formed a complex with the vitamin, and the complex was then excreted.

When experimental animals such as rats, guinea pigs or chicks are fed boric acid, they exhibit signs of borate toxicity which are minimized by supplementary riboflavin administration. For example, chicks receiving riboflavin in excess of their accepted growth requirements show a decreased incidence of borate toxicity when this chemical is added to their diet. Injection of $2\text{-}^{14}C$-riboflavin results in a significantly greater urinary excretion of labeled riboflavin in boric acid-fed animals than in controls for both rats and guinea pigs. *In vitro* it has been shown that the binding of riboflavin to serum proteins is reduced by borate even when it is present in low concentrations (Roe *et al.* 1972).

Studies are being carried out to find out whether cutaneous or intestinal absorption of boric acid can cause riboflavin depletion in man. It is known that borate is not absorbed through the intact skin, but only when the epidermal barrier is destroyed as in acute dermatitis.

NON-NARCOTIC ANALGESICS

Serum folate levels are known to be low in a high percentage of patients with rheumatoid arthritis. This observation was originally made by Gough *et al.* (1964), and subsequently by Deller *et al.* (1966) and Omer and Mowat (1968). Alter *et al.* (1971) found decreased serum folate levels in 71% of 51 patients with rheumatoid arthritis. They studied 11 of these patients intensively but all showed an abnormally rapid plasma clearance of tritium labeled pteroyl-glutamic acid. *In vitro* binding of tritiated folate was reduced in the sera of the patients with rheumatoid arthritis. All of these patients showing the reduced binding of labeled folate were on aspirin. Those rheumatoid arthritis patients not on aspirin did not show this change. When aspirin was added to normal sera, according to these authors, the binding of folate to the sera or serum proteins was reduced. The mean urinary excretion of orally administered tritiated folate was higher in patients with rheumatoid arthritis on aspirin than in three normal control subjects, but among both groups levels were within the reported normal range. The authors conclude from their studies that aspirin alters the transport of folate by competing for binding sites on serum proteins, but it is unclear whether this really results in hypervitaminuria. Further studies should be carried out to examine this possibility.

Coffey and Wilson (1975) have ascribed tissue depletion of ascorbic acid to numerous drugs and other foreign compounds including anorectic agents, alcohol, anticonvulsant drugs, oral contraceptives and tetracycline. They point out, quoting the work of Loh *et al.* (1971), that aspirin is the drug most likely to produce ascorbic acid tissue depletion in normal individuals. It is inferred that ascorbic acid depletion induced by aspirin could account for gastrointestinal hemorrhage due to malfunctioning of platelets. Caution should be exercised in accepting this premise because it is also known that aspirin can exert anticoagulant activity by a coumarin-like action.

Sahud and Cohen (1971) studied platelet and plasma ascorbic acid levels in 48 normal subjects and in 34 patients with rheumatoid arthritis (RA). Plasma ascorbic acid levels were abnormally low in patients with RA, unless supplementary vitamin C was taken. Low platelet levels of ascorbic acid were only found in RA patients on high doses of aspirin (12 or more tabs/day). In patients with RA, aspirin caused ascorbic acid depletion of tissues. The investigators cite evidence from earlier studies that aspirin blocks the uptake of ascorbic acid into blood platelets *in vitro* (Sahud 1970). Ascorbic acid in platelets reflect tissue stores. Normal platelet levels of ascorbic acid were found in RA patients not on aspirin. Two patients treated with indomethacin had low ascorbic acid levels in platelets. It is suggested that other anti-inflammatory agents may have a distinct effect on ascorbic acid levels in tissues (platelets). The authors advocate ascorbic acid supplements for patients with RA, receiving aspirin or other similar drugs.

Daniels and Everson (1936) many years ago showed that aspirin promotes the urinary excretion of ascorbic acid. They studied children between the ages of 4 and 6 with respect to their ascorbic acid excretion before and during aspirin intake. The dietary source of ascorbic acid was orange juice and intake was controlled. They were able to demonstrate clear cut increases in urinary ascorbic acid following each administration of aspirin.

BIBLIOGRAPHY

ALTER, H. J., ZVAIFLER, M. J., and RATH, C. E. 1971. Interrelationship of rheumatoid arthritis, folic acid and aspirin. Blood *38*, 405-416.
BAKER, L. R. I. *et al.* 1974. Iatrogenic osteomalacia and myopathy due to phosphate depletion. Brit. Med. J. *3*, 150-152.
BLOOM, W. L., and FLINCHUM, D. 1960. Osteomalacia with pseudofractures caused by the ingestion of aluminum hydroxide. J. Am. Med. Assoc. *174*, 1327-1330.
COFFEY, G., and WILSON, C. W. M. 1975. Ascorbic acid deficiency and aspirin-induced haematemesis. Brit. Med. J. *1*, 208.
DANIELS, A. L., and EVERSON, G. J. 1936-37. Influence of acetylsalicylic acid (aspirin) on urinary excretion of ascorbic acid. Proc. Soc. Exp. Biol. Med. *35*, 20-24.
D'ARCY, P. F., and GRIFFIN, J. P. 1972. Iatrogenic Diseases. Oxford Univ. Press, London and New York.
DEMARTINI, F. E., BRISCOE, A. M., and RAGAN, C. 1967. Effect of ethacrynic acid on calcium and magnesium excretion. Proc. Soc. Exp. Biol. Med. *124*, 320-324.
DENT, C. E., and WINTER, C. S. 1974. Osteomalacia due to phosphate depletion from excessive aluminum hydroxide ingestion. Brit. Med. J. *1*, 551-552.
DELLER, D. J. *et al.* 1966. Folic acid deficiency in rheumatoid arthritis. Relation of levels of serum folic acid activities to treatment with phenylbutazone. Brit. Med. J. *1*, 765-767.
DUARTE, G. C. *et al.* 1971. Thiazide-induced hypercalcemia. New Eng. J. Med. *284*, 828-830.
FELL, G. S. *et al.* 1973. Urinary zinc levels as an indication of muscle catabolism. Lancet *1*, 280-282.
GOUGH, K. R. *et al.* 1964. Folic acid deficiency in rheumatoid arthritis. Brit. Med. J. *1*, 212-217.
HANZE, S., and SEYBERTH, H. 1967. Investigation of the mechanism of action of the diuretic furosemide, ethacrynic acid and triamterene on the excretion of magnesium and calcium. Klin. Wschr. *45*, 313-314.
HARVEY, S. C. 1965. Gastric antacids and digestants. *In* The Pharmacological Basis of Therapeutics, 3rd Edition. L. S. Goodman, and A. Gilman (Editors). Macmillan Co., New York.
KUPFER, S., and KOSOVSKY, J. D. 1965. Effects of cardiac glycosides on renal tubular transport of calcium, magnesium, inorganic phosphate and glucose in the dog. J. Clin. Invest. *44*, 1132-1143.
LEE, D. B. N. *et al.* 1972. The adult Fanconi syndrome. Observations on etiology, morphology, renal function and mineral metabolism in three patients. Medicine *51*, 107-138.
LIM, P., and JACOB, E. 1972. Magnesium deficiency in patients on long-term diuretic therapy for heart failure. Brit. Med. J. *3*, 620-622.
LOH, H. S., and WILSON, C. W. M. 1971. Internat. J. Vit. Nutr. Res. *41*, 258; cited in Coffey and Wilson (1975).
LOTZ, M., ZISMAN, E., and BARTTER, F. C. 1968. Evidence for a phosphorus depletion syndrome in man. New Eng. J. Med. *278*, 409-415.

McCALL, J. T. *et al.* 1967. Comparative metabolism of copper and zinc in patients with Wilson's disease (hepatolenticular degeneration). Am. J. Med. Sci. *254*, 13-23.

MULTICENTRE TRIAL GROUP. 1973. Controlled trial of D (-) penicillamine in severe rheumatoid arthritis. Lancet *1*, 275-280.

OMER, A., and MOWAT, A. G. 1968. Nature of anaemia in rheumatoid arthritis. IX. Folate metabolism in patients with rheumatoid arthritis. Ann. Rheum. Dis. *27*, 414-424.

QUIGLEY, J. P., EINSEL, I. H., and MERSCHAN, I. 1939. Some effects produced in the normal stomach by the ingestion of moderate and massive quantities of aluminum hydroxide gel. J. Lab. Clin. Med. *24*, 485-494.

ROE, D. A., McCORMICK, D. B., and LIN, R.-T. 1972. Effects of riboflavin on boric acid toxicity. J. Pharm. Sci. *61*, 1081-1085.

SAHUD, M. A. 1970. Uptake and reduction of dehydroascorbic acid in human platelets. (Abst.) Clin. Res. *18*, 133.

SAHUD, M. A., and COHEN, R. J. 1971. Effect of aspirin ingestion on ascorbic-acid levels in rheumatoid arthritis. Lancet *1*, 937-938.

SUKI, W. N. *et al.* 1970. Acute treatment of hypercalcemia with furosemide. New Eng. J. Med. *283*, 836-840.

TAMBYAH, J. A., and LIM, M. K. L. 1969. Effect of furosemide on calcium excretion. Brit. Med. J. *1*, 751-752.

WANDS, J. R. *et al.* 1974. Chronic inorganic mercury poisoning due to laxative abuse. A clinical and ultrastructural study. Am. J. Med. *57*, 92-101.

WESTER, P. O. 1975. Zinc during diuretic treatment. Lancet *1*, 578.

CHAPTER 7

Antivitamins

In the processes of growth and cell division which occur in living organisms there is continuous chemical activity involving, for the most part, reactions between enzymes and metabolites. The enzymes remain unchanged in these reactions, and the metabolites are transformed into further metabolites. Whereas the enzymes are proteins, the metabolites are smaller molecules which either arise from the degradation of nutrients with or without biosynthesis, or are produced by biosynthetic processes occurring in the cell; i.e., the metabolites may be either exogenous in origin, or endogenous. Metabolites which participate in enzymatic reactions can be antagonized by substances having a chemically or physically similar structure but differing in some detail so that the enzymatic reaction is blocked. Side alteration in the chemical structure of a metabolite can result either in complete loss of its normal biological function, or diminution in such function. In nature, many physiological processes are regulated by pairs of analogous metabolites, as for example, the sex hormones, the porphyrins, and catecholamines. Enzyme systems consist of two parts; a protein component or apoenzyme, together with a coenzyme which is usually a fairly small molecule and often, as previously indicated, the active form of a vitamin. The coenzyme has such functions as transferring an electron from one metabolite to another, and this function can be repeated many times without destruction of the molecule in the process. Metabolite substrates which react with enzymes do so through several steps, the first of which is the formation of an enzyme-substrate complex. This enzyme complex in which the substrate is activated will then dissociate so as to yield the product of the enzymatic reaction. The enzyme is then freed to react again with further substrates.

Synthesis of structural analogs of vitamins began at a time when these nutrients were newly isolated, and it was considered desirable to define their molecular function. The early history of antivitamins is described by Woolley (1952).

Albert (1960) pointed out that metabolite analogs have been synthesized for almost every known vitamin. He makes the statement that "the molecular architecture (of antivitamins or antimetabolites) must be so similar to that of the substrate that the enzyme is deceived into taking up the foreign molecule in place of the substrate." In order to function as an antivitamin, a synthetic analog must be incapable of functioning as the natural substrate.

Baker (1959; 1962) has described two classes of compounds which function as antimetabolites or antivitamins. The first of these are considered as classical antimetabolites, and these are structurally similar to the metabolites which they block. There are also nonclassical antimetabolites or antivitamins, which are structurally different from the natural metabolites, but bear certain chemical groupings which bind to the active sites on the appropriate enzyme.

Whereas an antivitamin can interfere with normal metabolism by reacting with one or several components of a single biological system, it can also perform as a metabolic antagonist by impairing or arresting enzymatic function wherever the natural vitamin functions as a coenzyme. For a clear description of the chemistry of antivitamins and antimetabolites the reader is referred to the publication of Kaiser (1960).

Synthesis of antivitamins has either been purposeful or by chance, the latter occurring frequently in the history of modern pharmacology. Many early studies of the effects of drugs on nutrients and nutrient utilization were concerned with purposeful attempts to inhibit growth of pathogenic microorganisms by interfering with their nutrient requirements. Many antimicrobial drugs are antivitamins but their success therapeutically derives from the fact that the nutrition of bacteria or other microorganisms can be inhibited without affecting the nutrition of the host adversely. Cytotoxic agents which function as antivitamins have been used in experimental animals and in man for the control of neoplastic processes.

While pharmacologic agents which function as antivitamins have sometimes, as in the case of anticoagulants, been found accidentally, their continued use relates to their antagonistic effect on normal vitamin function. A wide range of drugs functioning therapeutically other than as antivitamins have been shown to exert vitamin antagonism either through classical or non-classical function on enzyme systems.

Drugs which inhibit vitamin metabolism in the animal body or in man are capable of inducing both acute toxic effects related to their nutrient antagonism, and also chronic toxic effects resulting from nutrient depletion because of non-utilization. Whether or not such adverse reactions occur depends not only on the chemical and pharmacological properties of the vitamin antagonist, but also on the dose, duration of administration, route of administration and perhaps more importantly, on the strength of binding of the vitamin antagonist to the enzyme complex. Since our further discussion of the acute and chronic nutritional effects of antivitamins will be mainly limited to those observed in human subjects, the reader is advised to consult other publications for those effects which have been seen and described in experimental and domestic animals (Broquist and Jukes 1968).

FOLIC ACID ANTAGONISTS

The synthesis of potent folic acid antagonists dates from the time when the role of the active form of folic acid in nucleic acid metabolism was first conceived. Interest in these compounds emanated from the belief that they might inhibit the growth of microorganisms as well as cell division in neoplastic tissues (Delmonte and Jukes 1962). A number of folic acid antagonists have been shown to inhibit the growth of bacteria and protozoa, and further, it has been known since 1948 that they can control the leukemic process to some extent. In that year, Ferber and his colleagues showed that remissions of acute leukemia in children could be brought about by administration of 4-aminopteroylglutamic acid, also known as aminopterin (Ferber *et al.* 1948). Two years later Nichols and Welch (1950) showed the mode of action of aminopterin. They demonstrated that, when this drug was injected into rats or added to *in vitro* liver preparations, it prevented the conversion of folic acid to reduced cofactor forms. It was shown by Broquist *et al.* (1951) that tetrahydrofolic acid could obviate the effects of aminopterin in mice, and these workers thought that the effect of the drug was to prevent the reduction of folic acid.

Subsequent work has pinpointed the site of action of folic acid antagonists. It has been shown that folic acid analogs are bound to a greater or lesser extent to the folic acid reductase enzyme, and that the degree of binding is related to the potency of the compound as a folate antagonist. Further, it has been shown that aminopterin and amethopterin (methotrexate) are very potent inhibitors of folate reductase both *in vivo* and *in vitro* (Werkheiser 1963).

Mice, given folic acid prior to treatment with aminopterin, are protected from the lethal effects of the drugs. After the drug has been given, folic acid no longer protects these animals, showing that the activity of folic acid requires the functioning of the folate reductase enzyme and that toxicity is related to its inhibition (Werkheiser 1961).

Gamble *et al.* (1960) stated that the analogs of folic acid which exhibit antifolic activity, while resembling the parent molecule in certain respects, have specific replacements in the molecule as follows: 1) the replacement of the 4-hydroxyl group in the pteridine ring by an amino group; 2) substitution of the 9- or 10-position; or 3) modification of the glutamic acid portion of the molecule or its replacement by other amino acids.

The most potent folic acid inhibitors used in clinical practice are methotrexate (4-amino-4-dioxy-10-methyl-folic acid, amethopterin) and the 2,4-diaminopyrimidines such as pyrimethamine (Franklin et al. 1949; Hitchings et al. 1954). Marked differences exist between bacterial and mammalian folate reductases with respect to their inhibition by folate-folic acid analogs (Burchall and Hitchings 1965). The structures of folic acid antagonists in comparison with that of folic acid are shown in Chapter 1, Fig. 1.9.

In the present context, we are interested in the toxicity of folate antagonists in relation to their clinical usage, and more particularly, we are concerned with the question as to whether these drugs can induce folate deficiency with long-term administration. The acute and chronic toxicity of folate antagonists is related to their capacity for preventing deoxyribonucleic acid (DNA) synthesis and rendering folic acid useless as a vitamin required for normal cell integrity and division, as well as maturation of blood cells. Under the effects of folate antagonists, tissues become deficient in tetrahydrofolic acid which is similar to the situation in nutritional folate deficiency, except that it may not be reversible by administration of folic acid. Depression in DNA synthesis and inhibition of cell division in microbial or mammalian cell systems brought about by folate antagonists can be explained. In the synthesis of DNA, deoxyuridylic acid (dUMP) is methylated to form thymidylic acid (dTMP) which is an essential component of DNA. Methylation is brought about by donation of a methyl group by the coenzyme N^5,N^{10}-methylene tetrahydrofolic acid, which is derived from tetrahydrofolic acid. Thus, impaired synthesis of tetrahydrofolic acid is directly related to the reduction in DNA biosynthesis. (See Chapter 1, Figure 1.8).

Folinic acid (citrovorum factor) can overcome the effects of folate antagonists because it can be transformed to N^5,N^{10}-methylene tetrahydrofolic acid (Connors 1970). The potency of known or suspected folic acid antagonists has been studied in human cells through their several effects; that is, by their inhibitory effect on tetrahydrofolic acid formation, their inhibition of dihydrofolate reductase, or by their interference with de novo synthesis of DNA-thymine from deoxyuridine using human bone marrow cultures (Waxman et al. 1969; Waxman et al. 1970). On the assumption that human cells are used for these in vitro studies, the potency of folate antagonists can be related to their toxicity in this manner, and also to their net effects on folate metabolism.

METHOTREXATE

Methotrexate (MTX) has been used in the treatment of malignant and benign diseases. It has been used in the treatment of leukemia, choriocarcinoma, advanced carcinoma, as a treatment or palliative, and very frequently in the treatment of psoriasis which has been resistant to other forms of therapy. It has also been occasionally used in the treatment of other cutaneous diseases such as pityriasis rubra pilaris. The toxicity of the drug and the special risk factors can better be evaluated from investigations and surveys of patients with psoriasis than they can from studies of patients with neoplastic disease whose health may already have been severely compromised. Gubner et al. (1951) observed that, when treating patients with rheumatoid arthritis using aminopterin, there was a marked remission of psoriasis in one subject. Following this, remissions of psoriasis were obtained in 13 patients, seven of whom also had arthritis. The dosages of aminopterin given to these patients were varied from 1.5 to 2.0 mg daily, the total dose varying from 14 to 140 mg in 10 days to 9 months. All of the patients developed toxic effects while the psoriasis was getting better. These toxic effects included ulceration of the mouth, diarrhea, abdominal pain, partial and temporary alopecia, erosions of the skin, especially about the genitalia, and delayed wound healing (Gubner 1951).

When Rees et al. (1955) used aminopterin to treat their patients with psoriasis, they decreased the dose used in earlier therapeutic trials, so that it did not exceed 6 mg for a single course of treatment, and they gave the drug over a period varying from 12–20 days (0.5 mg daily). They reported clearing of lesions in 80% of cases and toxicity in 8%, but they also stated that there were no delayed ill effects in six months after repeated courses of the drug.

The original 171 patients with psoriasis treated by Rees et al. (1955) were followed up and the data were analyzed on 158 additional patients, bringing the total to 329. It was again found that over 80% showed improvement or clearing of skin lesions lasting from a week up to several years, but toxic effects were found in about 20% of cases.

Edmonson and Guy (1958) first used methotrexate for the treatment of psoriasis, and compared their results with those using aminopterin. They either gave a tablet of aminopterin (0.5 mg) or of methotrexate (2.5 mg) daily for six days followed by a rest period of three days, and then a tablet daily for six days for a total of twelve doses. This course of treatment was repeated only after a rest of three months or more. They reported good results in 75% of 24 patients treated with aminopterin, and 13 treated with methotrexate. They said that toxic effects were uncommon.

Rees and Bennett (1961) again compared the effectiveness of aminopterin and methotrexate in psoriasis studying 37 patients. Two-thirds of the patients taking methotrexate had great improvement, and four-fifths of the patients taking aminopterin obtained similar benefits. However, the rate of toxicity was twice as high with aminopterin, even though they did not encounter severe reactions. Other workers, comparing the toxicity of these two drugs, have noted that aminopterin was far more toxic, side effects including aphthous lesions in the mouth, gastrointestinal cramps and leukopenia (Dobes 1963; Strakosch 1963). The inclusion of corticosteroids in the treatment schedule used by some of these workers may have contributed to the unfavorable reactions.

Rees et al. (1964) reported on their experiments with aminopterin and methotrexate, and they discussed in some detail the problems of using aminopterin in this disease, mentioning the lack of purity of the drug, its instability, its severe effects on bone marrow and on the gastrointestinal tract. They also note the development of anemia, granulocytopenia and thrombocytopenia.

Fry and McMinn (1966) studied the histological changes in the skin and intestinal mucosa as well as the clinical response to methotrexate in 12 subjects with psoriasis. The drug was administered intramuscularly in a dose of 0.5 mg/kg weekly. Skin biopsy specimens were obtained before treatment and after 3, 24 and 48 hours as well as 3 and 7 days post-treatment. Intestinal biopsy specimens were obtained before treatment and after 24 hours and 3 and 7 days. Mitotic counting was performed on skin sections and also on the crypt epithelium in the material from the small intestine. Patients responding to treatment showed a decrease in mitotic activity in the psoriatic epidermis and also a decrease in the mitotic activity within the intestinal epithelium. The fall in intestinal mitosis was marked at 24 hours, and this was followed by a trend toward normality, evident at 3 days, and complete at 7 days post-treatment. The authors believed that these results supported the hypothesis that the effect of methotrexate in psoriasis was a direct one to curb the excessive cellular activity and reproduction within the epidermis.

Acute toxicity from methotrexate is due to impaired DNA synthesis and non-utilization of folate. Diminution in cell replication during treatment with this drug affects all actively growing cells whether these are malignant, abnormal, or normal. This toxicity usually starts with loss of appetite, abdominal pain and nausea, and these symptoms are followed by ulceration in the mouth and pharynx. When diarrhea is present, this is considered to be a serious sign, sometimes associated with a fatal outcome unless the drug is discontinued at this stage. Leukopenia is frequently present with loss of neutrophils.

Transient alopecia and a characteristic dermatosis may be present (Chanarin 1969).

Baker (1970) discussed the morbidity and mortality associated with methotrexate therapy in psoriasis. He was able to find records of 18 deaths among patients with psoriasis which could be attributed to folate antagonists. In analyzing these case histories he attributed the deaths to the following causes: absolute overdosage (one case), relative overdosage (seven cases), absolute plus relative overdosage (four cases), and other causes (six cases). This author suggests that when patients receiving methotrexate have succumbed to doses of the drug which would not be fatal in other patients, they may have prior systemic disease including bone marrow hypoplasia, renal or hepatic dysfunction, an infection, or they may be receiving such drugs as aspirin which reduces the renal excretion and protein binding of the drug.

Methotrexate is readily absorbed from the intestine and quickly bound to the dihydrofolate reductase enzyme. It displaces folate from the enzyme and this is followed by an increased excretion of folate in the urine (Swenseid et al. 1952). Methotrexate does not inhibit folic acid absorption in man, and the increased urinary excretion of the vitamin has been attributed to its displacement from binding sites on the reductase molecule, and hence non-utilization as well as to renal changes brought about by the drug (Hoffbrand and Fry 1972).

In cases of acute methotrexate overdosage, the antidote is folinic acid since folic acid cannot be utilized, and the antidote has to be given within 4 hours of massive intake of the drug. Severe, acute toxicity with methotrexate has been encountered among women being treated for choriocarcinoma with high dosage parenteral treatment with this therapeutic agent. In order to reduce toxicity in these cases intermittent intramuscular injections of folinic acid have been given at a dose of 6-9 mg every 4-6 hours. The relief of toxicity has only been of temporary nature (Sullivan et al. 1959).

Harriman et al. (1964) investigated the relationship between serum folate levels and methotrexate toxicity in 18 patients with advanced carcinomata of the head and neck who were undergoing treatment with this drug. Low levels of folate in the serum before treatment appeared to predispose these patients to the toxic effect of the drug, though the folate levels were not related with the beneficial response to treatment. The authors comment that debilitated patients with cancer of the head and neck may have difficulty in swallowing, and therefore a folate deficiency on a nutritional basis. They particularly noted a correlation between the initial level of serum folate and the extent of bone marrow toxicity. After therapy with methotrexate, patients were found to have low levels of serum folate as determined by microbiological assay.

Moderate to severe encephalopathy has been encountered among patients with acute leukemia who have received intrathecal methotrexate therapy (Weiss *et al*. 1974).

Kay *et al*. (1972) believe that encephalopathy may be due to drug-induced folic acid deficiency. They have found that neurological disturbances were arrested when children treated with intrathecal methotrexate received systemic, folinic and folic acid. Whether or not intracerebral folate deficiency can account for methotrexate encephalopathy has not yet been confirmed.

Since in the treatment of psoriasis courses of methotrexate may be given over a period of many years, and since the intervals between treatments may be short, we are particularly concerned with the problems of chronic toxicity. In the literature there are very few recorded cases of folic acid deficiency associated with megaloblastic anemia which can be attributed to methotrexate. Ryan *et al*. (1964) reported a patient who developed a megaloblastic bone marrow during such treatment but the patient had no evidence of anemia, and treatment was continued without undue ill effects.

Borrie and Clark (1966) described a deaf and dumb man with psoriasis who received multiple courses of methotrexate at a level of 2.5 mg/day on alternate weeks for a period of one year and five months. During the course of treatment he had a tendency to develop stomatitis and balanitis, though apparently these side effects lessened as treatment continued. He had had a severe psoriasis which cleared with treatment. Two weeks after cessation of treatment the patient was seen when he complained of loss of appetite, tiredness, breathlessness on exertion, and edema of the ankles. He was found to have a severe megaloblastic anemia. Treatment was with folinic acid, 10 mg intramuscularly daily for ten days, and he made a complete recovery. Subsequent methotrexate therapy was given to this patient, and he showed a tendency towards macrocytosis, but the severe megaloblastic anemia did not recur. It is suggested by the authors that the drug has a cumulative effect. However, in this particular case, it is possible that an inadequate diet with respect to folic acid may have contributed to the outcome.

In the author's experience, macrocytosis is rather common in patients who have received repeated courses of methotrexate. A male patient, aged thirty-nine, who had had psoriasis for 18 years, was seen by the author, first in 1972. Before that time he had received methotrexate over a period of six years; that is, between 1966 and

1972, at a dose of 5 mg at 12 hour intervals for three doses each week. In February 1972 he developed megaloblastic anemia and also steatorrhea. The anemia was so severe that blood transfusions were required. The author saw this patient first in August 1972, at which time there was still a moderate megaloblastic anemia with changes in the polymorphonuclear neutrophils, characteristic of folate deficiency. The residual anemia and steatorrhea were successfully treated by oral administration of folic acid (5 mg three times daily for six weeks).

Anderson *et al.* (1966) described another case of megaloblastic anemia occurring following intensive methotrexate therapy. In this case the patient had cancer of the lung, and was treated with intravenous administration of 5-fluorouracil to a dose of 32,600 mg during 241 days, and methotrexate 90 mg during 55 days consecutively. It is questionable whether this case was actually one of folic acid deficiency, because, although a megaloblastic anemia was present, serum folate determination gave a value of 8 ng/ml and Schilling tests suggested a possible vitamin B_{12} deficiency. The authors suggest that the megaloblastic anemia was related to the administration of the antimetabolites and that the incomplete hemoglobin response to vitamin B_{12} suggests a toxic suppression of normal erythropoiesis. The low incidence of megaloblastic anemia following methotrexate therapy is remarkable. It is suspected by the author that such megaloblastic anemia exists, but has not been established by hematologic examinations. Development of radioassay methods for the determination of folate in serum, erythrocytes and tissues such as liver biopsies should facilitate the evaluation of the folate status of patients who have received methotrexate in whom microbiological assay of folate may give erroneous results. Among patients with benign diseases such as psoriasis, who may be given repeated courses of methotrexate, it is suggested that folate depletion should be a contraindication to further therapy using this drug.

Since Colsky *et al.* (1955) first reported hepatic fibrosis in children with acute leukemia receiving folic acid antagonists, there have been many published accounts of chronic hepatic disease following methotrexate therapy.

Hatler *et al.* (1960) analyzed clinical and autopsy records of 273 children with leukemia who were treated before and after chemotherapy was introduced. They found that there was a much higher incidence of hepatic fibrosis in children who received chemotherapy. In children and adult patients with leukemia, the incidence of hepatic fibrosis has been explained on the basis of such postulates as the idea that the drug might cause a replacement of leukemic infiltrates with fibrous connective tissue; that there might be a coincidental serum hepatitis; or that the drug might interfere with liver cell metabolism.

Since these reports appeared, hepatotoxicity has been recognized as a long-term side effect of methotrexate whether the drug is given for the treatment of malignant or benign disease. The incidence of hepatic fibrosis in patients who have received methotrexate varies in different reports, but it has been rather well recognized that such toxicity is dose-dependent. Though no close correlation exists between the total dosage of methotrexate and the severity of liver damage, there is strong support for the belief that if methotrexate is given too frequently, hepatotoxicity may supervene.

Dahl *et al.* (1972) studied 44 patients with post-methotrexate hepatic disease. Seventeen of these had received therapy by frequent small dosage technique, and two had received an intermittent larger dosage of the drug, the total milligrams of drug per month being the same in both groups. These workers caution others against using frequent small doses of methotrexate but they also believe that hepatic fibrosis may be inevitable if dosage is prolonged.

A variety of liver changes have been found in psoriatic patients who have received methotrexate, including fatty infiltration, toxic hepatitis, fibrosis and cirrhosis. Roenigk *et al.* (1971) have commented that there is no specific histological appearance characteristic of the liver in patients who have received this drug. They have made the suggestion that these patients have a nutritional cirrhosis, not related to methotrexate. This concept is difficult to accept in view of the earlier cases of leukemia who also showed methotrexate hepatotoxicity.

Several writers and editors have emphasized that patients whose alcohol intake has been excessive are predisposed to hepatic damage from methotrexate. Prior hepatic damage from other drugs, as well as the presence of diabetes mellitus and/or obesity, have also been mentioned as the predisposing factors to further liver damage from the drug (Zachariae and Schiødt 1971; Yearbook of Dermatology 1972; Yearbook of Dermatology 1973). Our concern is whether liver damage associated with methotrexate treatment is due in some manner to an interference with folate metabolism or, in other words, is due to a secondary folate deficiency. Methotrexate is concentrated in the liver where, in some species, it undergoes enzymatic oxidation. In man, liver metabolism of methotrexate is minimal, which may account for its chronic toxicity (Johns and Valerino 1971).

It has been suggested that when methotrexate is given repetitively over long periods without adequate rest periods, the drug gradually accumulates in the liver over time, until the dihydrofolate reductase reserves are saturated. This would prevent the formation of tetrahydrofolic acid needed for such reactions as the synthesis of purines, thymine and DNA. Coe and Bull (1968), who made this suggestion, have also postulated that this course of events may alter liver cell function to a point when cell death supervenes and is followed by stromal collapse and finally cirrhosis. However, there has been no experimental proof for these theories.

The teratogenic effects of methotrexate have been established in man as well as in experimental animals. This will be discussed in the section devoted to prenatal malnutrition produced by pharmacologic agents.

PYRIMETHAMINE

The chief uses of pyrimethamine are in the treatment of chloroquine-resistant malaria and ocular toxoplasmosis. In patients under treatment with pyrimethamine for these diseases, hematologic side effects have been observed which are due to folate deficiency (Hamilton *et al.* 1954; Tenpas and Abraham 1965).

Indeed, the concept that drugs might exert a selective antifolate effect was used in the development of pyrimethamine. It was reported in 1941 by Falco and his colleagues that 2,4-diaminopyrimidines were highly effective as folate antagonists in lactobacillus casei. This finding led to the evaluation of 2,4-diaminopyrimidines as antimalarials and marked activity was demonstrated (Falco *et al.* 1949). This drug is bound to the dihydrofolate reductase enzyme, thereby displacing folate and preventing its utilization. This binding of the drug to the dihydrofolate reductase is not selective for the enzyme within the malarial parasite, but also affects the enzyme in higher animal species including man. Thus pyrimethamine can be classified as a folate antagonist and can result in the development of folate deficiency with megaloblastic anemia in human subjects (Hamilton *et al.* 1952). Chanarin (1969), referring to the work of Myatt (1953), has commented that when pyrimethamine is used in malaria prophylaxis at a dose of 25 mg weekly, it is unlikely to produce folate deficiency except in those who are already folate deficient. Higher doses of pyrimethamine are likely to cause megaloblastic anemia and when the dose exceeds 25 mg daily, such an anemia becomes almost uniform in all treated patients. However, large doses of the drug are more commonly used in the treatment of toxoplasmosis or in the treatment of polycythemia rubra vera than in malaria (Perkins *et al.* 1956; Kaufman *et al.* 1960; Chanarin 1964). Akinyanju *et al.* (1973) reported a case of a 4-$^1/_2$-year-old girl who was given 25 mg pyrimethamine twice weekly over a period of six months as malaria prophylaxis. She developed severe megaloblastic anemia which was successfully treated by withdrawal of the drug and administration of folic acid orally at a dose of 10 mg daily. In severe megaloblastic anemia caused by pyrimethamine, the preferred treatment would be by administration of folinic acid which could be utilized when the metabolism of folic acid is blocked by the inhibition of the folate reductase enzyme.

Tong *et al.* (1970) carried out a study of the effects of folic acid and folinic acid as suppressants of the hematologic effects of pyrimethamine in military patients who were under antimalarial treatment in Viet Nam. All of these patients received chloroquine phosphate, pyrimethamine at a dose of 25 mg/8 hr for nine doses, and sulfisoxazole. Seventy-five patients receiving this combined antimalarial therapy were divided into three groups with 25 men in each group. One group received oral doses of 5 mg folic acid per day; the second group received 5 mg folinic acid per day, and the other men received a placebo. The study was carried out in a double-blind fashion for 12 days, commencing on the first day of antimalarial therapy. Those patients who were given either folic or folinic acid had a lower incidence of anemia than the control subjects. Neither the folic acid administration nor the administration of folinic acid had any deleterious effect on the clearing of the malarial parasites from the blood. The authors suggested that preformed folates were not utilized by the parasite. Unfortunately, no determinations were made in this study either of serum or of erythrocyte folate levels, nor were marrow biopsies studied. Since the antifolate effect of pyrimethamine has been fully corrected with folinic acid and partially with folic acid in human bone marrow culture systems (Waxman and Herbert 1969), it has been recommended that either folic or folinic acid should be given to patients when pyrimethamine is used in the doses commonly employed for the treatment of plasmodium falciparum malaria.

Waxman and Herbert (1969) studied a forty-five-year-old negro woman who received pyrimethamine as treatment for diffuse bilateral chorioretinitis. She had a positive tuberculin reaction and was therefore treated with anti-tuberculous drugs. Her chorioretinitis progressed in spite of eight months treatment with isonicotinic acid hydrazide (INH), para-aminosalicylic acid (PAS) and prednisone. She was then given pyrimethamine (Daraprim), 25 mg/day, sulfisoxazole (Gantrisin), 2 gm/day, and prednisone, 40 mg every-other day. Six weeks later, while she was still receiving these drugs, she showed mild hematologic changes including slight leukopenia, hypersegmentation of neutrophils, occasional nucleated circulating red blood cells, and a megaloblastic bone marrow picture. Reversal of these changes followed discontinuation of drug therapy. The mechanism of action of pyrimethamine was studied using samples of this patient's bone marrow which were prepared for short-term *in vitro* culture to evaluate effective DNA synthesis from deoxyuridine. Defective deoxyuridine suppression of thymidine-^{3}H-methyl(^{3}HTdR) into DNA was found in the pyrimethamine-induced megaloblastic bone marrow in this case, but was absent from the recovered marrow. Further, this DNA lesion could be reproduced by the *in vitro* addition of pyrimethamine to the patient's recovered marrow. The deranged DNA synthesis in the bone marrow was corrected completely by addition of folinic acid but only partially corrected by folic acid. The lower ability of pyrimethamine-treated patients to utilize folic acid is taken to indicate defective folate reduction which is due to the block of dihydrofolate reductase.

PENTAMIDINE

Pentamidine isethionate has been used for about 30 years as a preventive drug and treatment for African trypanosomiasis. It has also been used in the therapy of leishmaniasis. Ivady and Paldy (1958) first used pentamidine in the treatment of infants with *Pneumocystis carinii* pneumonia. Later, Robbins *et al.* (1965) described a case of pneumocystis pneumonitis in an eight-year-old girl with congenital hypogammaglobulinemia in whom the disease was successfully treated with pentamidine. Bone marrow smears obtained before therapy and on the 7th, 11th and 14th days of therapy showed the gradual development of erythroid hypoplasia with marked megaloblastic changes. In the peripheral blood there were occasional hypersegmented neutrophils and macro-ovalocytes. The authors found serum folate levels of less than 1 ng/ml. However, we are not told at what stage of therapy the serum folate determinations were made, nor whether the authors studied the problem of whether the microbiological assay of folate was impaired by the presence of the drug in the circulation. Pentamidine was discontinued after the hematologic changes were detected.

In a survey of 164 patients who had received pentamidine for suspected or proven pneumocystis pneumonia, Weston *et al.* (1970) described the occurrence of depressed serum folate levels in two patients who did not show megaloblastic changes in the peripheral blood.

TRIAMTERENE

Triamterene, a drug which has structural similarities to folic acid, has been extensively used as a diuretic. Lieberman and Bateman

(1968) reported on patients with alcoholic cirrhosis who developed megaloblastic anemia while taking this drug, and they believed that there could be a causal relationship. Megaloblastosis developing in patients receiving this drug has been believed to be due to inhibition of the dihydrofolate reductase enzyme, and this has been proven *in vitro* as well as *in vivo*.

Corcino *et al.* (1970) described a thirty-five-year-old alcoholic woman with cirrhosis of the liver who developed megaloblastosis after receiving triamterene for two weeks. Short-term human bone marrow cultures showed that triamterene interfered with the *de novo* DNA-thymine synthesis from dU and that this interference was completely corrected by folinic acid, but only partially by folic acid. The authors make the important comment that this drug should be used with great caution in patients who may have depleted folate stores, such as alcoholics and pregnant women.

A male patient, aged seventy-two, who was under treatment with triamterene was found by the author to have developed megaloblastic anemia after he had received the drug over a two-year period. This anemia was successfully treated with folic acid in the dose of 5 mg three times a day, and the anemia has not recurred, although the drug has been continued. When folate supplements are discontinued in this patient, macrocytosis rapidly supervenes (Roe, D. A., unpublished).

TRIMETHOPRIM

This drug is being extensively used as a potentiator of sulfonomides in the therapy of bacterial infection. In chronic toxicity tests in animals, the drug has been shown to cause depression and maturation defects of hemopoiesis as indicated by falls in the concentration of hemoglobin, the number of erythrocytes, neutrophils, lymphocytes, and platelets. These effects have been noted in dogs and monkeys receiving high dose intake. In combination with sulfonamides, its chemotherapeutic effectiveness includes that against such organisms as Proteus, Bordetella, Hemophilus, and Neisseria. It is believed that its primary site of action is by inhibition of bacterial dihydrofolate reductases. It acts as an inhibitor of folate utilization, and the sulfonamides which are given concomitantly inhibit the biosynthesis of folic acid in the target organism (Bushby and Hitchings 1968).

There has been some dispute as to whether this drug offers a risk with respect to induction of folate deficiency in human subjects. According to Kahn *et al.* (1968), minimal folate deficiency may appear in human subjects after long term, high dosage of trimethoprim, and this folate deficiency may be reversed by administration of folinic acid.

Girdwood *et al.* (1973) studied 28 patients who were undergoing long term treatment with trimethoprim for chest infections. They were given 160 mg trimethoprim and 800 mg sulphamethoxazole twice daily, as well as ampicillin in a dose of 500 mg twice daily. Long term results were obtained for 17 patients who received this drug combination for six months, and 11 who received it for a year. No depression of serum or erythrocyte folate levels were found, nor were the platelet counts depressed. There was no significant fall in hemoglobin, white cell or vitamin B_{12} levels. Six other patients were described who were supposed to have developed megaloblastic anemia following treatment over a short period of trimethoprim. In four of these, the real diagnoses were found to be pernicious anemia, regional enteritis, gluten-sensitive enteropathy, and a complex form of anemia of 11-years duration that finally responded to a splenectomy.

Of the other two patients, one had had various drugs, some of which are supposed to cause megaloblastic anemia, and a three months course of trimethoprim given later did not cause folate depletion. For the other patient it is suggested that folate deficiency arose from chronic illness, and it is described that a later course of trimethoprim did not cause any anemia. These authors do not believe that there is a high risk of folate deficiency from trimethoprim, but they do emphasize that if a patient is already folate-depleted, the risk of this drug might be increased with respect to its effects in causing folate deficiency.

ANTIMETABOLITES CAUSING MACROCYTOSIS

A number of drugs other than folate antagonists have been shown capable of producing macrocytosis. Increase in erythrocyte size has been described in patients on cytosine arabinoside, 6-azouridine triacetate (Azaribine), cyclophosphamide (Cytoxan), and azathioprin (Imuran). 6-Mercaptopurine has also been shown to cause megaloblastosis (Talley and Vaitkevicius 1963; Klippel and Decker 1974; Bethell and Thompson 1954).

It has been suggested by Vilter *et al.* (1950) that DNA deficiency might be responsible for megaloblastosis. As pointed out by Talley and Vaitkevicius (1963), these drugs which produce macrocytosis increase the intermitotic phase of cell growth and inhibit cell division. Thus the cell is permitted to increase in size at the expense of cell division. Cells other than erythrocytes may be involved in the macrocytic phenomenon.

VITAMIN B₆ ANTAGONISTS

Vitamin B_6 antagonists such as deoxypyridoxine have been synthesized in order to study the functions of this vitamin and also in an attempt to produce agents which could inhibit growth of neoplasms. In addition, a number of drugs of differing chemical structure and pharmacologic action have been found to produce antagonism to vitamin B_6 during their clinical usage. Rosen *et al.* (1964) have summarized the types of compounds which interfere with vitamin B_6 metabolism as follows: 1) structural analogs of pyridoxine which are substrates for pyridoxal kinase. This group would include 4-deoxypyridoxine; 2) compounds that inhibit pyridoxal kinase, preventing the formation of the cofactor; 3) analogs of pyridoxal phosphate which can compete with the cofactor; and 4) compounds that combine with pyridoxal phosphate such as isonicotinic acid, hydralazine, other hydrazides, and penicillamine. This group now includes L-dopa (Rosen *et al.* 1964). (See Chapter 1, Fig. 1.5).

Syndromes of vitamin B_6 deficiency induced by decreased intake of the vitamin or by administration of the various pyridoxine antagonists differ from one another with respect to biochemical and clinical effects. Braunstein (1964) pointed out that all enzymatic functions conditional upon the presence of pyridoxine do not decrease at equal rates as a result of vitamin B_6 depletion induced by diet or one or another of these drugs. The evolution of the syndromes of vitamin B_6 deficiency is as yet not always predictable because specific differences in the linkage of the coenzymes to the various apoenzymes, the location and role of functional groups of the apoenzymes involved in the promotion of different reactions between coenzyme and substrate, remains to be elucidated in relation to vitamin B_6.

The succession of effects of drugs on vitamin B_6 metabolism differ according to the precise site or sites of action of the particular drug, but in general, states of vitamin B_6 depletion are produced which follow roughly those found in experimental pyridoxine deficiency. Wiss and Weber (1964) have pointed out that various pyridoxal phosphate enzymes are affected to a different extent by vitamin B_6 depletion. Early effects tend to be on the degradation pathway of tryptophan and sulfur-containing amino acids, followed by effects on B_6-dependent pathways in the brain, and lastly, effects on the B_6-dependent locus in heme synthesis. Transaminases are more resistant to vitamin B_6 depletion, and it has been observed in connection with the latter that nitrogen balance is only disturbed with severe vitamin B_6 deficiency.

Drugs which have been proven to produce vitamin B_6 deficiency in man include hydrazide drugs such as INH and hydralazine, cycloserine, pyrazinamide, ethionamide, thiosemicarbizones, penicillamine, and L-dopa. Hydrazide drugs such as thiosemicarbizide and INH, as well as other hydrazides, form hydrazone complexes with pyridoxal phosphate, and in this way inactivate the coenzyme. The reduction of pyridoxal phosphate availability by formation of hydrazone derivatives with INH has been described by Braunstein (1960).

After the initial recognition that INH and other hydrazides form hydrazones with vitamin B_6, it was postulated that vitamin B_6 depletion resulted from hyperexcretion of the INH-B_6 complex in the urine. Biehl and Vilter (1954) demonstrated that there was an increased vitamin B_6 excretion in the urine of patients receiving INH, this effect being dose dependent.

Levy (1969) carried out a metabolic study of human volunteers with respect to their vitamin B_6 metabolism during administration of INH. His subjects consisted in two slow and one rapid inactivator of isoniazid. An increased urinary excretion of microbiologically-active forms of vitamin B_6 was demonstrated in these three subjects, but changes in vitamin B_6 balance were not uniform. Prior to INH administration a positive B_6 balance was found in all three subjects, but during the period of drug administration this balance became rather less positive in one of the slow inactivators and increased slightly in the other two subjects. This author did not think that his findings indicated that the loss of vitamin B_6 from the body during INH administration at high dosage was sufficient to support the theory that the drug produces vitamin B_6 deficiency through hyperexcretion of the drug vitamin complex.

In order to gain insight into the range of toxic effects associated with drug or diet induced pyridoxine deficiency, it is necessary to examine the facts relating to interaction between pyridoxal phosphate or derivatives of pyridoxine and the various apoenzymes. Each apoenzyme which is vitamin B_6-dependent has multipoint attachments to the coenzyme. Interactions between coenzyme and apoenzyme vary from one enzyme to another in the extent of conformational change induced by the interaction, in the structure of segments of the coenzyme binding site, in the type of optical activity induced in the coenzymes by binding to the apoenzyme, and in the effectiveness of pyridoxal phosphate analogs or drugs as substitutes for the natural coenzyme. Conformational changes in the apoenzyme protein are prerequisites for normal activity. Pyridoxal phosphate participates in controlling the structure of the holoenzyme molecule by maintaining the apoenzyme in the conformation required for activity. Some vitamin B_6-dependent enzymes can function in the presence of minimal amounts of the vitamin, or perhaps independently of the vitamin, whereas in the case of other enzymes, activity is markedly stimulated by the presence of the vitamin in its coenzyme form. Enzymes of the cell sap are far more sensitive to pyridoxine deficiency whether produced by diet or drugs than are those associated with particulate fractions of the cell such as the mitochondria (Chatagner 1970).

Most of the drugs with which we will be concerned as vitamin B_6 antagonists are weak in the sense that whenever there is sufficient pyridoxal phosphate present, their adverse effects are not observable. Many enzymes have been shown to be protected by pyridoxal phosphate against inactivation. However, an absolute pyridoxine deficiency or an inhibition of enzymes concerned in the metabolism of pyridoxine and its derivatives leads to a spectrum of effects which not only vary with the severity and rate of production of the deficiency, but also vary within species and between animal species (Coursin 1969). Species variability in the manifestations of pyridoxine deficiency may be related to enzyme variability and structure.

In human infants, dietary B_6 deficiency as described by Snyderman *et al.* (1950; 1953) is associated with failure to gain weight, abnormal tryptophan metabolism, and convulsions.

In mice, dietary deprivation of vitamin B_6 induces weight loss and anemia which varies in severity with the degree of deprivation (Mirone and Jackson 1959). Vilter *et al.* (1953) studied 50 patients who were given the B_6 antagonist deoxypyridoxine (DOP) with or without a low pyridoxine intake. Among 34 of these subjects who developed symptoms and signs of pyridoxine deficiency, the progress of the toxic signs was as follows: early there appeared seborrheic dermatitis and/or glossitis, stomatitis, cheilosis and conjunctivitis, and later severe sensory neuritis. Symptoms suggestive of pellagra appeared in some patients before the termination of the experiment. All of these symptoms were relieved by pyridoxine, pyridoxamine or pyridoxal. Mild anemia occurred in five of the patients who developed vitamin B_6 deficiency as a result of the DOP-low B_6 dietary treatment.

Harriss *et al.* (1965), who studied the effects of DOP on mice, also followed the effects of antituberculous drugs in these animals. Whereas a combination of INH, cycloserine, pyrazinamide and para-aminosalicylic acid did not produce anemia in the mice, abnormal sideroblasts were found in the bone marrow and an elevated number of siderocytes and hypochromic cells in the circulating blood. These hematological effects were induced by INH and cycloserine in combination, but either of these drugs given alone produced less severe effects. Pyrazinamide and para-aminosalicylic acid did not produce any hematologic changes. INH and cycloserine, given singly or in combination, to guinea pigs at various dose levels and with varying iron load, produce hypochromic anemia with ring sideroblasts and other hematologic features observed in human sideroblastic anemia.

INH alone, with or without iron load, produced no anemia until a lethal dose level was reached. Cycloserine, given alone, in large dosages produced mild anemia in iron-loaded animals.

Experimental sideroblastic anemia induced by antituberculous drugs has been further studied recently by Tanaka and Bottomly (1974). They produced such an anemia in guinea pigs by giving INH and cycloserine in combination with or without an iron load. Associated with the anemia there was low blood pyridoxal phosphate and also a diminished bone marrow delta-aminolevulinic acid synthetase activity, that was only partly corrected by pyridoxal phosphate in $vitro$. The authors suggest that in this experimental drug-induced vitamin B_6 deficiency the function of Δ-aminolevulinic acid synthetase is depressed.

As indicated earlier, vitamin B_6 antagonists tend not to have a marked effect on mitochondrial enzymes such as Δ-aminolevulinic acid synthetase. Relative lack of inhibition of this enzyme by the B_6 antagonists accounts for the uncommonness of sideroblastic anemia induced by drugs or other foreign compounds in this category. In particular, drugs such as INH, given alone (that is, without other antituberculous drugs which are also B_6 antagonists) do not induce anemia unless the patient already has a genetically determined trait for pyridoxine responsive anemia (McCurdy and Donohoe 1966).

On the other hand, if antituberculous drugs which are B_6 antagonists are given in combination, there is a risk that sideroblastic or pyridoxine deficiency anemia will ensue. Verwilghen et $al.$ (1965) described five cases of such anemia in patients with pulmonary tuberculosis treated with INH, cycloserine, and pyrazinamide. Anemia in these patients disappeared completely when the cycloserine or the pyrazinamide were discontinued, though INH and in some patients, other antituberculous drugs such as PAS, were continued. It is suggested that cycloserine and pyrazinamide act synergistically with INH to cause sideroblastic anemia. It is possible, as already indicated, that these various B_6 antagonists act at different sites.

The common therapeutic practice of using antituberculosis drugs in combination for effective treatment of the disease may result either in a high risk of B_6 deficiency, or, as indicated elsewhere in this text, in other vitamin deficiencies such as niacin and folate deficiency.

Hydrazide drugs, other than INH, as well as hydrazides used industrially, have the capacity to produce vitamin B_6 deficiency. A characteristic pyridoxine deficiency neuropathy has been reported in patients receiving high doses of the antihypertensive drug, hydralazine. In two patients reported by Kirkendall and Paige (1958), there is evidence that polyneuritis developed while patients were receiving hydralazine may have been precipitated both by the high level of intake of the drug, and also a prior low dietary intake of pyridoxine. Killam and Bain (1957) reported that thiosemicarbazide, furfural hydrazide, as well as INH, could inhibit vitamin B_6-dependent enzyme systems *in vitro*. Convulsions produced in animals by these compounds were therefore believed to be due to inhibition of one or more of the enzyme systems requiring pyridoxal phosphate as a cofactor.

In 1963, Medina reported that convulsions produced in experimental animals by hydrazine could be inhibited by pyridoxine, but not by pyridoxal. Hydrazine, and more particularly the methyl substituted hydrazines, have been used extensively as rocket fuels. As with INH, these compounds can form hydrazones with vitamin B_6 and can inhibit the function of vitamin B_6-dependent enzyme systems. Such hydrazones are toxic and it is believed that this fact may be important in explaining the *in vivo* toxic responses to various industrial hydrazines. In mice, convulsive seizures can be induced by 1,1-dimethylhydrazine (UDMH), or by monomethylhydrazine (MMH), or by the corresponding hydrazones (Furst and Gustavson 1967).

In the rat all forms of vitamin B_6 are partially effective against the convulsive effects of hydrazine, the sparing effects of the vitamin being dependent upon the amount administered (Cornish 1969). Species differences in the toxicity of UDMH and MMH have been observed as well as a differential response to pyridoxine vitamers. In addition to its capacity for producing acute vitamin B_6 deficiency with convulsions, MMH causes hypoglycemia. In order to prevent convulsions in monkeys, and this may also be true in man, pyridoxine is required as well as IV glucose (Bach 1970).

Chabner *et al.* (1969) reported that in mice, intraperitoneal injection of procarbazine (N-isopropyl-α-(2-methylhydrazino)-p-toluamide hydrochloride), a derivative of methyl hydrazine, produced a depression in plasma levels of pyridoxal phosphate. They postulated that the neurotoxic side effects of this antitumor agent might be partially due to pyridoxal phosphate depletion. Their reasoning was based on the idea that methylhydrazine may be a metabolite of procarbazine and that pyridoxal methylhydrazine formation may occur causing a B_6 deficiency. However, pyridoxal phosphate has been used in attempts to combat procarbazine-induced neuropathy and confusional states and has been shown to be ineffective (Falkson *et al.* 1965; Samuels *et al.* 1969). These negative reports have laid doubt on the role of procarbazine as a B_6 antagonist (Weiss *et al.* 1974).

Penicillamine has been used since 1956 in the treatment of patients with Wilson's disease (hepatolenticular degeneration), because of the drug's copper-chelating properties (Walshe 1956). Effective treatment of acute copper poisoning, gold dermatitis and lead intoxication also depend upon the chelating properties of this drug (Goldberg *et al.* 1963; Aposhian 1961; Davis 1969). In rats, oral or intramuscular administration of N-acetylpenicillamine has been found to protect rats against the lethal effects of intoxication by mercuric chloride (Aposhian and Aposhian 1959).

The use of penicillamine has been advocated in a number of diverse clinical conditions other than those in which its chelating properties are being utilized. As a sulfhydryl reducing agent, penicillamine can break the disulfide bonds of certain high molecular weight proteins and amino acids (Deutsch and Morton 1957). This effect of the drug has led to clinical trials of its effectiveness in macroglobulinemia and cystinuria (Ritzmann *et al.* 1960; Crawhall *et al.* 1963). Penicillamine has been used successfully in the treatment of cystinuria and during this treatment with the drug there is excretion of soluble, mixed disulfide products of cystine and penicillamine. The excretion of these soluble products reduces the risk of cystine stone formation (Crawhall and Watts 1968).

When the effects of penicillamine on the macroglobulin of rheumatoid arthritis (rheumatoid factor) was studied, it was noticed that prolonged administration of penicillamine led to a decrease in the level of the rheumatoid factor and also a fall in the erythrocyte sedimentation rate, as well as the C-reactive protein (Jaffe 1963A; 1963B).

Evidence has been presented that D-penicillamine reduces the rate of collagen biosynthesis and maturation. On the basis of these findings the drug has been advocated for use in the treatment of patients with scleroderma (systemic sclerosis), a disease in which patients may show increased collagen formation (Uitto *et al.* 1970). Benefits, if any, to patients with scleroderma who have received penicillamine have been offset by the common appearance of the side effects (Bluestone *et al.* 1970).

The L-isomer of penicillamine was first shown to exert an antagonistic effect to vitamin B_6 in the rat, though in this animal the D-form was believed to be devoid of this property (Wilson and duVigneaud 1950). Subsequently Asatoor (1964) found that the D-isomer of penicillamine also possessed vitamin B_6 antagonism in the rat. Evidence has also been obtained by Jaffe (1969) that D-penicillamine, in doses given therapeutically to man, can produce biochemical changes indicative of impaired vitamin B_6 metabolism; that is, increased xanthurenic acid and kynurenine excretion after a tryptophan load.

In a 1964 review of penicillamine as a copper chelating agent (Council on Drugs), hypochromic anemia is mentioned as an occasional side effect. Though the authors of this article do not mention the question, it is possible that this anemia could be due to vitamin B_6 deficiency. Reversible optic neuritis observed by Tu *et al.* (1963) in patients receiving D-L-penicillamine has been attributed to pyridoxine deficiency.

It has been shown that both L-penicillamine and D-penicillamine form thiazolidine compounds with pyridoxal-6-phosphate (Heyl *et al.* 1948; Ueda *et al.* 1960).

Hollister *et al.* (1966) treated 13 schizophrenic patients with D-penicillamine on the assumption that this might prove to be a useful therapeutic agent. They based this treatment regimen on two hypotheses: that the drug might decrease copper oxidase activity, said to be increased in schizophrenia, and on the idea that the drug might decrease the level of S19 macroglobulins which have also been found to be increased in this disease (Shiller *et al.* 1961; Fessel 1962). Daily doses of 1000 mg D-penicillamine or more were given during the major portion of the treatment program. The antipyridoxine effect of the drug was demonstrated by increased urinary excretion of xanthurenic and kynurenic acids following a tryptophan load. Six of the 13 patients showed abnormal excretions of these tryptophan metabolites during the fourth week of therapy. After six weeks of treatment, neither the serum macroglobulin levels nor the serum copper oxidase activity were consistently changed. Eleven other schizophrenic patients were also treated with D-penicillamine in doses of 750 or 1500 mg daily over a period of four weeks with no added pyridoxine and then for three weeks with the addition of 100 mg pyridoxine per day. The tryptophan load test was carried out before treatment, during treatment without pyridoxine, and again after supplementation with pyridoxine. All of these patients showed evidence of an antipyridoxine effect induced by the drug which was reversed by the pyridoxine supplement. It was suggested by these authors that during D-penicillamine therapy routine pyridoxine supplements should be given (Hollister *et al.* 1966).

Sternlieb and Scheinberg (1964) reported on a series of 33 patients with Wilson's disease who were treated either with D-L-penicillamine or with D-penicillamine. The drugs were administered in divided oral doses from 1 up to 4 gm being given daily. All of their patients who were taking D-L-penicillamine received 50 mg pyridoxine daily, and it is stated that none of these patients showed either symptoms or signs of pyridoxine deficiency. The authors do not make it clear what was the outcome of treatment with respect to vitamin B_6 status of the patients who were given D-penicillamine, nor did they investigate the antipyridoxine effect of these drugs by tryptophan load test.

For discussion of the effects of L-dopa and also contraceptive steroids on vitamin B_6 metabolism, the reader is referred to other sections of the text.

Although contraceptive steroids have been shown to induce biochemical evidence of vitamin B_6 depletion, there is no evidence as yet that these drugs act as vitamin B_6 antagonists in the sense that they form complexes with pyridoxal phosphate or with other pyridoxine derivatives, or that they inhibit B_6-dependent enzyme systems.

The antipyridoxine effect of certain drugs has been used experimentally in animals and in man to inhibit tumor growth. It was found by Littman et al. (1963) that pyridoxamine dihydrochloride accelerates the growth of ascitic Sarcoma 180 in CF_1 mice, and that this form of vitamin B_6 decreases the life span of such tumor-bearing animals. The pyridoxamine also increased the rate of growth of the solid form of this tumor, which is believed indicates that the tumor system has a strong affinity for vitamin B_6. In support of this theory, it was shown that a diet deficient in vitamin B_6 will retard the growth of the solid form of the tumor, while pyridoxamine obviates this effect. L-Penicillamine was shown to decrease the rate of growth of the solid form of Sarcoma S180.

The effect of L-penicillamine on growth of this tumor was enhanced by maintaining the mice on a pyridoxine deficient diet. It was found that the D-, L-, and DL forms of penicillamine were all active in retarding the growth of sarcoma, but that the L-form was the most active (Littman et al. 1963).

Another vitamin B_6 antagonist, which has been shown to inhibit tumor growth in experimental animals and in man, is the drug N-dichloroacetyl-DL-serine (FT-9045). This drug bears structural relationships to chloramphenicol, a drug which is an inhibitor of protein synthesis. FT-9045 has been shown to inhibit the growth of Sarcoma-37 in mice (Levi et al. 1960).

Blondal et al. (1961) also found that FT-9045 has an inhibitory effect on the growth of Walker-256 tumors in rats, though this effect is weaker than the effect of the drug on the growth of Sarcoma-37. Among 25 patients with advanced carcinoma or sarcoma treated by Blondal with FT-9045, as well as by other cancer chemotherapeutic agents, 19 developed a neuropathy. Symptoms included paresthesias of the hands and feet, gross tremors, diplopia, slurred speech and also ataxia. Some of the patients showed an absence of knee and ankle reflexes, as well as absent plantar responses. The neuropathy which developed rather suddenly resembled, in many respects, that seen in patients on INH. Five of the patients who developed severe neuropathy were treated by pyridoxine in doses of 150–250 mg given intravenously, and the vitamin induced a remarkable amelioration of their symptoms. In one patient in whom the xanthurenic acid levels in the urine were measured, these were found to be abnormally high.

VITAMIN K AND THE ANTICOAGULANTS

In the last five years, our knowledge of the functions of vitamin K in the clotting mechanism has greatly increased, and with this new information has come insight into the mechanism by which anticoagulants function. The problem which until recently has been a challenge to investigators is whether vitamin K controls the rate of synthesis of prothrombin and the other K-dependent clotting factors, or if it functions so as to convert a precursor protein to the active clotting factors such as prothrombin. Extensive evidence has now been presented to support the latter hypothesis. On the basis of many investigations in the laboratory, Suttie (1973) has postulated that a precursor protein or perhaps precursor proteins exist in the liver which are converted to their active forms such as prothrombin in a step requiring vitamin K. He further believes that the precursor proteins are continually produced, but do not build up if the vitamin is present. It has been suggested that the vitamin K-dependent step either involves production or the attachment of an unknown prosthetic group to the precursor protein, or the modification of that protein so that calcium binding sites are available. Such calcium binding sites would be required for normal activation in the clotting mechanism. Biologically inactive prothrombins have been found in the plasma of human subjects and of cattle that have been given coumarin anticoagulants. In addition it is known that the precursor proteins or inactive precursor proteins are present in the plasma of vitamin K-deficient warfarin-treated rats. There are inactive prothrombin molecules in the plasma of people given coumarin anticoagulants, and it appears that these inactive proteins are released from the liver following the administration of anticoagulants such as dicumarol, when the precursor protein cannot be normally completed.

Bell et al. (1972) have found that in warfarin-treated rats a major part of the vitamin K in the liver is present as the 2,3-epoxide, also called vitamin K oxide. It is their suggestion that coumarin anticoagulants work through the build-up of this metabolite which may act as an inhibitor of the parent vitamin. Bell's group found that warfarin blocks the normal conversion of vitamin K oxide to vitamin K_1 (Fig. 16). However, vitamin K_1 can counteract the effect of warfarin and the separate effects of vitamin K_1 and warfarin on prothrombin synthesis are non-competitive. In a later study, Bell and Caldwell (1973) found that in warfarin-resistant rats, a mutation exists such that the conversion of vitamin K oxide to K_1 is no longer inhibited by warfarin. Their work has suggested that in warfarin-resistant animals the enzyme responsible for catalyzing the conversion of vitamin K oxide to K_1 is less effective, and that this may account for the high vitamin K requirements in this strain. It is supposed, but presently unproven, that in warfarin-resistant families a similar situation may exist.

Shah and Suttie (1973) who have also studied warfarin-resistant rats are of the opinion that there may be several biochemical alterations in this strain, and they do not believe that the defect has been adequately explained by current research.

Koch-Weser and Seller (1971) reviewed drugs which interact with coumarin anticoagulants, and it is pointed out that there are a number of drugs which differ from one another, not only chemically but in pharmacological action, which share the common property of potentiating coumarin anticoagulant function in human subjects. These authors give a detailed discussion of the effects of coumarin anticoagulants on vitamin K-dependent clotting factors II, VII, IX, and X. They state that the degree of depression of synthesis of these clotting factors at any time depends on the plasma coumarin concentration. Recognizing the antagonistic effect of vitamin K on coumarin action, they comment that during anticoagulant treatment the amount of vitamin K available at the synthetic site must influence the rate of synthesis of these clotting factors. In their discussion of individual drugs or drug groups which act synergistically or interact with anticoagulants to increase their action, they lay emphasis on the role of antibiotics which may influence the rate of intestinal K synthesis, thus altering the availability of the vitamin. Although, as pointed out by Koch-Weser and his colleague, it has been suggested that broad spectrum antibiotics may cause hypoprothrombinemia, in practice this has rarely been observed, probably because in man the synthesis of vitamin K by the intestinal microflora may not be such an important source of this vitamin.

Other drugs which have been cited as having the property of potentiating the action of coumarin anticoagulants include chloral hydrate, which causes a decrease in coumarin-albumin binding; chloramphenicol, which inhibits coumarin metabolism; clofibrate, which may possibly decrease coumarin-albumin binding; dextrothyroxine, in which the action with respect to vitamin K is unknown; mefenamic acid, which decreases coumarin-albumin binding; neomycin, which decreases vitamin K absorption, oxyphenbutazone, which causes a decrease in coumarin-albumin binding; phenylbutazone, which may act similarly; phenyramidol, which inhibits coumarin metabolism; quinidine, which may cause a decrease in clotting factor synthesis; and salicylate, which may possibly have similar properties (Koch-Weser and Sellers 1971).

Deykin (1970) has classified drugs which interact with coumarin anticoagulants into four major categories as follows: 1) drugs that bind vitamin K or prevent its absorption by trapping bile salts. This would include cholestyramine; 2) those drugs that displace anticoagulants such as warfarin from their binding sites on albumin, so increasing the concentration of the free anticoagulant, and thus augmenting the anticoagulant response. Within this group are included clofibrate and phenylbutazone; also according to Deykin, indomethacin and certain acidic sulfonamides such as sulfisoxazole; 3) another group of drugs are those which compete with anticoagulants such as warfarin at their sites of degradation within the endoplasmic reticulum. Drugs included in this group are tolbutamide and diphenylhydantoin which are metabolized by the same enzymes that break down warfarin. If one of these drugs is given with warfarin, then the rate of degradation of the anticoagulant is slowed and the anticoagulant function is prolonged within the patient. Conversely, the rate of degradation of drugs given such as diphenylhydantoin will also be slowed under these circumstances. Chloramphenical also inhibits the metabolism of anticoagulants such as warfarin, but this is by direct suppression of the degradative enzymes; and 4) certain drugs increase the affinity of the receptor site for warfarin. These drugs definitely include quinidine and may possibly include clofibrate, dextrothyroxine, and anabolic steroids. In this group the action of the anticoagulant or the sensitivity to the drug is greatly increased. In Table 7.1 drugs are listed that potentiate the response to anticoagulants and their function, if known, is also summarized.

There have been a number of review articles pertaining to the effect of drugs in diminishing the effectiveness of anticoagulants, but as this is not a subject for review in this text, readers are referred to the works of MacDonald and Robinson (1968), O'Reilly and Aggeler (1970), and Sigell and Flessa (1970) for further information.

Drugs such as barbiturates and other hepatic microsomal enzyme inducers have the capacity to increase the metabolism of coumarin anticoagulants when they are given concurrently. However, when the enzyme inducer is withdrawn, the anticoagulant action of the coumarin is suddenly markedly increased and this has been shown to incur a very severe risk of bleeding episodes in the patient (Burns

TABLE 7.1

DRUGS WHICH POTENTIATE VITAMIN K "DEFICIENCY"
INDUCED BY COUMARIN ANTICOAGULANTS IN MAN

Mechanism of Action	Drugs
1. Microbial synthesis of $K_2\downarrow$	Tetracyclines Other broad spectrum antibiotics
2. K_1 absorption$\downarrow$	Mineral oil Cholestyramine Neomycin Colchicine? Vitamin E?
3. Coumarin-albumin binding$\downarrow$	Chloral hydrate Clofibrate Mefenamic acid Ethacrynic acid Nalidixic acid Oxyphenbutazone Phenylbutazone Indomethacin Salicylates
4. Synthesis of K-dependent clotting factors$\downarrow$	Salicylates Quinidine Quinine Cinchophen Ethanol Anabolic steroids? Dextrothyroxine?
5. Inhibition of coumarin metabolism	Chloramphenicol Phenyramidol Disulfiram Tolbutamide Diphenylhydantoin
6. Catabolism of vitamin K dependent clotting factors$\uparrow$	Anabolic steroids?$\uparrow$

1964; Cucinell *et al.* 1965; Burns and Conney 1965; Cohen and
Catalano 1967).

BIBLIOGRAPHY

AKINYANJU, O., GODDELL, J. C., and AHMED, I. 1973. Pyrimethamine
poisoning. Brit. Med. J. *4*, 147–148.
ALBERT, A. 1960. Selective Toxicity. John Wiley & Sons, New York.
ANDERSON, J. M., SMITH, M. D., and HUTCHISON, J. 1966. Megaloblastic
anemia and methotrexate therapy. Brit. Med. J. *2*, 641–642.
ANON. 1972. Yearbook of Dermatology. Yearbook Med. Publ., Chicago.
ANON. 1973. Yearbook of Dermatology. Yearbook Med. Publ., Chicago.
APOSHIAN, A. H. V. 1961. Biochemical and pharmacological properties of
the metal-binding agent, penicillamine. Fed. Proc. *20*, Suppl. 10, 185–188.

APOSHIAN, H. F., and APOSHIAN, M. M. 1959. N-acetyl-dl-penicillamine, a new oral protective agent against the lethal effects of mercuric chloride. J. Pharm. Exp. Therap. *126*, 131-135.
ASATOOR, A. M. 1964. Pyridoxine deficiency in the rat produced by D-penicillamine. Nature *203*, 1382-1383.
BACH, K. C. 1970. Aerospace toxicology. I. Propellant toxicology. Fed. Proc. *29*, 2000-2005.
BAKER, B. R. 1959. The case for irreversible inhibitors as anticancer agents, an essay. Cancer Chemotherapy Rep. No. 4, 1-10.
BAKER, B. R. 1962. Non-classical antimetabolites. VIII. The bridge principle of specificity with exo-alkylating irreversible inhibitors. Biochem. Pharmacol. *11*, 1155-1161.
BAKER, H. 1970. Some hazards of methotrexate treatment of psoriasis. Trans. St. John's Hosp. Dermat. Soc. *56*, 111-116.
BELL, R. G., and CALDWELL, P. P. 1973. Mechanism of warfarin resistance. Warfarin and the metabolism of vitamin K_1. Biochem. *12*, 1759-1762.
BELL, R. G., SADOWSKI, J. A., and MATSCHINER, J. T. 1972. Mechanism of action of warfarin. Warfarin and metabolism of vitamin K_1. Biochem. *11*, 1959-1961.
BETHELL, S. H., and THOMPSON, D. S. 1954. Treatment of leukemia and related disorders with 6-mercaptopurine. Ann. N. Y. Acad. Sci. *60*, 436-438.
BIEHL, J. P., and VILTER, R. W. 1954. Effect of iso-niazid on vitamin B_6 metabolism; its possible significance in producing isoniazid neuritis. Proc. Soc. Exp. Biol. Med. *85*, 389-392.
BLONDAL, H., LEVI, I., LATOUR, J. P. A., and FRASER, W. D. 1961. Observations on the antitumor effect of N-dichloroacetyl-DL-serine (FT-9045). Radiology *76*, 945-959.
BLUESTONE, R., GRAHAME, R., HOLLAWAY, V., and HOLT, P. J. L. 1970. Treatment of systemic sclerosis with D-penicillamine. Ann. Rheumat. Dis. *29*, 153-158.
BORRIE, P., and CLARK, P. A. 1966. Megaloblastic anaemia during methotrexate treatment of psoriasis. Brit. Med. J. *1*, 1339.
BRAUNSTEIN, A. E. 1960. Pyridoxal phosphate. *In* The Enzymes, 2. P. D. Boyer, H. Lardy, and K. Myrback (Editors). Academic Press, New York.
BRAUNSTEIN, A. E. 1964. Binding and reactions of the vitamin B_6 coenzyme in the catalytic center of aspartate transaminase. *In* Vitamins and Hormones, R. S. Harris, P. L. Munson, and E. Diczfalusy (Editors). *22*, 451-484. Academic Press, New York and London.
BROQUIST, H. P., *et al.* 1951. "Citrovorum factor" activity of tetrahydropteroylglutamic acid. J. Am. Chem. Soc. *73*, 3535-3536.
BROQUIST, H. P., and JUKES, T. H. 1968. Antimetabolites—effect on nutrition. *In* Modern Nutrition in Health and Disease, M. G. Wohl, and R. S. Goodhart (Editors). Lea and Febiger, Philadelphia.
BURCHALL, J. J., and HITCHINGS, G. H. 1965. Inhibitor binding analysis of dihydrofolate reductases from various species. Mol. Pharmacol. *1*, 126-136.
BURNS, J. J. 1964. Implications of enzyme induction for drug therapy. Am. J. Med. *37*, 327-331.
BURNS, J. J., and CONNEY, A. H. 1965. Enzyme stimulation and inhibition in the metabolism of drugs. Proc. Roy. Soc. Med. *58*, 955-960.
BUSHBY, S. R. M., and HITCHINGS, G. H. 1968. Trimethoprim, a sulfonamide potentiator. Brit. J. Pharm. Chemotherap. *33*, 72-90.
CHABNER, B. A., DeVITA, V. T., CONSIDINE, N., and OLIVERIO, V. T. 1969. Plasma pyridoxal phosphate depletion by the carcinostatic procarbazine. Proc. Soc. Exp. Med. Biol. *132*, 1119-1122.
CHANARIN, I. 1964. Studies in drug-induced megaloblastic anaemia. Scand. J. Hemat. *1*, 280-288.
CHANARIN, I. 1969. The Megaloblastic Anaemias. Blackwell Scientific Publishers, Oxford and Edinburgh.

CHATAGNER, F. 1970. Influence of pyridoxine derivatives on the biosynthesis and stability of pyridoxal phosphate enzymes. *In* Vitamins and Hormones, R. S. Harris, P. L. Munson, and E. Diczfalusy (Editors). *28*, 291-302. Academic Press, New York and London.

COE, R. O., and BULL, F. E. 1968. Cirrhosis associated with methotrexate treatment of psoriasis. J. Am. Med. Assoc. *206*, 1515-1520.

COHEN, S. I., and CATALANO, P. M. 1967. Griseofulvin-warfarin antagonism. J. Am. Med. Assoc. *199*, 582-584.

COLSKY, J., GREENSPAN, E. M., and WARREN, P. N. 1955. Hepatic fibrosis in children with acute leukemia after therapy with folic acid antagonists. Arch. Path. *59*, 198-206.

CONNORS, T. A. 1970. Mechanism of action of cytotoxic agents. Trans. St. John's Hosp. Dermat. Soc. *56*, 100-110.

CORCINO, J., WAXMAN, S., and HERBERT, V. 1970. Mechanism of triamterene-induced megaloblastosis. Ann. Intern. Med. *73*, 419-424.

CORNISH, H. H. 1969. The role of vitamin B_6 in the toxicity of hydrazine. *In* Vitamin B_6 in Metabolism of the Nervous System. Ann. N. Y. Acad. Sci. *166*, 136-145.

COUNCIL ON DRUGS—The American Medical Association. 1964. A copper chelating agent—penicillamine (Cuprimine). J. Am. Med. Assoc. *189*, 847-848.

COURSIN, D. B. 1969. Vitamin B_6 and brain function in animals and man. *In* Vitamin B_6 in Metabolism of the Nervous System. Ann. N.Y. Acad. Sci. *166*, 7-15.

CRAWHALL, J. C., SCOWEN, E. F., and WATTS, R. W. E. 1963. Effect of penicillamine on cystinuria. Brit. Med. J. *1*, 588-590.

CRAWHALL, J. C., and WATTS, R. W. E. 1968. Cystinuria. Am. J. Med. *45*, 736-755.

CUCINELL, S. A. *et al.* 1965. Drug interactions in man. I. Effect of phenobarbital on plasma levels of bishydroxycoumarin (Dicumarol) and diphenylhydantoin (Dilantin). Clin. Pharmacol. Therap. *6*, 420-429.

DAHL, M. G. C., GREGORY, M. M., and SCHEUER, P. J. 1972. Methotrexate hepatotoxicity in psoriasis: Comparison of different dose regimens. Brit. Med. J. *1*, 654-656.

DAVIS, C. M. 1969. D-Penicillamine for the treatment of gold dermatitis. Am. J. Med. *46*, 472-474.

DELMONTE, L., and JUKES, T. H. 1962. Folic acid antagonists in cancer chemotherapy. Pharm. Rev. *14*, 91-135.

DEUTSCH, H. F., and MORTON, J. I. 1957. Dissociation of human macroglobulin. Science *125*, 600-601.

DEYKIN, D. 1970. Warfarin therapy (second of two parts). New Eng. J. Med. *283*, 801-803.

DOBES, W. L. 1963. Use of folic acid antagonists and steroids in treatment of psoriasis. Southern Med. J. *56*, 187-192.

EDMONSON, W. F., and GUY, W. B. 1958. Treatment of psoriasis with folic acid antagonists. A. M. A. Arch. Derm. *78*, 200-203.

FALCO, E. A. *et al.* 1949. Antimalarials as antagonists of purines and pteroylglutamic acid. Nature *164*, 107-108.

FALKSON, G., deVILLIERS, P. C., and FALKSON, H. C. 1965. N-isopropyl-α-(2-methylhydrazino)-p-toluamide hydrochloride) (NSC-77,213) for treatment of cancer patients. Cancer Chemother. Rep. *46*, 7-26.

FERBER, S., *et al.* 1948. Temporary remissions in acute leukemia in children produced by folic acid antagonists, 4-aminopteroylglutamic acid (aminopterin). New Eng. J. Med. *238*, 787-793.

FESSEL, W. J. 1962. Blood proteins in functional psychoses: a review of the literature and unifying hypothesis. Arch. Gen. Psychiat. *6*, 132-148.

FRANKLIN, A. L., BELT, M., STOKSTAD, E. L. R., and JUKES, T. H. 1949. Biological studies with 4-amino-10-methyl pteroylglutamic acid. J. Biol. Chem. *177*, 621-629.

FRY, L., and McMINN, R. M. H. 1966. Action of methotrexate on skin and intestinal epithelium in psoriasis. Arch. Dermat. *93*, 726-730.

FURST, E. A., and GUSTAVSON, W. 1967. A comparison of alkylhydrazines and their B_6 hydrazones as convulsive agents. Proc. Soc. Exp. Biol. Med. *124*, 172-175.

GAMBLE, D. F., BOND, H. W., and BURGER, A. 1960. Chemotherapy of neoplastic diseases. *In* Medicinal Chemistry, 2nd Edition, A. Burger (Editor). Interscience Publishers, New York.

GIRDWOOD, R. H., DA COSTA, A. J., and SAMSON, R. R. 1973. Co-trimoxazole as a possible cause of folate depletion. Brit. J. Haematol. *25*, 279-280.

GOLDBERG, A., SMITH, J. A., and LOCHHEAD, A. C. 1963. Treatment of lead-poisoning with oral penicillamine. Brit. Med. J. *1*, 1270-1275.

GUBNER, R. 1951. Effect of "aminopterin" on epithelial tissues. A.M.A. Arch. Derm. Syph. *64*, 688-699.

GUBNER, R., AUGUST, S., and GINSBERG, V. 1951. Effect of aminopterin in rheumatoid arthritis and psoriasis. Am. J. Med. Sci. *220*, 176-182.

HAMILTON, L. *et al.* 1952. Hematological effect of certain 2,4-diamino-pyrimidine antagonists of folic acid. Abst. Fed. Proc. *11*, 225.

HAMILTON, L. *et al.* 1954. Hematological effects of certain 2,4-diamino-pyrimidines, antagonists of folic acid metabolism. Blood *9*, 1062-1081.

HARRIMAN, S., IANNOTTI, A. T., and BERTINO, J. R. 1964. Determinations of the levels of serum folate in patients with carcinoma of the head and neck treated with methotrexate. Cancer Res. *24*, 105-110.

HARRISS, E. B., MACGIBBON, B. H., and MOLLIN, D. L. 1965. Experimental sideroblastic anaemia. Brit. J. Haematol. *11*, 99-106.

HEYL, D., HARRIS, S. A., and FOLKERS, K. 1948. The chemistry of vitamin B_6. VI. Pyridoxylamino acids. J. Am. Chem. Soc. *70*, 3429-3431.

HITCHINGS, G. J., ELION, G. B., and SINGER, S. 1954. Derivatives of condensed pyrimidine systems as metabolites. *In* Chemistry and Biology of Pteridines. J. & A. Churchill, London.

HOFFBRAND, A. V., and FRY, L. 1972. Effect of methotrexate on the absorption of folates. Lancet *2*, 1025.

HOLLISTER, L. E., MOORE, F. F., FORREST, F., and BENNETT, J. L. 1966. Antipyridoxine effect of D-penicillamine in schizophrenic men. Am. J. Clin. Nutr. *19*, 307-312.

HUTTER, R. V. P. *et al.* 1960. Hepatic fibrosis in children with acute leukemia. Cancer *13*, 288-307.

IVADY, G., and PALDY, L. 1958. A new form of treatment of interstitial plasma-cell pneumonia in premature infants with pentavalent antimony and aromatics diamidines. Mschr. Kinderheilk *106*, 10-14.

JAFFE, I. A. 1963A. Comparison of effect of plasmapheresis and penicillamine on level of circulating rheumatoid factor. Ann. Rheum. Dis. *22*, 71-76.

JAFFE, I. A. 1963B. Proc. 5th European Congr. of Rheumatic Diseases, Stockholm, August.

JAFFE, I. A. 1969. Antivitamin B_6 effect of D-penicillamine. *In* Vitamin B_6 in Metabolism of the Nervous System. Ann. N. Y. Acad. Sci. *166*, 57-60.

JOHNS, D. G., and VALERINO, D. M. 1971. Metabolism of folate antagonists. *In* Folate Antagonists as Chemotherapeutic Agents. Ann. N. Y. Acad. Sci. *186*, 378-386.

KAHN, S. B., FEIN, S. A., and BRODSKY, I. 1968. Effects of trimethoprim on folate metabolism in man. Clin. Pharmacol. Therap. *9*, 550-560.

KAISER, C. 1960. Metabolite Antagonism in Medicinal Chemistry, 2nd Edition. A. Burger (Editor). Interscience Publishers, New York.

KAUFMAN, H. E., and GEISLER, P. H. 1960. The hematologic toxicity of pyrimethamine (daraprim) in man. Arch. Ophthal. *64*, 140-146.

KAY, H. E. M. *et al.* 1972. Encephalopathy in acute leukaemia associated with methotrexate therapy. Arch. Dis. Child *47*, 344-354.

KILLAM, K. F., and BAIN, J. A. 1957. Convulsant hydrazide. I. *In vitro* and *in vivo* inhibition of vitamin B_6 enzymes by convulsant hydrazide. J. Pharmacol. Exp. Therap. *119*, 255-262.

KIRKENDALL, W. M., and PAGE, E. B. 1958. Polyneuritis occurring during hydralazine therapy: Report of two cases and discussion of adverse reactions to hydralazine. J. Am. Med. Assoc. *167*, 427-432.

KLIPPEL, J. H., and DECKER, J. L. 1974. Relative macrocytosis in cyclophosphamide and azathioprine therapy. J. Am. Med. Assoc. *229*, 180-181.

KOCH-WESER, J., and SELLERS, E. M. 1971. Drug interactions with coumarin anticoagulants. New Eng. J. Med. *285*, 487-498; 547-558.

LEVI, I., BLONDAL, H., and LOZINSKI, E. 1960. Serine derivative with antitumor activity. Science *131*, 666.

LEVY, L. 1969. Mechanism of drug induced vitamin B_6. *In* Vitamin B_6 in Metabolism of the Nervous System. Ann. N. Y. Acad. Sci. *166*, 184-191.

LIEBERMAN, F. L., and BATEMAN, J. R. 1968. Megaloblastic anemia possibly induced by triamterene in patients with alcoholic cirrhosis. Ann. Intern. Med. *68*, 168-173.

LITTMAN, M. L., TAGUCHI, T., and SHIMIZU, Y. 1963. Acceleration of growth of Sarcoma 180 with pyridoxamine and retardation with penicillamine. Proc. Soc. Exp. Biol. Med. *113*, 667-674.

MAASS, A. R. *et al.* 1967. Effect of triamterene on folic reductase activity and reproduction in the rat. Toxicol. Appl. Pharmacol. *10*, 413-423.

MacDONALD, M. B., and ROBINSON, D. S. 1968. Clinical observations of possible barbiturate interference with anticoagulation. J. Am. Med. Assoc. *204*, 95-100.

McCURDY, P. R., and DONOHOE, R. F. 1966. Pyridoxine-responsive anemia conditioned by isonicotinic acid hydrazide. Blood *27*, 352-362.

MEDINA, M. A. 1963. The *in vivo* effects of hydrazines and vitamin B_6 in the metabolism of gamma-amino butyric acid. J. Pharmacol. Exp. Therap. *140*, 133-137.

MIRONE, L., and JACKSON, C. D. 1959. The development and cure of pyridoxine deficiency symptoms in weanling mice. J. Nutr. *67*, 167-180.

MYATT, A. V., HERNANDEZ, T., and COATNEY, G. R. 1953. Studies in human malaria. 33. The toxicity of pyrimethamine (Daraprim) in man. Am. J. Trop. Med. *2*, 788.

NICHOLS, C. A., and WELCH, A. D. 1950. On the mechanism of action of aminopterin. Proc. Soc. Exp. Biol. Med. *74*, 403-411.

O'REILLY, R. A., and AGGELER, P. M. 1970. Determinants of the response to oral anticoagulant drugs in man. Pharmacol. Rev. *22*, 35-96.

PERKINS, E. S., SMITH, E. H., and SCHOFIELD, P. B. 1956. Treatment of uveitis with pyrimethamine (Daraprim). Brit. J. Ophthal. *40*, 577-586.

REES, R. B., and BENNETT, J. H. 1959. Further observations on aminopterin for psoriasis. J. Invest. Dermat. *32*, 61-66.

REES, R. B., and BENNETT, J. H. 1961. Methotrexate vs. aminopterin for psoriasis. Arch. Derm. *83*, 970-972.

REES, R. B., BENNETT, J. H., and BOSTICK, W. L. 1955. Aminopterin for psoriasis. A. M. A. Arch. Derm. *72*, 133-143.

REES, R. B., BENNETT, J. H., HAMLIN, E. M., and MAIBACH, H. I. 1964. Aminopterin for psoriasis. Arch. Derm. *90*, 544-552.

RITZMANN, S. E., COLEMAN, S. L., and LEVIN, W. C. 1960. The effect of some mercaptanes upon macrocryogelglobulin modification induced by cysteamine, penicillamine and penicillin. J. Lab. Clin. Invest. *39*, 1320-1329.

ROBBINS, J. B., MILLER, R. H., AREAN, V. M., and PEARSON, H. A. 1965. Successful treatment of pneumocystis carinii pneumonitis in a patient with congenital hypogammaglobulinemia. New Eng. J. Med. *272*, 708-713.

ROENIGK, H. H. *et al.* 1971. Hepatotoxicity of methotrexate in the treatment of psoriasis. Arch. Derm. *103*, 251-261.

ROSEN, F., MIHICH, E., and NICHOL, C. A. 1964. Selective metabolic and chemotherapeutic effects of vitamin B_6 antimetabolites. *In* Vitamins and Hormones, R. S. Harris, I. G. Wool, and J. A. Loraine (Editors). *22*, 609-641. Academic Press, N. Y. and London.

ROSENTHALE, M. E., and VAN ARMAN, C. G. 1963. A pteridine diuretic, WY-3654. J. Pharmacol. Exp. Therap. *142*, 111-121.

RYAN, T. J. *et al.* 1964. The treatment of psoriasis with folic acid antagonists. Brit. J. Derm. *76*, 555-564.

SAMUELS, M. L., LEARY, W. V., and HOWE, C. D. 1969. Procarbazine (NSC-77213) in the treatment of advanced bronchogenic carcinoma. Cancer Chemotherap. Rep. *53*, 135-145.

SHAH, D. V., and SUTTIE, J. W. 1973. The chloroanalog of vitamin K: Antagonism of vitamin K action in normal and warfarin-resistant rats. Proc. Soc. Exp. Biol. Med. *143*, 775-779.

SHILLER, M., *et al.* 1961. Oxidase activity and cupremia in the course of high doses of chlorpromazine and levomepromazine. J. Brasil. Psiquiat. *10*, 53.

SIGELL, L. P., and FLESSA, H. C. 1970. Drug interactions with anticoagulants. J. Am. Med. Assoc. *214*, 2035-2038.

SNYDERMAN, S. E., CARRETERO, R., and HOLT, L. E. JR. 1950. Pyridoxine deficiency in the human being. Fed. Proc. *9*, 371-372.

SNYDERMAN, S. E., HOLT, L. E. JR., CARRETERO, R., and JACOBS, K. 1953. Pyridoxine deficiency in the human infant. J. Clin. Nutr. *1*, 200-207.

STERNLIEB, I., and SCHEINBERG, I. H. 1964. Penicillamine therapy for hepatolantricular degeneration. J. Am. Med. Assoc. *189*, 748-754.

STRAKOSCH, E. A. 1963. Study of folic acid antagonists in treatment of psoriasis (aminopterin vs. methotrexate vs. aminopterin anticorticosteroids). Dermatologica *126*, 259-267.

SULLIVAN, R. D., MILLER, E., and SIKES, M. P. 1959. Antimetabolite-metabolite combination cancer chemotherapy. Effects of intra-arterial methotrexate-intramuscular citrovorum factor therapy in human cancer. Cancer *12*, 1248-1262.

SUTTIE, J. W. 1973. Vitamin K and prothrombin synthesis. Nutr. Rev. *31*, 105-109.

SWENSEID, M. E., SWANSON, A. L., MILLER, S., and BETHELL, F. H. 1952. The metabolic displacement of folic acid by aminopterin. Studies in leukemia patients. Blood 7, 302-306.

TALLEY, R. W., and VAITKEVICIUS, V. K. 1963. Megaloblastosis produced by a cytosine antagonist, 1-β-D-arabinofuranosylcytosine. Blood *21*, 352-362.

TANAKA, M., and BOTTOMLY, S. S. 1974. Bone marrow delta-aminolevulinic acid synthetase activity in experimental sideroblastic anemia. J. Lab. Clin. Med. *84*, 92-98.

TENPAS, A., and ABRAHAM, J. P. 1965. Hematological side effects of pyrimethamine in treatment of ocular toxoplasmosis. Am. J. Med. Sci. *249*, 448-453.

TONG, M. J., STRICKLAND, T., VOTTERI, B. A., and GUNNING, J-J. 1970. Supplemental folates in the therapy of plasmodium falciparum malaria. J. Am. Med. Assoc. *214*, 2330-2333.

TU, J.-B., BLACKWELL, R. Q., and LEE, P.-F. 1963. D,L-Penicillamine as a cause of optic axial neuritis. J. Am. Med. Assoc. *185*, 83-86.

UEDA, K., HITOSHI, A., and MASAM, S. 1960. Intestinal absorption of amino acids. IV. Participation of pyridoxal phosphate in the active transport of L-amino acids through the intestinal wall. J. Biochem. (Tokyo) *48*, 584-592.

UITTO, J., HELIN, P., RASMUSSEN, O., and LORENZEN, I. 1970. Skin collagen in patients with scleroderma: biosynthesis and maturity *in vitro* and effect of D penicillamine. Ann. Clin. Res. *2*, 228-234.

VERWILGHEN, R., REYBROUCK, G., CALLENS, L., and COSEMANS, J. 1965. Antituberculous drugs and sideroblastic anemia. Brit. J. Haemat. *11*, 92-98.

VILTER, R. W. *et al.* 1950. Studies on the relationships of vitiamin B_{12}, folic acid, thiamin, uracil, and methyl group donors in persons with pernicious anemia and related megaloblastic anemias. Blood *5*, 695–717.

VILTER, R. W. *et al.* 1953. The effect of vitamin B_6 deficiency induced by desoxypyridoxine (DOP) in human beings. J. Lab. Clin. Med. *42*, 335–357.

WALSHE, J. M. 1956. Penicillamine: A new oral therapy for Wilson's disease. Am. J. Med. *21*, 487–495.

WAXMAN, S., CORCINO, J. J., and HERBERT, V. 1970. Drugs, toxins and dietary amino acids affecting vitamin B_{12} or folic acid absorption or utilization. Am. J. Med. *48*, 599–607.

WAXMAN, S., and HERBERT, V. 1969. Mechanism of pyrimethamine-induced megaloblastosis in human bone marrow. New Eng. J. Med. *280*, 1316–1319.

WAXMAN, S., METZ, J., and HERBERT, V. 1969. Effective DNA synthesis in human megaloblastic bone marrow; effects of homocysteine and methionine. J. Clin. Invest. *48*, 284–289.

WEISS, H. B., WALKER, M. D., and WIERNIK, P. H. 1974. Neurotoxicity of commonly used antineoplastic agents. New Eng. J. Med. *291*, 75–81, 127–133.

WERKHEISER, W. C. 1961. The relation of folic acid reductase to aminopterin toxicity. J. Pharmacol. Exp. Therap. *137*, 167–172.

WERKHEISER, W. C. 1963. The biochemical, cellular and pharmacological action and effects of the folic acid antagonists. Cancer Res. *23*, 1277–1285.

WESTON, K. A., PERERA, D. R., and SCHULTZ, M. G. 1970. Pentamidine isethionate in the treatment of pneumocystis carinii pneumonia. Ann. Intern. Med. *73*, 695–702.

WILSON, J. E., and DUVIGNEAUD, V. 1950. Inhibition of the growth of the rat by L-penicillamine and its prevention by aminoethanol and related compounds. J. Biol. Chem. *184*, 63–70.

WISS, O., and WEBER, F. 1964. Biochemical pathology of vitamin B_6 deficiency. *In* Vitamins and Hormones *22*, 495–501, Academic Press, New York and London.

WOOLLEY, D. W. 1952. A Study of Antimetabolites. John Wiley & Sons, New York.

ZACHARIAE, H., and SCHIØDT, T. 1971. Liver biopsy in methotrexate treatment. Acta Dermat. Venereol. *51*, 215–220.

CHAPTER 8

Fetal Malnutrition, Abnormal Development, and Growth Retardation

Drugs and other foreign compounds have been believed to stunt the growth of infants as well as the developing fetus. Children have often been forbidden to drink tea or coffee because it might impair their growth. Similarly it has been suspected that pregnant women who are alcoholics may have abnormally small infants, and that if children drink alcoholic beverages they might fail to grow normally. There is now evidence from animal and human studies that this is not all folklore, and that many drugs are, in fact, capable of interfering with growth by one mechanism or another.

Despite extensive evidence that foreign compounds can impair normal fetal development, women continue to take drugs during pregnancy, even if these are not justified by the presence of physical illness. The following reasons are usually given to account for the taking of pharmacologic agents during gestation: 1) to maintain the pregnant state; 2) to induce abortion; 3) to treat disease associated with pregnancy; 4) to treat or control acute or chronic disease unrelated to pregnancy; and 5) to relieve various symptoms which may or may not be related to physical illness.

ADVERSE EFFECTS OF DRUGS FOR THE DEVELOPING FETUS

Forfar and Nelson (1973) studied drug consumption during pregnancy among 911 women. Drugs had been prescribed for 82% of these women during pregnancy, and the average number of drugs prescribed was four. Drugs taken as self-medication involved 65% of the mothers, and the average number of non-prescription drugs taken was 1.5. The duration of drug therapy for the various categories of drugs ranged from 10 to 125 days. Some of these drugs were administered early in pregnancy, some late, and some throughout pregnancy. In this study the five most common classes of drugs taken throughout pregnancy were iron preparations, analgesics, vitamins, antacids, and barbiturates. Among the drugs prescribed for medical purposes, analgesics were given much more frequently than any other drugs. Certain drugs were used chiefly in the first trimester of pregnancy including antiemetics. Most of the drugs used were given as symptomatic treatment rather than as specific therapy for defined diseases. In comparing prescription drugs used commonly by the

Edinburgh population studied by these authors, and a population studied ten years earlier in Oakland, California by Peckham and King (1963), it was found that the same drug groups were taken frequently, these being, apart from iron and vitamins, sedatives, antidepressants, tranquilizers and stimulants, antibiotics and sulfonamides, diuretics, antiemetics, analgesics and antacids.

Mirkin (1973) has reviewed the transplacental transfer of drugs and their distribution within the fetus. Placental transfer of drugs varies with specific drug characteristics such as their lipid solubility, their degree of ionization at a physiological pH, and their molecular weight, and also such properties of the placenta as its ability to metabolize the drugs and the age of the placenta. Whereas it has been found that, in general, drug distribution within the fetus may be similar to that within the mother, there is evidence for specific tissue concentration of drugs within the fetus.

Teratogenic drugs exert their adverse effects during the period of active embryogenesis, but many other drugs lacking specific teratogenic potential can impair the later development and maturation of the fetus by interfering in one way or another with its growth. Fetal malnutrition may be associated with fetal malformations or with impaired fetal growth, both conditions being inducible by drugs and/or by other environmental foreign compounds. Relationships between drug administration and fetal malnutrition have been studied in laboratory animals on many occasions, though it is difficult to extrapolate such data to human subjects. Major species differences exist between the teratogenic potential of drugs for different animals, and between laboratory animals and man. These differences may relate in part to differing nutritional requirements of these species as well as to such factors as the rate and mode of fetal development. It is often difficult to ascribe the teratogenic properties of drugs to their effects on fetal nutrition, because drugs may have other intrinsic toxic properties unrelated to their nutritional effects.

In order to understand the relationships between drug-induced fetal malnutrition and the production of fetal abnormalities, it is necessary to know the key nutrients for embryogenesis and also the nutrients that are required during the period of fetal maturation. To develop normally the fetus must synthesize proteins, including nucleoproteins. Whereas nucleic acids may be synthesized from certain small molecules within the fetus, protein synthesis requires the availability of essential amino acids derived from the maternal blood. Among the key nutrients derived from the mother, which are required for the synthesis of desoxyribonucleic acid and ribonucleic acid, none is probably as important as folic acid. Whereas many other macro and micronutrients including vitamins and minerals are necessary to fetal development, supply is usually sufficient for fetal demand, a situation which may not pertain with respect to folic acid. Severe folate deficiency during the period of embryogenesis is known from studies of experimental animals to both interfere with normal development and to promote the production of malformations. Prenatal cellular growth is dependent upon an adequate supply of riboflavin, and when this vitamin is in very short supply fetal malformations may occur. After the early period of embryogenesis, the critical nutrients are those concerned with brain development, bone maturation and the laying down of nutrient stores. Normal structural and functional development of the fetal brain requires the presence of pyridoxine which is necessary to protein synthesis and also in the production of neurotransmitters. Adequate placental transfer of vitamins A and D as well as sulfate, derived from sulfur-containing amino acids, is necessary for normal maturation of the fetal skeleton. An extensive review of the nutritional requirements of the fetus has been given by Giroud (1973).

Wilson (1973) has reviewed the literature in which evidence is presented of drugs which have a detrimental effect on human intrauterine development. He divides these drugs into four categories, as follows: 1) those positively implicated as being teratogenic; 2) those suspected to have some teratogenic potential; 3) those which may be teratogenic under specific conditions; and 4) those which do not have a teratogenic potential under the common conditions of usage. In these categories he lists, among other drugs, those which have been shown to have effects on fetal nutrition. Thus, among the teratogenic drugs, the folic acid antagonists figure prominently. Anticonvulsants, oral hypoglycemic agents and alkylating agents are considered as drugs suspected of teratogenic potential, and antituberculous drugs among those drugs which may be teratogenic under certain conditions.

FOLATE ANTAGONISTS

Early studies of folate antagonists in laboratory animals showed that these drugs were commonly lethal to the embryo. Indeed, these findings led to the use of folate antagonists to induce abortions (Thiersch 1952; 1956).

Nelson (1963) fed a folate-deficient diet containing 1% succinylsulphathiazole and 0.5% x-methyl-pteroylglutamic acid to rats for varying periods during pregnancy. Malformations occurred in the young, their incidence and types being dependent upon the time that folate deficiency was induced, as well as upon the duration and severity of such deficiency. The folate deficiency induced by this method of using a folate-deficient diet with a folate antagonist caused changes in the embryo when this regime was instituted during the critical period of organogenesis in the second week of pregnancy. Defects represented both retardation or stopping of development and also abnormal patterns of development. Malformations in the rat fetuses included defects of the urinary system, defects of the palate and face, with a high incidence of cleft palate, defects of the eyes and of the brain. In the discussion of Nelson's paper, Thiersch (1952) described a woman who received 10 mg of aminopterin in divided doses over two days between the 49th and 51st days of pregnancy. She aborted the fetus about 17 days after aminopterin administration and it was found to have an advanced meningoencephalocele and multiple malformations of the face. Several others have reported on malformations occurring in infants whose mothers took aminopterin early in pregnancy. In each of these cases, multiple defects in the osseous development of the skull have been described (Warkarny et al. 1959; Meltzer 1956).

Schorr and Steinbach (1968) described a female infant born to a woman who attempted abortion by ingesting aminopterin through the 58th day of pregnancy. This infant weighed 1750 gm at birth. The skull was almost uncalcified except at the base, and there were multiple bony abnormalities including very short forearms and legs. Although the chances of survival seemed poor, and also the chances for mental and physical development, this child did, in fact, thrive. A follow-up on this child was reported by Schorr (1972) when the girl was between eight and a half and nine years of age. At this time, cranial calcification was normal except for prominent bosses in the frontal area. The mandible was unusually short, and the teeth were crowded together and protuberant. The relative shortness of the arms and legs was not as noticeable as at the earlier time. Extension of the right elbow was limited. However, her mental development was normal for her age, or possibly very slightly retarded by the Stanford Binet score.

Chepenik and Moseley Waite (1973) studied the effect of a folate antagonist on the synthesis of subcellular organelles in the fetal rat. Maternal rats were fed a folate-deficient diet containing 9-methyl-pteroylglutamic acid from the eleventh to the fourteenth day of gestation. They found that the folate antagonist, or perhaps the combined impairment of folate metabolism by diet and the antagonists, stimulated lysosomal synthesis and depressed nuclear synthesis in the fetus. They also found disturbances in the chemical composition of various intraembryonic subcellular membranes.

Pyrimethamine used in the control of malaria and in the treatment of toxoplasmosis has been found to be teratogenic. The teratogenicity of this drug varies with animal species, and it has been shown to be much less teratogenic to hamsters than rats. In the rat, intraperitoneal injection of folinic acid given to the dam lessens the teratogenic risk (Sullivan and Takacs 1971). The danger of pyrimethamine to the human fetus has been considered when women are treated with high doses of the drug for toxoplasmosis during early pregnancy (Frenkel 1967). Since, however, toxoplasmosis itself presents a severe danger to the developing infant, it is recommended that pyrimethamine be given with added folinic acid.

ANTICONVULSANTS

Anticonvulsants are believed to be teratogenic under certain conditions. Diphenylhydantoin, phenobarbital, and primidone have all been shown to cross the placenta, though the degree of placental transfer varies with the stage of gestation (Melchior et al. 1967; Mirkin 1971A; Martinez and Snyder 1973; Stevens and Harbison 1974).

According to Speidel (1973), anticonvulsants known to impair folate metabolism may exert a teratogenic action through this effect on fetal nutrition. Two questions have be be answered: firstly, what evidence do we have that anticonvulsants are teratogenic in man, and secondly, what evidence do we have that any such teratogenic potential may be associated with the induction of folate deficiency in the fetus. Mirkin (1971B) studied three epileptic women who were receiving diphenylhydantoin throughout pregnancy, and these women gave birth to children with cleft lip or cleft palate. The association of maternal intake of anticonvulsant drugs and fetal abnormalities has also been noted by Pashayan et al. (1971) and McMullin (1971).

Martinez and Snyder (1973), who studied the transplacental passage of primidone, found that newborn infants from mothers receiving this drug had abnormal tremulousness but no congenital abnormalities were defined. Fedrick (1973), in his report from analysis of the Oxford Record Linkage Study showed that there are highly significant increases of congenital abnormalities among infants born to epileptic mothers. No relationships were found between the frequency in which the mother had fits, nor the length of time that she had had epilepsy, and the tendency for defects to occur in the offspring, except in the cases of two mothers who developed epilepsy in the first trimester of pregnancy, both of whose infants had severe malformations. Statistical evidence was produced in this study suggesting that anticonvulsant drugs were important in the association with malformations. Epileptic women who were taking diphenyl-hydantoin seemed more likely than those taking phenobarbitone to produce children with defects, but if these two drugs were taken together, the chances of malformations occurring in the infants were more evident. Women whose epilepsy was well-controlled so that no seizures occurred had as great a risk of having a child with a malformation as women who had frequent fits. Fedrick reported a wide range of congenital defects either noted at birth in the offspring of women who had received anticonvulsants during pregnancy, or noted at a later hospital admission or at the time of death. Many of these abnormalities were related to the skeletal system, and there were several cases of congenital heart disease. The reported defects do not appear to be similar to those observed in animals on folate-deficient diets with added anti-folate agents, or to those found in women who have taken aminopterin.

In view of the known effects of the anticonvulsant drugs on folate and vitamin D metabolism, it is possible that some malformations occurring in the offspring of mothers receiving these drugs may be due to nutritional deficiencies in the fetus, but other defects may be due to chromosomal effects of these drugs, or to effects of these drugs on hormone metabolism. Presently, however, there is no definitive evidence that congenital defects found in the children of epileptic women on anticonvulsants are due to the nutritional side effects of these drugs.

Apart from the structural malformations which have been found in the children of women taking such drugs as diphenylhydantoin and phenobarbitone, hemorrhagic episodes have been reported in such infants. Mountain et al. (1970) reported on a neonatal coagulation defect present in infants of women who received anticonvulsant agents during pregnancy. Evans et al. (1970) similarly reported neonatal hemorrhages in children of women taking diphenylhydantoin, phenobarbital and primidone. The coagulation defect found in these children is similar to that associated with vitamin K deficiency and is prevented by the administration of vitamin K. Conney and Burns (1972) believed that vitamin K deficiency occurring in neonates from women on anticonvulsant drugs may occur because these drugs are inducers of hepatic microsomal enzymes, and this may lead to an increased metabolism and catabolism of vitamin K in the fetus.

HYPOGLYCEMIC AGENTS

Oral hypoglycemic agents are now included among those drugs suspected of having teratogenic potential in man. Malformed infants have been born to women who have taken sulfonylurea compounds, such as tolbutamide, throughout pregnancy to control diabetes. Campbell (1961) and Larsson and Sterky (1961) were the first authors to report on the abnormalities of infants of women who had taken these drugs through pregnancy. Later authors have also reported on the teratogenic effects of sulfonylurea drugs in the infants of diabetic women. However, no syndrome of defects has been established, nor is it known that the association between intake of these drugs and malformations is nutritional in origin. On the other hand, there is evidence from animal studies that sulfonylureas do possess teratogenic potential, and that they specifically impair skeletal development. Smithberg (1960) and Smithberg and Runner (1963) found that in certain strains of mice there were embryonic defects involving the skull, ribs and vertebral column. These changes occurred after the dam had received single 20 mg doses of tolbutamide on day nine of gestation.

Because tolbutamide had been found to produce these fetal malformations in mice, Robertson (1968) decided to study the effect of the drug on sulfur metabolism in the developing mesenchyme-cartilage-bone system. He injected two strains of mice with sodium-^{35}S-sulfate on days 9, 10, 11 and 12 of gestation, or, in other groups he injected ^{35}S-methionine. Experimental animals were also given a teratogenic dose (10 mg sodium tolbutamide). There was a significant reduction in the uptake of radiosulfate in the experimental groups of both strains, but the level of uptake of ^{35}S-methionine was similar for control and drug-treated groups. The author proposed that tolbutamide may interfere with sulfate metabolism during the formation of sulfated mucopolysaccharides, vital to the formation of skeletal tissue. Tolbutamide may interfere with the synthesis of sulfated mucopolysaccharides or their precursors. Conceivably, as Robertson suggests, this could arise because of decreased formation or impaired formation of chondroitins which are dependent on normal carbohydrate metabolism. It is thought that drugs, such as tolbutamide, affect chondroitin formation by altering metabolism of carbohydrates and inducing relative or absolute hypoglycemia. Another suggestion has been that the drug interferes with the sulfation of acceptor molecules, presumably those of the mucopolysaccharides. Under normal conditions, sulfate is readily taken up by the developing fetus and is concentrated in tissues synthesizing sulfated mucopolysaccharides, particularly in the latter part of gestation. It is of particular interest that normally the sulfate which passes from the maternal organism to the fetus is derived from sulfur-containing amino acids in the diet of the dam or mother.

ANALGESICS

One of the most common classes of drugs taken by pregnant women, the analgesics, have been implicated as causing impairment of fetal development. Epidemiological evidence has been supplied by Richards (1969), who showed that more women giving birth to defective children had taken salicylate drugs during the first trimester of pregnancy than had women delivering normal children. Nelson and Forfar (1971), in a somewhat similar study of 458 women who bore deformed infants, showed that analgesics, including aspirin, were taken by more women with such infants than by those who had normal babies. It has been shown that salicylic acid inhibits the biosynthesis of mucopolysaccharide sulfates in cartilage and the cornea (Whitehouse and Bostrom 1962).

Another analgesic drug, salicylamide, has been shown by Lapointe and Harvey (1964) to induce fetal abnormalities of the skeleton as well as the circulatory and nervous systems of the rat and golden hamster when the drug is administered at high dosage. McGarry and Roe (1973) used salicylamide in rat studies in order to find the extent to which fetal development is affected by administration of compounds excreted as sulfoconjugates in the urine. Salicylamide is excreted both as a sulfate and as a glucuronide. Salicylamide was found to cause a significant reduction in the passage of radiosulfate to the rat fetus. The drug-induced reduction found in fetal and placental retention and maternal liver and serum retention of radiosulfate corresponded to an increase in the fraction of the injected dose of radiosulfur excreted as ester sulfate. While retention of radiosulfate by the dam was independent of the stage of pregnancy, the portion of the dose of the radiosulfate transferred to the fetus increased with increasing fetal age. Similar studies were carried out using indole as an endogenous compound undergoing sulfation with rather similar results. It therefore appears that accretion of sulfate by the maturing rat fetus is depressed by foreign compounds excreted as sulfoconjugates.

A later study in this series was carried out by Roe and Menges (1973) to show how maternal protein restriction, salicylamide or combined drug and diet treatments, would affect the fetal tissue distribution of radiosulfate. After injection of labeled sulfate, the highest concentration of the radioisotope was found in the fetal skeletons, followed by skin, intestine, brain, and liver, respectively. This was true in experimental and control groups. Protein restriction increased radiosulfate retention, and salicylamide impaired radiosulfate retention, by these fetal tissues as well as by the placenta. Drug-induced changes in radiosulfate concentration were significantly greater in the skeleton, skin, brain and intestine than in the liver or placenta. Urinary excretion of labeled sulfate in the ester form was increased in salicylamide-fed animals. It is postulated that mandatory sulfoconjugation of salicylamide may divert sulfate away from fetal tissues synthesizing sulfomucopolysaccharides or sulfolipids. Whether these effects account for malformations found in the fetuses from salicylamide-treated animals is not known at the present time, nor is it known whether salicylamide is a drug which can impair development of skeletal tissues in human subjects.

APPETITE SUPPRESSANTS

Anorectic agents such as dextroamphetamine may be teratogenic to animals such as mice and also in human subjects. This has been shown in the studies of Nora *et al.* (1965), Nora *et al.* (1967), and also in a survey by Nelson and Forfar (1971). There is no solid evidence to suggest that fetal malformations, either in experimental animals or in man, induced by anorectic agents, occur because of diminished nutrient intake by the maternal organism.

ALCOHOL

The infants of women who are chronic alcoholics have been shown to exhibit growth deficiency with lower birth weight and length than children from women who are not alcoholics. Jones *et al.* (1974) showed that not only does maternal alcoholism affect the physical growth of the fetus, but also the offspring may show abnormal features, including deficient intellectual performance. Perinatal mortality among the infants of alcoholic women is unusually high.

Observations of late dysmaturity and growth failure in six infants of alcoholic mothers led Ulleland (1972) to study institutional records on small-for-date infants and alcoholic mothers at the University of Washington's Harborview Medical Center, which serves a low income population. During the 18-month period of review, 1,594 babies were delivered at that hospital and of these, 2.9% were undersized. Thirty-seven infants (2.3%) of non-alcoholic mothers were small-for-dates, and 10 out of 12 infants (83.3%) of alcoholic mothers. Three of the alcoholic mothers had liver-biopsy proven alcoholic cirrhosis. The diets during their pregnancies of seven of the alcoholic women were studied, and also parameters of their nutritional status. Dietary histories indicated that five of these women had diets low in protein, calories, or both, during pregnancy. Laboratory tests showed that one woman had a hypoalbuminemia and another a low serum folate value. These findings suggest that growth failure in the infants of alcoholic women is multifactorial, being related not only to drinking habits but also to inadequacies of maternal diet.

ILLICIT DRUGS

Poland *et al.* (1972) studied the neonatal infants of teenagers who took illicit drugs either during a part of pregnancy or throughout pregnancy. Low birth weight infants were significantly more common among those women who continued drug intake throughout pregnancy. It is suggested that the occurrence of low birth weight infants may be multifactorial but that impaired food intake was certainly contributory.

In this study it is unfortunate that no attempt was made to identify whether hallucinogenic drugs, stimulants such as amphetamines or methylphenidate, barbiturates or narcotics were influencing the prevalence of small-for-dates babies.

Naeye *et al.* (1973) studied the adverse fetal effects of maternal heroin addiction. They reviewed the records of 82 drug-addicted women who had taken heroin through pregnancy, as well as the records of their offspring. The neonates whose mothers used heroin throughout pregnancy were small-for-dates. Since it was found in autopsy material on the neonates that growth retardation was due, at least in part, to a subnormal cell number in various tissues, it is suggested by the authors that the infantile dysmaturity was initiated by the heroin early in gestation. Their data suggest that heroin does have a direct adverse effect on antenatal growth, though other factors present in the addicted mothers may contribute to prenatal growth retardation. Such factors include maternal undernutrition, antenatal infection, low serum growth hormone concentrations in the fetus, as well as the effects of periodic episodes of heroin withdrawal during gestation. One or more of these factors, as well as the direct toxic effects of the heroin, may contribute to fetal malnutrition in the offspring of heroin-addicted women.

EFFECTS OF STIMULANT DRUGS ON GROWTH

It has long been suggested that many drugs cause growth impairment among children because of their anorectic effects. While it is true that in rodents such as the weanling laboratory rat, growth retardation may occur when any of a wide range of foreign compounds are added to the animals' diet, and that this is due in many instances to diminished food intake, such observations cannot be extrapolated to human subjects who do not usually take their drugs mixed with food. There are drugs, however, which have a primary effect as appetite suppressants, and these have been shown to impair the growth of young children. Several reports have indicated that when hyperactive children are given stimulant drugs to control their behavior, initial weight loss occurs, this weight loss being usually only of transitory duration (Knights and Hinton 1969; Eisenberg *et al.* 1963).

Safer *et al.* (1972) reported growth retardation in a group of hyperactive children also receiving stimulant drugs. They first studied data pertaining to 20 children in elementary school who were either taking methylphenidate or dextroamphetamine. The children's records were studied during the school year and then again when they returned to school after a summer vacation, during which time 13 of the children had discontinued intake of these stimulants. The second series of nine children studied by these workers had been taking stimulant drugs for the control of hyperactivity continuously for two or more years. Among these 29 children, it was found that dextroamphetamine in the dose of 10–15 mg/day or methylphenidate in the dose of 30–40 mg/day induced a suppression of weight gain. The children who discontinued intake of stimulants during the summer vacation gained more weight than expected for their ages, while those who continued on medication during the summer had an abnormally low weight gain. Among the set of nine children who had been on medication for two or more years, it was found that growth retardation in terms of diminished weight gain continued with the long use of medication. There was considerable variability in linear growth among the children. However, it was found that the percentile height changes correlated significantly with the weight changes, and that those children who were continuously on stimulant drugs showed a diminished linear growth as compared with hyperactive children who are not on medication. These authors concurred with the opinion of others (Silverstone and Stunkard 1968) that the growth retardation with respect to weight gain may be secondary to appetite suppression.

Partial support for this hypothesis was gained by Safer and his group who observed that more of the children on stimulants than other children had poor intake during a school lunch period. However, this is hardly enough to support such a conclusion. After this paper of Safer's was submitted for publication, he and his colleagues studied data on a further 49 children who had been on stimulants for two or more years, and in this study they confirmed that dextroamphetamine depressed growth, both in weight and height, as compared to controls, and that the growth retardation in children on dextroamphetamine was greater than that of children on methylphenidate (Addendum above paper of Safer *et al.* 1972). In an editorial (Nutrition Reviews 1973) describing this work of Safer *et al.* it is pointed out that further studies are required to corroborate the findings However, it is suggested that in all children on chronic stimulant therapy, anthropometric measurements should be made regularly, and that these drugs might be discontinued during vacation periods in order to induce catch-up growth.

In a follow-up study by Safer *et al.* (1975) it was shown that in hyperactive children, catch-up growth occurs with cessation of stimulant drug therapy. The degree of growth rebound appears to be proportional to the extent of drug-induced growth suppression. Growth rebound as well as growth suppression are greater with dextroamphetamine than with methylphenidate. However, if dextroamphetamine is stopped only over the summer while the child is out of school, the subsequent growth spurt does not fully compensate for growth retardation induced by stimulant drugs given throughout the school year.

There have been many reports in the literature of growth retardation associated with long term administration of glucocorticoids. In 1952, the author first saw a young boy who had had severe atopic dermatitis and asthma, whose growth was virtually stopped during a period of high level cortisone administration. Blodgett *et al.* (1956) described the adverse effects of cortisone intake on growth and skeletal maturation. Niermann and VanMetre (1958) described growth depression among the side effects induced by methylprednisolone in 47 cases of asthma that were studied. Suppression of growth was found in 4 out of 8 children who received methylprednisolone for 6 months or a greater length of time. Those patients who received an average daily dose of less than 5 mg/sq meter of body surface per day for up to 6 months or possibly longer, grew at a normal rate, while those who received higher doses of methylprednisolone showed diminished growth rates. Children who received 7.1 mg or more of methylprednisolone per sq meter/day had a growth rate which was from 17–60% of that predicted. These effects of methylprednisolone on growth were compared with a study conducted in 1957, at which time prednisone was administered, and no significant differences were found between the effects of the two drugs on growth rate.

As first noted by Blodgett *et al.* (1956) when corticosteroid drugs are withdrawn from children who have been on long-term therapy, a growth spurt tends to occur. Frantz and Rabkin (1964) described a standard test of growth-hormone secretory capacity which was based on radioimmunoasay of plasma growth hormone after insulin hypoglycemia. With insulin-induced hypoglycemic stimulation there was, as is now well known, a rise in the blood levels of growth hormone in normal subjects, whereas in patients receiving corticosteroids the growth hormone response was inhibited, the amount of inhibiting being proportional to the drug dosage. The inhibitory effect of large doses of corticosteroids on growth hormone release has also been demonstrated by Hartog et al. (1964).

Knowing that corticosteroids may retard growth, and also that in high dosage they inhibit the release of growth hormone, Matiasevic and Gershberg (1966) administered human growth hormone to two children receiving large doses of corticosteroids as long-term treatment, in the one case for asthma, and in the other for the hypoplastic anemia. Growth rate in these children, which initially was at a very slow rate, increased to a normal level during the treatment with the growth hormone preparation. When treatment with growth hormone was discontinued, the level of growth returned to the former rate. Urinary hydroxyproline excretion increased when growth hormone was given, and decreased when this hormone was stopped. The authors note a certain resemblance between children on chronic corticosteroid treatment and hypopituitary dwarfs, particularly with respect to growth rates which may be increased by human growth hormone, and also with respect to the changes in hydroxyproline excretion.

BIBLIOGRAPHY

ANON. 1973. The growth of children given stimulant drugs. Nutr. Rev. 31, 91-92.

BLODGETT, F. M. et al. 1956. Effects of prolonged cortisone therapy on the statural growth, skeletal maturation, and metabolic status of children. New Eng. J. Med. 254, 636-641.

CAMPBELL, G. D. 1961. Possible teratogenic effect of tolbutamide in pregnancy. Lancet 1, 891-892.

CHEPENEK, K. P., and MOSELEY WAITE, B. 1973. Incorporation of a phospholipid precursor into the subcellular organelles of 9-methyl-pteroylglutamic acid-treated rat embryos. Teratology 8, 175-190.

CONNEY, A. H., and BURNS, J. J. 1972. Metabolic interactions among environmental chemicals and drugs. Science 178, 576-586.

EISENBERG, L. et al. 1963. A psychopharmacologic experiment in a training school for delinquent boys: Methods, problems, findings. Am. J. Orthopsychiat. 33, 431-447.

EVANS, A. R., FORRESTER, R. M., and DISCOMBE, C. 1970. Neonatal hemorrhage following maternal anticonvulsive therapy. Lancet 1, 517-518.

FEDRICK, J. 1973. Epilepsy and pregnancy: A report from the Oxford Record Linkage Study. Brit. Med. J. 2, 442-448.

FORFAR, J. O., and NELSON, M. M. 1973. Epidemiology of drugs taken by pregnant women: Drugs that may affect the fetus adversely. Clin. Pharmacol. Therap. 14, 632-642.

FRANTZ, A. G., and RABKIN, M. T. 1964. Human growth hormones. Clinical measurements, response to hypoglycemia and suppression by corticosteroids. New Eng. J. Med. *271*, 1375-1381.

FRENKEL, J. K. 1967. Toxoplasmosis. *In* Comparative Aspects of Reproductive Failure, K. Benirschke (Editor). Springer-Verlag, New York.

GIROUD, A. 1973. Nutritional Requirements of the embryo. *In* World Review of Nutrition and Dietetics, Basel Karger, *18*, 195-262.

HARTOG, M., GAAFAR, M. A., and FRASER, R. 1964. Effect of corticosteroids on serum growth hormone. Lancet *2*, 376-378.

JONES, K. L., SMITH, D. W., STREISSGUTH, A. P., and MYRIANTHOPOULOS, N. C. 1974. Outcome of offspring of chronic alcoholic women. Lancet *1*, 1076-1078.

KNIGHTS, R. M., and HINTON, G. G. 1969. The effects of methylphenidate (Ritalin) on the motor skills and behavior of children with learning problems. J. Nerv. Ment. Dis. *148*, 643-653.

LAPOINTE, R., and HARVEY, E. B. 1964. Salicylamide induced anomalies in hamster embryos. J. Exp. Zool. *156*, 197-199.

LARSSON, Y., and STERKY, G. 1961. Possible teratogenic effects of tolbutamide in a pregnant pre-diabetic. Lancet *2*, 1424-1425.

MARTINEZ, G., and SNYDER, R. D. 1973. Transplacental passage of primidone. Neurology *23*, 381-383.

MATIASEVIC, D., and GERSHBERG, H. 1966. Studies on hydroxyproline excretion and corticosteroid-induced dwarfism: treatment with human growth hormones. Metabolism *15*, 720-729.

McGARRY, P. C., and ROE, D. A. 1973. Development of sulfur depletion in pregnant and fetal rats: Interaction of protein restriction and indole or salicylamide administration. J. Nutr. *103*, 1279-1290.

McMULLIN, G. P. 1971. Teratogenic effects of anticonvulsants. Brit. Med. J. *4*, 430.

MELCHIOR, J. C., SVENSMARK, O., and TROLLE, D. 1967. Placental transfer of phenobarbitone in epileptic women, and elimination in newborns. Lancet *2*, 860.

MELTZER, H. J. 1956. Congenital anomalies due to attempted abortion with 4-aminopteroglutamic acid. J. Am. Med. Assoc. *161*, 1253.

MIRKIN, B. L. 1971A. Diphenylhydantoin: Placental transport, fetal localization, neonatal metabolism and possible teratogenic effects. J. Pediat. *78*, 329-337.

MIRKIN, B. L. 1971B. Placental transfer and neonatal elimination of diphenylhydantoin. Am. J. Obstet. Gynecol. *109*, 930-933.

MIRKIN, B. L. 1973. Maternal and fetal distribution of drugs in pregnancy. Clin. Pharmacol. Therap. *14*, 643-647.

MOUNTAIN, K. R., HIRSH, J., and GALLUS, A. S. 1970. Neonatal coagulation defect due to anticonvulsant drug treatment in pregnancy. Lancet *1*, 265-268.

NAEYE, R. L. *et al.* 1973. Fetal complications of maternal heroin addiction: Abnormal growth, infections, and episodes of stress. J. Pediat. *83*, 1055-1061.

NELSON, M. M. 1963. Teratogenic effects of pteroylglutamic acid deficiency in the rat. *In* Ciba Foundation Symposium on Congenital Malformations, G. E. W. Wolstenholme, and C. M. O'Connor (Editors). Little, Brown and Co., Boston.

NELSON, M. M., and FORFAR, J. O. 1971. Associations between drugs administered during pregnancy and congenital abnormalities of the fetus. Brit. Med. J. *1*, 523-527.

NIERMANN, W. A., and VANMETRE, T. E. JR. 1958. Efficacy of Medrol in treatment of bronchial asthma in children. Metabolism *7*, 473-476.

NORA, J. J., McNAMARA, D. G., and FRAZIER, S. C. 1967. Dexamphetamine sulfate and human malformations. Lancet *1*, 570-571.

NORA, J. J., TRASLER, G., and FRAZIER, F. C. 1965. Malformations in mice induced by dexamphetamine sulfate. Lancet 2, 1021-1022.

PASHAYAN, H. H., PRUZANSKY, D., and PRUZANSKY, S. 1971. Are anticonvulsants teratogenic? Lancet 2, 702-703.

PECKHAM, C. H., and KING, R. W. 1963. A study of intercurrent conditions observed during pregnancy. Am. J. Obstet. Gynecol. 87, 609-624.

POLAND, B. J., WOGAN, L., and CALVIN, J. 1972. Teenagers, illicit drugs and pregnancy. Canad. Med. Assoc. J. 107, 955-958.

RICHARDS, L. D. G. 1969. Congenital malformations and environmental influences in pregnancy. Brit. J. Prev. Soc. Med. 23, 218-225.

ROBERTSON, D. W. 1968. The effect of sodium tolbutamide on the uptake of sodium-S^{35}-sulfate and ^{35}S-methionine in inbred strains of mice. Teratology 1, 387-392.

ROE, D. A., and MENGES, J. 1973. Distribution of ^{35}S-sulfate in fetal rats from dams fed salicylamide. Fed. Proc. 32, 746 (Abst.).

SAFER, D., ALLAN, R., and BARR, E. 1972. Depression of growth in hyperactive children on stimulant drugs. New Eng. J. Med. 287, 217-220.

SAFER, D. J., ALLAN, R. P., and BARR, E. 1975. Growth rebound after termination of stimulant drugs. J. Pediat. 86, 113-116.

SCHORR, E. B., and STEINBACH, H. L. 1968. Aminopterin-induced fetal malformation: Survival of infant after attempted abortion. Am. J. Dis. Child 115, 477-482.

SCHORR, E. B. 1972. Fetal damage due to maternal aminopterin ingestion. Am. J. Dis. Child 124, 93-94.

SILVERSTONE, J. T., and STUNKARD, A. J. 1968. The anorectic effect of dexamphetamine sulfate. Brit. J. Pharmacol. Chemotherap. 33, 513-522.

SMITHBERG, M. 1960. Teratogenic effects of some hypoglycemic agents in mice. Anat. Rec. 136, 280 (Abst.).

SMITHBERG, M., and RUNNER, M. N. 1963. Teratogenic effects of hypoglycemic treatments in in-bred strains of mice. Am. J. Anat. 113, 479-489.

SPEIDEL, B. D. 1973. Folic acid deficiency and congenital malformation. Develop. Med. Child Neurol. 15, 81-83.

STEVENS, M. W., and HARBISON, R. D. 1974. Placental transfer of diphenylhydantoin: Effects of species, gestational age and route of administration. Teratology 9, 317-326.

SULLIVAN, G. E., and TAKACS, E. 1971. Comparative teratogenicity of pyrimethamine in rats and hamsters. Teratology 4, 205-210.

THIERSCH, J. B. 1952. Therapeutic abortions with a folic acid antagonist, 4-aminopteroylglutamic acid (4-amino-P.G.A.) administered by the oral route. Am. J. Obstet. Gynecol. 63, 1298-1304.

THIERSCH, J. B. 1956. The control of reproduction in rats with the aid of antimetabolites and early experiments with antimetabolites as abortifacient agents in man. Acta Endocrinol., Suppl. 28, 23, 37-45.

ULLELAND, C. N. 1972. The offspring of alcoholic mothers. Ann. N.Y. Acad. Sci. 197, 167-169.

WARKANY, J., BEAUDRY, P. H., and HORNSTEIN, S. 1959. Attempted abortion with aminopterin. Am. J. Dis. Child 98, 274-281.

WHITEHOUSE, M. W., and BOSTROM, H. 1962. The effect of some anti-inflammatory (antirheumatic) drugs on the metabolism of connective tissue. Biochem. Pharmacol. 11, 1175-1201.

WILSON, J. G. 1973. Present status of drugs as teratogens in man. Teratology 7, 3-16.

CHAPTER 9

Alcohol and Alcoholism

While Leevy (1972) emphasized that obesity occurs in those who add calories from alcohol to a normal food intake, it is also true that the social and psychological maladjustments which lead people to indulge in alcohol may lead them to eat excessively with the result that they put on excessive weight and may become grossly obese. It has been the experience of the author and of other nutritionists that inability to relate dietary recall of caloric intake to weight gain in obese persons may be due to unreported caloric gain from alcoholic beverages.

Mitchell (1935) found that when alcohol was ingested by people on an adequate caloric intake, nitrogen excretion was decreased, suggesting that alcohol has a sparing action on protein utilization. More recently, Sardesai and Walt (1969) found that moderate amounts of alcohol may also spare fat and carbohydrates, thus accounting for observed weight gain in social drinkers.

Prevalence of malnutrition among alcoholics varies with socioeconomic status, with their dietary intake, the pattern of their drinking, as well as with the presence or absence of alcoholic liver disease (Vitale and Coffey 1971). It has been traditionally believed that excessive alcohol intake is inevitably associated with malnutrition. While it is still true that alcoholism is a codeterminant of malnutrition, the prevalence of avitaminoses and other nutritional deficiencies among indigent alcoholics has decreased since the Second World War. Bean et al. (1949) reported that there had been a decrease from 1940 onwards in the number of cases of pellagra among alcoholics admitted to a Cincinnati general hospital. They attributed this change to the improved economic situation of the population beginning with world War II, and to rationing which made nutritious foods available on a per capita basis.

Figueroa et al. (1953) reported that in screening 16,000 inmates of the House of Correction in Chicago they found very few cases of overt nutritional disease among alcoholics, and they only found seven men with a specific nutritional disease, and another seven with neuropathies of nutritional origin. The authors attributed the paucity of cases of malnutrition among the alcoholics to the success of cereal fortification with B vitamins and other nutrients. Neville et al. (1968) reported their studies of a group of chronic alcoholics at the Saint

Margaret's Memorial Hospital and the Nutrition Clinic of Falk Clinic at the University of Pittsburgh Medical Center. There was considerable divergence in physical condition, dietary history and life history within the group. They examined 34 alcoholics with respect to general physical condition and status for thiamin, riboflavin and niacin. Frank nutritional deficiency was found in only one subject. They considered that among their subjects the nutritional status was not markedly inferior to that of non-alcoholics, and that this was particularly true if persons of similar economic and health history were compared.

The etiology of malnutrition in alcoholics is complex. Whereas it is true that certain groups of alcoholics may have an inadequate nutrient intake, a primary factor which will explain in large part the nutritional deficiencies which are encountered is the fact that alcohol has a primary toxic effect on the gastrointestinal tract, the pancreas, the liver, the bone marrow and also other tissues such as the myocardium (Myerson 1973). Rubin and Lieber (1974) have shown that in primates the whole spectrum of liver disease can be produced in the absence of impaired nutrient intake. In a recent report, alcohol, 4.5–8.3 gm/kg as caloric substitution for carbohydrates, was fed by these workers to 13 baboons from nine months to four years. In these animals, alcoholic liver injury was produced, including fatty liver in all animals, alcoholic hepatitis in four, and cirrhosis in two. Their data suggest that a nutritious diet could not and will not prevent the development of alcoholic liver disease.

Lindenbaum and Lieber (1969) studied the hematological effects of alcohol in man in the situation where nutritional deficiency was not a factor. They administered alcohol to nine adult volunteers including eight men and one woman with a history of chronic alcoholism. The protein and vitamin intake of these subjects was maintained by feeding an adequate diet supplemented by vitamins including daily doses of 5 mg riboflavin, 2 μg vitamin B_{12}, 30 mg iron, 1 mg pyridoxine, 100 mg ascorbic acid, and 200 μg folic acid, except in four subjects who were given larger doses of folic acid (1200 μg folic acid by mouth daily). Two of the four subjects receiving the high intake of folic acid, i.e. 1200 μg daily, were also given 30 mg folic acid parenterally. Protein intake comprised 12.5% of total calories in five subjects, and 25% in four. When these subjects were given alcohol they developed bone marrow changes with vacuolation of promyelocytes. The presence of vacuolation of promyelocytes was dose-related. The bone marrow changes occurred in spite of the excellent diet and the administration of large doses of folic acid. Several other studies document the fact that high alcohol intake produces changes in the blood that may be due to direct toxic action of the alcohol on the bone marrow (McCurdy *et al.* 1962; Douglass and Twomey 1970).

Wu *et al.* (1974) studied 63 patients who on a chronic basis had been consuming more than 80 gm of ethanol daily. Macrocytosis was present in 89% of the subjects, but in only a few was this associated with anemia. Megaloblastic changes were found in about one-third of the bone marrow samples. Decreases in the serum, erythrocyte and liver folate levels were found in approximately one-third of the patients also. Macrocytosis was reversed when alcohol was withdrawn, but persisted when the subjects were given folate supplements if alcohol intake was not also stopped. The authors comment that "macrocytosis is one of the commonest abnormalities in alcoholics in the U.K." They believe that this is due to the direct action of alcohol on developing red cells, and that it is not necessarily due to folate deficiency.

In a nutrition and health study of 469 low income women carried out by the author in 1971, case histories included documentation of alcohol intakes. Complete blood counts were obtained for this sample. Whereas one might be skeptical about the accuracy with which these women reported their intakes of alcoholic beverages, it was found that the mean corpuscular volume of the red cells was directly related to alcohol intakes. The Pearson's correlation (r) between mean corpuscular volume and alcohol intake was 0.183, p < .001 (Roe and Eickwort 1973).

Malabsorption of vitamins has been documented among alcoholics. This malabsorption is associated with active or binge consumption of alcohol. Tomasulo *et al.* (1968) carried out a controlled study of thiamin absorption in severe alcoholics who had been consuming alcohol just prior to the study. They found a significant impairment of thiamin absorption in the alcoholic subjects in contrast to the controls. It was the opinion of the authors that the malabsorption of thiamin is responsible, at least in good part, for the thiamin deficiency which is found among alcoholic persons.

Thompson *et al.* (1968) were able to induce thiamin malabsorption in healthy volunteers by giving them large doses of alcohol at the same time as the test dose of thiamin.

Halsted *et al.* (1971) demonstrated that the jejunal uptake of tritiated folic acid was decreased among actively drinking alcoholics. When these patients were staying in the hospital and were not allowed access to alcoholic beverages, their jejunal uptake of tritiated folate returned to normal levels, i.e., levels found in control subjects. The authors consider this finding to reflect the poor diet of the alcoholics prior to hospital admission. However, it could also be explained in terms of a direct toxic effect of the ethanol on the intestinal absorptive mucosa which would then not be capable of absorbing folate in the normal manner. It has further been shown that binge drinking alcoholics have a decreased absorption of fat and also of D-xylose (Small *et al.* 1959; Mezey *et al.* 1970). These findings, taken collectively, add further support to the concept of the primary effects of alcohol on the intestine and it seems that malnutrition may follow malabsorption.

Alcohol has a direct toxic effect on the pancreas, producing acute pancreatitis and hyperglycemia which may be activated by binge drinking (Oakley 1968). Chronic pancreatitis is common in alcoholics (Feres *et al.* 1968). It has been postulated that certain of the nutritional effects of alcohol, notably malabsorption of certain nutrients such as amino acids and fat, may be secondary to maldigestion due to impaired production of pancreatic enzymes (Myerson 1973).

It has been pointed out by Wallgren (1971) that the consequences of excessive or chronic intake of alcohol can be classified into those changes which are due to the direct action of the toxin and those which are a consequence of nutritional imbalance. Whereas this generalization can perhaps be accepted, the very fact that alcohol has a primary toxic effect on tissues can lead to malnutrition because the affected tissues cannot utilize nutrients or are unable to store nutrients in the physiological manner. In the chronic alcoholic whose liver function is depressed, by alcoholic hepatitis or Laennec's cirrhosis, the stores of vitamins in the liver are depleted. This depletion of vitamins may be due to an inability of the hepatocytes to store vitamins. The impairment of vitamin storage may not be confined to the liver, but may also include other tissues, probably nervous tissue (Leevy and Baker 1968). It has been shown by Eichner (1973) that if alcoholic subjects are placed on a low folate diet they will develop megaloblastic hemopoiesis more rapidly than normal subjects. This finding has been explained on the basis of depleted body folate stores which are found in alcoholics who have been consuming alcohol on a very chronic basis.

Signs and symptoms of vitamin A deficiency may occur in alcoholics with cirrhosis (Patek 1939). These may variously be attributed to malabsorption (Sun *et al.* 1967), to impaired hepatic storage of vitamin A, or to competitive utilization of alcohol dehydrogenase for alcohol metabolism over the conversion of retinol to retinal, which is required in vitamin A-dependent visual and testicular function (Koen and Shaw 1966).

The relative unresponsiveness of alcoholics to therapeutic vitamin intake has been documented. Sullivan and Herbert (1964) studied the effects of alcohol ingestion in subjects maintained on a diet containing 5 μg of total folate daily over a period of several months. The authors found the hemopoietic response to administered folate, and they demonstrated that in those patients who were folate-deficient and also receiving alcohol, the response to adequate supplements of folic acid (i.e., supplements which could be used in normal subjects) was suppressed. The effect of alcohol in suppressing the hemopoietic response to folic acid could be overcome by eliminating intake of alcohol.

It has been accepted that a number of neurological syndromes occurring in chronic alcoholics can be attributed to vitamin deficiencies. Among these are Wernicke's disease, Korsakoff's syndrome and peripheral neuropathy, Morel's corticoid sclerosis, the Marchiafava-Bignami's disease, and cerebellar degeneration. At the present time, it is not clear whether one or more of these diseases is clearly nutritional in origin, or whether each is produced by primary toxic effect of ethanol on which nutritional impairment is imposed at the tissue level. By analogy with the effects of ethanol, which we have described in other tissues, it is possible that the effects of ethanol on the central and peripheral nervous systems are primarily toxic, and that then the tissues lose their ability to utilize nutrients in the normal way. Taking the example of Wernicke's disease, it is known that patients with this encephalopathy respond variably to therapeutic doses of thiamin, suggesting that the disease is not entirely nutritional in origin (Victor 1960; Allsop and Turner 1966; French 1971).

It has been demonstrated that alcohol increases the urinary excretion of magnesium and zinc. On the basis of several studies, it has been proposed that magnesium depletion arising from prolonged alcohol intake can be responsible for the symptoms of delirium tremens.

Patients with alcoholic cirrhosis are known to have low serum and hepatic zinc levels (Vallee et al. 1956; Vallee et al. 1957). Sullivan and Lankford (1965), who reported zincuria in 124 chronic alcoholics, found that excessive zinc excretion disappeared in one to two weeks following abstention from alcohol and an adequate diet. A defined symptomatology associated with zinc depletion has not been established in alcoholics, though Flink (1971) has pointed out the requirement for zinc in tissue repair processes, and presumably zinc depletion could retard repair of liver damage. Asymptomatic hypercalciuria and hypocalcemia have been demonstrated following ingestion of alcohol. Chronic alcoholism with pancreatitis may also be associated with hypocalcemia, but, in this condition, tetany may supervene, requiring intravenous calcium salts. Flink, who has reviewed the effects of alcohol on calcium status, has tentatively suggested that osteoporosis in alcoholics could be due to prolonged hypercalciuria (Flink 1971).

The nutritional problems of the alcoholic are more complex than those found in any other single group of subjects. Factors responsible include socioeconomic problems leading to impaired nutrient intake, psychological problems, and psychoses which again may alter appetite or food intake, perversion of eating habits, as well as the disease-related problems which have been discussed. In Table 9.1 and 9.2 the nutritional problems of the alcoholic are summarized and their interrelationships indicated.

It is important to remember that among malnourished peoples the excessive intake of alcohol may be the one factor which precipitates clinical vitamin deficiencies. Indeed, among populations with a limited diet, ariboflavinosis (Rosenthal *et al.* 1973) and scurvy (Lester *et al.* 1960) are more common among alcoholics than among other people. In previously endemic areas of pellagra, the people who still have this disease are often alcoholics (Roe 1973).

The risks of nutritional deficiency induced by medications are often markedly increased, when concurrently there is excessive intake of alcohol or when prior alcoholism has depleted nutrient stores (Kirk-

TABLE 9.1

ETIOLOGICAL FACTORS LEADING TO MALNUTRITION
IN ALCOHOLISM

1) Decreased or sporadic food intake
    Inebriation
    Indigence
    Appetite perversion
    Anorexia
    Psychoses
2) Increased nutrient losses
    Fecal
        a. Maldigestion due to pancreatitis
        b. Malabsorption due to GI effects of ethanol
    Urinary
    Toxic effects of ethanol on the kidney
3) Decreased nutrient stores
    Alcoholic hepatitis ⟍
                ⟍ decreased cell uptake of nutrients
    Laennec's cirrhosis ⟋
    Decreased nutrient intake (see also 1 and 2)
4) Impaired nutrient utilization—defective metabolism
                       —end organ refractoriness
    Alcoholic liver disease
    Toxic effects of ethanol on bone marrow

TABLE 9.2

CLASSIFICATION OF NUTRIENT DEPLETION
IN ALCOHOLISM

1) *Vitamin depletion* Folic acid Thiamin Riboflavin Niacin Ascorbic acid Vitamin B_6 Vitamin B_{12} 2) *Mineral depletion* Magnesium Zinc 3) *Protein depletion*

endall and Page 1958; Klipstein *et al.* 1967). However, in circumstances in which ethanol increases the metabolism of other drugs, it may exert a sparing effect on potential drug-induced vitamin depletion (Hansten 1973; Kater *et al.* 1969).

BIBLIOGRAPHY

ALLSOP, J., and TURNER, B. 1966. Cerebellar degeneration associated with chronic alcoholism. J. Neurol. Sci. *3*, 238–258.

BEAN, W. B., VILTER, R. W., and BLANKENHORN, M. A. 1949. Incidence of pellagra. J. Am. Med. Assoc. *140*, 872–873.

DOUGLASS, C. C., and TWOMEY, J. J. 1970. Transient stomatocytosis with hemolysis: A previously unrecognized complication of alcoholism. Ann. Intern. Med. *72*, 159–164.

EICHNER, E. R., and HILLMAN, R. S. 1973. Effect of alcohol on serum folate level. J. Clin. Invest. *52*, 584–591.

FERES, A., ORREGO, H., and NAVIA, E. 1968. Effect of chronic administration of ethanol on the incorporation of ^{14}C-amino acids into pancreatic proteins. Arch. Biol. Med. Exper. *5*, 62–67.

FIGUEROA, W. G., SARGENT, F., INPERIALE, L. *et al.* 1953. Lack of avitaminosis among alcoholics. Its relation to fortification of cereal products and the general nutrition of the population. J. Clin. Nutr. *1*, 179–199.

FLINK, E. B. 1971. Mineral metabolism in alcoholism. *In* The Biology of Alcoholism, Vol. 1, Biochemistry, B. Kissin, and H. Beglerter (Editors). Plenum Press, New York and London.

FRENCH, S. W. 1971. Acute and chronic toxicity of alcohol. *In* The Biology of Alcoholism, Vol. 1, Biochemistry, B. Kissin, and H. Beglerter (Editors). Plenum Press, New York and London.

HALSTED, C. H., ROBLES, E. A., and MEZEY, E. 1971. Decreased jejunal uptake of labeled folic acid (^{3}H-PGA) in alcoholic patients: Roles of alcohol and nutrition. New Eng. J. Med. *285*, 701–706.

HANSTEN, P. D. 1973. Drug Interactions, 2nd Edition. Lea and Febiger, Philadelphia.

KATER, R. M. H., ROGGIN, G., TOBORN, F. *et al.* 1969. Increased rate of clearance of drugs from the circulation of alcoholics. Am. J. Med. Sci. *258*, 35–39.

KIRKENDALL, W. M., and PAGE, E. B. 1958. Polyneuritis occurring during hydralazine therapy. J. Am. Med. Assoc. *167*, 427-432.

KLIPSTEIN, F. A., BERLINGER, F. G., and JUDEN REED, L. 1967. Folate deficiency associated with drug therapy for tuberculosis. Blood *29*, 697-711.

KOEN, A. L., and SHAW, C. R. 1966. Retinol and alcohol dehydrogenases in retina and liver. Biochem. Biophys. Acta *128*, 48-54.

LEEVY, C. M. 1972. Physiological and nutritional interrelationships in alcoholism. *In* Proc. Western Hemisphere Nutrition Congress III, Futura Publishing Co., Mount Kisco, N.Y.

LEEVY, C. M., and BAKER, H. 1968. Vitamins and alcoholism. Am. J. Clin. Nutr. *21*, 1325-1328.

LESTER, D., BUCCINO, R., and BIZZOCCO, D. 1960. The vitamin C status of alcoholics. J. Nutr. *70*, 278-282.

LINDENBAUM, J., and LIEBER, C. S. 1969. Hematologic effects of alcohol in man in absence of nutritional deficiency. New Eng. J. Med. *281*, 333-338.

McCURDY, P. R., PIERCE, L. E., and RATH, C. E. 1962. Abnormal bone-marrow morphology in acute alcoholism. New Eng. J. Med. *266*, 505-507.

MEZEY, E., JOW, E., SLAVIN, R. E. *et al.* 1970. Pancreatic function and intestinal absorption in chronic alcoholism. Gastroenterology *59*, 657-664.

MITCHELL, H. H. 1935. The food value of ethyl alcohol. J. Nutr. *10*, 311-335.

MYERSON, R. M. 1973. Metabolic aspects of alcohol and their biological significance. Med. Clin. N. Am. *57*, 925-940.

NEVILLE, J. N., EAGLES, J. A., SAMSON, G. *et al.* 1968. Nutritional status of alcoholics. Am. J. Clin. Nutr. *21*, 1329-1340.

OAKLEY, W. G. 1968. *In* Clinical Diabetes and Its Biochemical Basis, W. G. Oakley, D. A. Pyke, and K. W. Taylor (Editors). Blackwell Scientific Publishers, Oxford.

PATEK, A. J., JR. and HAIG, C. 1939. The occurrence of abnormal dark adaptation and its relation to vitamin A metabolism in patients with cirrhosis of the liver. J. Clin. Invest. *18*, 609-616.

ROE, D. A. 1973. A Plague of Corn. The Social History of Pellagra. Cornell Univ. Press, Ithaca, N. Y.

ROE, D. A., and EICKWORT, K. R. 1973. Health and nutritional status of working and non-working mothers in poverty groups. Manpower Administration, USDL Contract no. 51-36-71-02, Final Report. Addendum.

ROSENTHAL, W. S., ADHAM, N. F., LOPEZ, R. *et al.* 1973. Riboflavin deficiency in complicated chronic alcoholism. Am. J. Clin. Nutr. *26*, 858-860.

RUBIN, E., and LIEBER, C. S. 1974. Fatty liver, alcoholic hepatitis and cirrhosis produced by alcohol in primates. New Eng. J. Med. *290*, 128-135.

SARDESAI, V. M., and WALT, A. J. 1969. Biochemical and Clinical Aspects of Alcohol Metabolism, V. M. Sardesai (Editor). Charles C. Thomas, Springfield, Ill.

SMALL, M., LONGARINI, A. and ZAMCHECK, N. 1959. Disturbances of digestive physiology following acute drinking episodes in "skid row" alcoholics. Am. J. Med. *27*, 575-585.

SULLIVAN, J. F., and LANKFORD, H. G. 1965. Zinc metabolism and chronic alcoholism. Am. J. Clin. Nutr. *17*, 57-63.

SULLIVAN, L. W., and HERBERT, V. 1964. Suppression of hematopoiesis by ethanol. J. Clin. Invest. *43*, 2048-2062.

SUN, D. C., ALBACETE, R. A., and CHEN, J. K. 1967. Malabsorption studies in cirrhosis of the liver. Arch. Intern. Med. *119*, 567-572.

THOMSON, A., BAKER, H., and LEEVY, C. M. 1968. Thiamine absorption in alcoholism. Am. J. Clin. Nutr. *21*, 537-538.

TOMASULO, P. A., KATER, R. M. H., and IBER, F. L. 1968. Impairment of thiamine absorption in alcoholism. Am. J. Clin. Nutr. *21*, 1340-1344.

VALLEE, B. L. *et al.* 1956. Zinc metabolism in hepatic dysfunction. 1. Serum zinc concentrations in Laennec's cirrhosis and their validation by sequential analysis. New Eng. J. Med. *255*, 403-408.

VALLEE, B. L. *et al.* 1957. Zinc metabolism in hepatic dysfunction. II. Correlation of metabolic patterns with biochemical findings. New Eng. J. Med. *257*, 1055–1065.
VICTOR, M. 1960. The role of nutrition in the alcoholic neurologic diseases. J. Clin. Invest. *39*, 1037–1038.
VITALE, J. J., and COFFEY, J. 1971. Alcohol and vitamin metabolism. *In* The Biology of Alcoholism, Vol. 1. Biochemistry, B. Kissin, and H. Beglerter (Editors). Plenum Press, New York and London.
WALLGREN, H. 1971. Effect of ethanol on intracellular respiration and cerebral function. *In* The Biology of Alcoholism, Vol. 1. Biochemistry, B. Kissin, and H. Beglerter (Editors). Plenum Press, New York and London.
WU, A., CHANARIN, I., and LEVI, A. J. 1974. Macrocytosis of chronic alcoholism. Lancet *1*, 829–830.

CHAPTER 10

Nutritional Effects of Anticonvulsants

The anticonvulsant drugs, diphenylhydantoin, phenobarbital and primidone have been shown to be capable of inducing a biochemical or clinical folate deficiency or of inducing vitamin D deficiency as evidenced by rickets or osteomalacia.

EFFECTS OF ANTICONVULSANTS ON FOLATE STATUS

Folate deficiency or depletion may result from chronic intake of anticonvulsants. Numerous reports and reviews have appeared since Mannheimer *et al.* (1952) first showed that megaloblastic anemia might be a complication of anticonvulsant therapy. For reasons of common drug usage, most of the published reports of folate deficiency due to anticonvulsants are concerned with epileptic patients though other patients taking anticonvulsants may also exhibit folate deficiency (Haghshenass and Rao 1973). The prevalence of megaloblastic anemia in persons taking anticonvulsants has been found to vary from 0.15 to 0.75%. Reynolds (1972) has noted that this anemia appears to be more common in the United Kingdom, where 47 of the first 58 published cases were reported.

The frequency of hematologic and biochemical evidences of folate deficiency in patients receiving anticonvulsants has been emphasized by a number of authors. In a survey carried out by Hawkins and Meynell (1958) it was found that 20 out of 72 epileptic patients receiving these drugs had a mean red cell volume greater than 94 cu. μ, whereas this was so in only one out of 30 nonepileptic persons who were resident in the same institution where the survey was carried out. Klipstein (1964) carried out hematologic studies and microbiological assays of serum folate levels in 60 subjects receiving anticonvulsant drug therapy, and in five epileptics who were receiving no treatment. Subnormal serum folate levels, (that is, levels less than 5.0 ng/ml) were found in 58% of 53 subjects receiving diphenylhydantoin, and in one of seven patients on other anticonvulsant agents. The incidence of subnormal serum folate values was greater in subjects who had been taking diphenylhydantoin for periods greater than five years, but there did not appear to be any correlation with drug dosage. Slight or moderate macrocytosis was observed in 71% of patients receiving diphenylhydantoin who had subnormal serum folate levels and in 18% of subjects with normal levels.

Reynolds and his co-workers (1966) carried out a study of the effects of anticonvulsant therapy on epileptics and control subjects. The treated epileptics were an unselected group of 54 persons (mean age 33) among whom there were 31 males and 23 females. The control group was made up of eight patients with a mean age of 21 who had come to the out-patient department of the National Hospital, Queen's Square, London, and they had been diagnosed as having epilepsy but had not received any drug therapy. In this group there were four males and four females. The authors state in their report that a detailed diet history was obtained from all of these patients, and that they were taking a good or adequate diet with the exception of one patient who had a poor appetite and ate very little meat, vegetables or fruit. All of the patients, except one who was being treated with chlordiazepoxide alone, were taking phenobarbital, diphenylhydantoin or primidone, either singly or in various combinations. None of the treated patients were anemic. Hematologic changes found in this group included seven who showed macrocytosis and five who showed hypersegmentation of neutrophils in the peripheral blood. In 17 of the 45 subjects in whom the bone marrow was examined, megaloblastic hemopoiesis was found and when folic acid was given to seven of these patients, normoblastic hemopoiesis was restored. Serum folate levels were subnormal in 76% of the treated patients. The mean serum folate concentration for all the treated epileptics was 3.7 ng/ml and the mean value for the untreated control subjects was 6.4 ng/ml, these differences being highly significant. These authors were unable to demonstrate a definite relationship between serum folate concentrations and duration of drug therapy, and they noted that there was an occurrence of low folate concentrations and megaloblastic marrows in the early years of therapy. Because of the high incidence of subnormal serum folate levels in the epileptics receiving the major anticonvulsant drugs, it was suggested by these authors that the therapeutic and antifolate actions of the drugs might be related.

Folic acid is a convulsant when given intraventricularly to dogs and to rats (Hayashi 1959; Noell et al. 1960; Hommes and Obbens 1972). Baxter et al. (1973) compared folic acid and some known convulsants with respect to their actions following intracerebral ventricular and intravenous injection in mice. By either route the convulsion pattern produced in mice by folic acid resembled that with all other convulsants except strychnine and ouabain. The convulsant activity of folic acid was greater after injection into the ventricles than after intravenous administration, which the authors suggest may reflect either greater metabolism of folate or poorer brain penetration following the intravenous injections. It is suggested that high localized folate concentrations in the brain could form epileptic foci. In several cases there have been reports of increased fit frequency and in one instance of the evolution of status epilepticus when folic acid has been given in therapeutic amounts for the treatment of diphenyl-hydantoin-induced folate deficiency (Chanarin *et al*. 1960; Reynolds 1967; Wells 1968).

While increases in the number and frequency of fits may occur when folic acid is given in large doses to epileptics receiving anticonvulsants, this course of events is not uniform. Further, it is as yet quite unclear whether folic acid has any convulsant properties in man; indeed, the literature might suggest the reverse. Pharmacologic doses of folic acid do not appear to influence the mood or behavior of epileptic patients or normal control subjects. In experiments on Beagle dogs, Moir *et al*. (1971) showed that the administration of folic acid was without effect on the concentration of homovanillic acid, 5-hydroxy-indolacetic acid, and also the folate activity in the cerebrospinal fluid of these animals. According to the authors, these findings would be against the proposed central toxic action for folic acid.

Chanarin *et al*. (1974) injected intravenously a dose of tritiated methyltetrahydrofolic acid and then obtained cerebrospinal fluid samples either 4 or 24 hours later. They found that a significant amount of the labelled folate appeared in the cerebrospinal fluid samples. The highest proportion of the dose was found 4-5 hours after the injections, and lower levels 24 hours later. These results suggest that there is a considerable circulation of methyltetrahydro-folate between the plasma and the cerebrospinal fluid.

Mattson *et al*. (1973) investigated a group of epileptic patients with low serum and cerebrospinal fluid folate levels. These subjects were treated in a double-blind control study over a six month period, either with folic acid at a dose of 15 mg per day or with placebo material. Although there was some individual variation in seizure frequency and severity among the control and treated subjects, there were no significant intergroup differences. During the course of the study serum and cerebrospinal fluid levels of diphenylhydantoin and of phenobarbital increased in the control group and decreased in the experimental group; this was especially true for phenobarbital levels. All of the subjects treated with folic acid had a marked rise in serum folate concentrations but there was no similar increase in the cere-brospinal fluid folate levels. Since the cerebrospinal folate levels failed to increase during the six months of folic acid treatment, it was postulated that the anticonvulsants might be interfering with the conversion of folic acid to 5-methyltetrahydrofolate, and that this drug-induced effect prevented the entry of folate into the central nervous system. In order to test this hypothesis, six adult epileptic patients with cerebrospinal fluid folate levels below 20 ng/ml were selected for a three month trial of 5-formyltetrahydrofolate (leucovorin). Four of these patients had been treated with folic acid for six months in the first part of the study without a rise in cerebrospinal fluid folate. The other two had not been treated previously with any form of folate. All six patients showed a marked rise in cerebrospinal fluid folate levels when samples were taken for analysis three months after the initiation of the trial. There were no gross changes in seizure frequency or severity during the period of the test.

Several very interesting comments are made by these authors. They consider that anticonvulsant drugs interfere with the conversion of folic acid to 5-methyltetrahydrofolate, and that this accounts for their inability to demonstrate a rise in cerebrospinal fluid folate levels after folic acid administration. They also believe that, since folic acid decreased the cerebrospinal fluid content of the anticonvulsants, this may account for the increased frequency and severity of seizures which have been demonstrated by other authors in patients receiving anticonvulsants. Other authors have shown that folic acid decreases the blood levels of diphenylhydantoin (Bayless et al. 1971; Jenson and Oleson 1970). It has been suggested that folic acid alters the metabolism of diphenylhydantoin, but the indications that there is an altered parahydroxylation of diphenylhydantoin have not been confirmed (Buch Andreasen et al. 1971).

In spite of the risk of reducing cerebrospinal fluid and presumably brain levels of anticonvulsants by administration of large doses of folic acid, there is ample justification for the administration of small amounts of folic acid to correct folate deficiency in epileptics on drug treatment. Severe folate deficiency may cause neurological deficits (Reynolds et al. 1973). When Neubauer (1970) gave both folic acid and vitamin B_{12} to epileptic children with folate deficiency there was an improvement in their mental condition. However, their treatment was not uniformly successful and this may be due to the fact that the dose of folic acid in some instances was as high as 15 mg/day, and in others as low as 5 mg/week. All of the patients had been treated with anticonvulsant drugs for several years.

Many hypotheses have been put forward to account for the effects of anticonvulsants on folate metabolism. Diphenylhydantoin has been supposed to impair food folate absorption by inhibiting intestinal conjugase (polyglutamate hydrolase) (Hoffbrand and Necheles 1968). However, more recently Perry and Chanarin (1972) have convincingly shown that diphenylhydantoin does not interfere with the absorption of either mono- or polyglutamate forms of folate. Further, *in vitro* studies have produced no evidence that this drug inhibits conjugases in human intestine, liver, or brain (Baugh and Krumdieck 1969). Reverting to the assertion by Perry and Chanarin, that diphenylhydantoin does not affect the absorption of folate, certain comments with respect to their methodology should be mentioned. They pre-saturated their healthy volunteers with 15 mg folic acid, given by the oral route 36 hours before each test. An oral test dose of pteroylmonoglutamic acid or of yeast polyglutamate with or without 100 mg of diphenylhydantoin was then administered. Peak serum folate levels were measured as well as the urinary excretion of folate. The urinary excretion of folate was not significantly different in persons given the anticonvulsant drug and those who received the folate alone.

Gerson *et al.* (1972) studied the effects of diphenylhydantoin on the absorption of tritiated pteroylglutamic acid with a triple lumen perfusion system in nine healthy volunteers. There was a significant reduction in tritiated folic acid absorption when diphenylhydantoin was added to the perfusion solution. In some subjects this inhibition of folate absorption was sustained for as long as two hours. If diphenylhydantoin slows the absorption of folate into the intestinal mucosal cells but does not impair release of the active form of the vitamin from the liver into the blood, then the apparent contradiction between the findings of Gerson and those of Perry and Chanarin would be removed. According to Benn *et al.* (1971) the administration of folic acid in the monoglutamic form with either sodium bicarbonate or diphenylhydantoin results in lower serum levels of folic acid than when the vitamin is administered alone. These workers believe that the diphenylhydantoin, like the bicarbonate, increases the intraluminal pH of the gut, and that this effect is responsible for the impaired absorption of folic acid.

Anticonvulsants have been termed "antifolates," but this is misleading. *In vitro* studies have failed to show any effect of these drugs on the growth of folate-dependent mutant bacteria, nor do these drugs inhibit the function of dihydrofolate reductase, 5,10-methylenetetrahydrofolate dehydrogenase or tetrahydrofolate formylase (Hamfelt and Wilmanno 1965).

Folate may be required as a co-factor in hydroxylation of foreign compounds. It has been suggested that prolonged administration of drugs such as diphenylhydantoin, capable of inducing microsomal drug-metabolizing enzymes, will therefore increase the demand for folate and could cause deficiency. Maxwell *et al.* (1972) studying a group of 75 children with epilepsy found that their degree of folate deficiency was significantly related to increased hepatic microsomal enzyme activity as assessed from an increased urinary excretion of D-glucaric acid. Richens and Waters (1971) also suggested that enzyme induction could be an etiological factor in anticonvulsant-induced folate deficiency. In a later comment Richens (1972) points out that it is still not clear whether measurements of urinary D-glucaric acid offer a precise method for the study of hepatic enzyme induction.

From the files of the Oxford Record Linkage Study in the United Kingdom, Fedrick (1973) has abstracted information on infants born to epileptic women and control subjects. The mothers of the children included in this study were matched exactly for social class, civil status, age, parity, hospital and year of delivery. There was a very significant excess of congenital abnormalities among the infants born to epileptic mothers. Neither the frequency of fits nor the length of time that the women had had epilepsy bore any relationship to the frequency of defects in the offspring, except in two cases of women who developed epilepsy in the first trimester of pregnancy. Both of the infants of these women had major abnormalities. The information obtained suggested that anticonvulsant drugs might be responsible for producing the malformations; more particularly, diphenylhydantoin or a combination of diphenylhydantoin and another anticonvulsant required, such as phenobarbital. Since folate deficiency is known to induce these malformations, at least in certain animal species, it has been inferred that perhaps epileptic women receiving anticonvulsants developed a folate deficiency which leads to fetal malformations.

Vitamin B_{12}

While certain authors have shown that anticonvulsants may impair vitamin B_{12} absorption, most writers studying epileptic patients on these drugs have not shown that their vitamin B_{12} status is decreased (Lees 1961; Reynolds et al. 1965). In the study by Reynolds et al. (1966) of epileptics receiving anticonvulsants and a control group, serum vitamin B_{12} levels were nearly always within the normal range and there were no intergroup differences.

In a study by Leary (1973), serum vitamin B_{12} levels of treated epileptic children were found to be significantly lower than those in a control group who were attending a hospital in Cape Town for the treatment of minor traumatic lesions. Hunter et al. (1969) gave folic acid at a dose of 15 mg/day over a period of three months to 31 patients on long-term anticonvulsant medication who had reduced serum folate levels at the beginning of the study. Serum vitamin

B_{12} levels were measured in this experimental group before and after treatment and also in a control group of 21 persons. After administration of the folic acid the mean serum B_{12} level fell by almost half, and there were very marked and significant differences in the post-treatment vitamin B_{12} levels of the experimental group after treatment as contrasted with the control group. The authors note that in cases of pernicious anemia, treatment with folic acid leads to a further fall in serum vitamin B_{12}, an effect which has been attributed to the utilization of depleted vitamin B_{12} stores in hemopoiesis. There appears to be a risk that large doses of folic acid given to patients on anticonvulsants could precipitate clinical vitamin B_{12} deficiency, more particularly if prior malabsorption was present, or vitamin B_{12} status was already impaired by some other mechanism.

In the management of epileptics, serum and erythrocyte folate levels, serum vitamin B_{12} levels, and hematologic profiles should be carried out, before treatment is initiated and thereafter at regular intervals. The administration of folic acid should be such as to overcome the increased folate requirement induced by the anticonvulsant drugs. The effects of folate supplementation should always be carefully followed from a hematologic and biochemical standpoint.

Vitamin D

Vitamin D deficiency, associated with intake of anticonvulsants, has already been discussed in relation to drug-induced malabsorption. In view of the importance of this subject, a summary of our current state of knowledge is in order, as also an indication of the major gaps in our understanding of the mechanisms whereby anticonvulsants impair vitamin D status. Indications for the effectiveness of vitamin D supplementation in epileptic patients on anticonvulsants will also be discussed. Clinical rickets and osteomalacia are uncommon complications of long-term anticonvulsant therapy. In large groups of epileptic patients on these drugs a subclinical abnormality of calcium metabolism has commonly been found, with low serum calcium levels occurring in 20–30% of such patients and raised serum alkaline-phosphatase levels in 25–30% of the patients. Radiological bone changes indicative of rickets or osteomalacia occur in 15% up to 80%, and reduced bone mineral content which has been measured by proton absorptiometry in all patients examined. In this summary, which is extracted from an article by Bowden (1974), it is pointed out that most group studies have been carried out on institutionalized epileptic patients who have been treated for many years with combinations of anticonvulsant drugs, but that in non-institutionalized outpatients the results are similar.

Factors conducive to the development of rickets or osteomalacia in epileptic patients on anticonvulsant drugs relate to prior impairment of vitamin D status by inadequate dietary intake of vitamin D and/or low exposure to ultraviolet light, so that there is inadequate synthesis of vitamin D in the skin.

Clinical reports since 1962 reveal that both rickets and osteomalacia are common among immigrant Asians, particularly Pakistanis in Britain. The high frequency of these forms of vitamin D deficiency among Asians in Britain has been explained both by their low intake of vitamin D and their inadequate exposure to sunlight (Hodgkin et al. 1973). A recent report suggests that a moderate form of subclinical vitamin D deficiency may not be uncommon in Britain, not only among immigrants but also among other children. When Cooke et al. (1974) gave calciferol therapy for a year to white, Asian, and West Indian school children, there was a highly significant increase in height and weight when compared to other school children who were not so treated. Dietary studies on a sub-sample of the total survey population showed a low average intake of vitamin D. Estimates of 25-hydroxycholecalciferol levels on a sub-sample of the children studied were low, particularly among the Asian population. The authors conclude that there is a significant problem of vitamin D deficiency, both among Asian and West Indian young people, and that white children may also be affected to some degree.

There is as yet no comparable study of children or adolescents in the U.S. to demonstrate whether or not similar conditions pertain, particularly in inner-city populations. However, this possibility cannot be dismissed. In view of the British findings there is a real likelihood that epileptics who are put onto anticonvulsants may have an impaired vitamin D status prior to treatment. Thus, while Bowden suggests that biochemical screening of persons on anticonvulsants should be restricted to those who are at risk, this seems to be a rather limited and perhaps inadequate approach. He has considered that at risk are those who have dark skins, children and pregnant women whose diet and exposure to sunlight may be inadequate, and patients on chronic high dose of multiple drug anticonvulsant therapy.

Hypomagnesemia, as well as hypocalcemia, has been found in epileptics on anticonvulsant drugs. On the assumption that abnormal levels of calcium and magnesium might increase fit frequency, Christiansen et al. (1974) administered vitamin D_2 or a placebo to epileptic patients on anticonvulsant drugs. The number of fits was reduced during treatment with vitamin D_2 but not with the placebo, this effect being unrelated to changes in serum calcium or magnesium. It is suggested that epileptics should be treated prophylactically with vitamin D, though this general viewpoint is not accepted by all other authors. Variability has been shown in the response of anticonvulsant rickets to vitamin D or its metabolite.

In a survey of 134 institutionalized patients on anticonvulsants (these were all children), it was found by Lifschitz and MacLaren (1973) that eight had radiological evidence of rickets. These eight patients, who were between the ages of three and nine years, had severe cerebral palsy, lived indoors most of the time, and also had some chronic recurrent infections. They had been treated for more than three years with combinations anticonvulsant therapy including diphenylhydantoin, primidone and phenobarbital. Rickets persisted with daily supplements of 8-2000 units of vitamin D. The disease also persisted in three patients who were receiving less than 6000 units of vitamin D daily, one of whom received 6000 daily for 10 months. One patient in this series responded to 15,000 of vitamin D daily for 10 weeks and two responded to a single oral dose of 600,000 units. However, oral daily doses of 50 units of 25-hydroxycholecalciferol produced rapid healing in five patients. The rapid response to this hepatic vitamin D metabolite has suggested that the mechanism for anticonvulsant rickets induction is that of interference with vitamin D metabolism at the stage of hepatic conversion from cholecalciferol to 25-hydroxycholecalciferol. As soon as 25-hydroxycholecalciferol is available in quantity it would appear to be the treatment of choice in patients who have actually developed rickets or osteomalacia as a result of intake of anticonvulsants.

BIBLIOGRAPHY

BAUGH, C. M., and KRUMDIECK, C. L. 1969. Effects of phenytoin on folic-acid conjugases in man. Lancet 2, 519-521.
BAXTER, M. G., MILLER, A. A., and WEBSTER, R. A. 1973. Some studies on the convulsant action of folic acid. Brit. J. Pharm. 48, 350P-351P.
BAYLIS, E. M. et al. 1971. Influence of folic acid on blood-phenytoin levels. Lancet 1, 62-64.
BENN, A. et al. 1971. Effect of intraluminal pH on the absorption of pteroyl-monoglutamic acid. Brit. Med. J. 1, 148-150.
BOWDEN, A. M. 1974. Anticonvulsants and calcium metabolism. Develop. Med. Child Neurol. 16, 214-217.
BUCH ANDREASEN, P. et al. 1971. Folic acid and the half-life of diphenyl-hydantoin in man. Acta Neurol. Scand. 47, 117-119.
CHANARIN, I., LAIDLOW, J., LOUGHRIDGE, L. W., and MOLLIN, D. L. 1960. Megaloblastic anaemia due to phenobarbitone. The convulsant action of therapeutic doses of folic acid. Brit. Med. J. 1, 1099-1102.
CHANARIN, I., PERRY, J., and REYNOLDS, E. H. 1974. Transport of 5-methyltetrahydrofolic acid into the cerebrospinal fluid in man. Clin. Sci. Molec. Med. 46, 369-373.
CHRISTIANSEN, C., RØDBRO, P., and SJO, O. 1974. "Anticonvulsant action" of vitamin D in epileptic patients? A controlled pilot study. Brit. Med. J. 2, 258-259.

COOKE, W. T. *et al.* 1974. Rickets, growth and alkaline phosphatase in urban adolescents. Brit. Med. J. *2*, 293-297.
FEDRICK, J. 1973. Epilepsy and pregnancy: a report from the Oxford record linkage study. Brit. Med. J. *2*, 442-448.
GERSON, C. D. *et al.* 1972. Inhibition by diphenylhydantoin of folic acid absorption in man. Gastroenterology *63*, 246-251.
HAGHSHENASS, M., and RAO, D. B. 1973. Serum folate levels during anticonvulsant therapy with diphenylhydantoin. J. Am. Geriat. Soc. *21*, 275-277.
HAMFELT, A., and WILMANNO, S. 1965. Inhibition studies on folic acid metabolism with drug suspected to act on the myeloproliferative system. Clin. Chem. Acta *12*, 144-152.
HAWKINS, C. F., and MEYNELL, M. J. 1958. Macrocytosis and macrocytic anaemia caused by anticonvulsant drugs. Quart. J. Med. *27*, 45-63.
HAYASHI, T. 1959. Neurophysiology and Neurochemistry of Convulsion. Dainihon-Tosho Co., Tokyo.
HODGKIN, P. *et al.* 1973. Vitamin D deficiency in Asians at home and in Britain. Lancet *2*, 167-172.
HOFFBRAND, A. V., and NECHELES, P. F. 1968. Mechanism of folate deficiency in patients receiving phenytoin. Lancet *2*, 528-530.
HOMMES, O. R., and OBBENS, E. A. M. T. 1972. The epileptogenic action of NA-folate in the rat. J. Neurol. Sci. *16*, 271-281.
HUNTER, R., BARNES, J., and MATTHEWS, D. M. 1969. Effect of folic acid supplements on serum-vitamin-B_{12} levels in patients on anticonvulsants. Lancet *2*, 664-667.
JENSEN, O. N., and OLESEN, O. V. 1970. Subnormal serum folate due to anticonvulsive therapy: A double-blind study of the effect of folic acid treatment in patients with drug-induced subnormal serum folates. Arch. Neurol. *22*, 181-182.
KLIPSTEIN, F. A. 1964. Subnormal serum folate and macrocytosis associated with anticonvulsant drug therapy. Blood *23*, 68-86.
LEARY, P. M. 1973. Folate studies in underprivileged children with epilepsy. S. Afric. Med. J. *47*, 2245-2246.
LEES, F. 1961. Radioactive vitamin B_{12} absorption in the megaloblastic anemia caused by anticonvulsant drugs. Quart. J. Med. N.S. *30*, 231-248.
LIFSHITZ, F., and MACLAREN, N. 1973. Vitamin D_2, dihydrotachysterol (DHT) and 25-hydroxycholecalciferol (25-OHCC) treatment of vitamin D dependency rickets associated with anticonvulsants. Fed. Proc. *32*, 918.
MANNHEIMER, E., PAKESCH, F., REIMER, E. E., and VETTER, H. D. 1952. Hematologic complications of epilepsy treated with a systemic hydantoin. Med. Klin. *47*, 1397-1401.
MATTSON, R. H., GALLAGHER, B. B., REYNOLDS, E. H., and GLASS, D. 1973. Folate therapy in epilepsy. A controlled study. Arch. Neurol. *29*, 78-81.
MAXWELL, J. D. *et al.* 1972. Folate deficiency after anticonvulsant drugs: An effect of hepatic enzyme induction. Brit. Med. J. *1*, 297-299.
MOIR, A. T. B., HALLIDAY, J., and WILLIAMS, I. R. 1971. Lack of effect of folic acid administration on cerebral metabolism. Lancet *2*, 798-800.
NEUBAUER, C. 1970. Mental deterioration in epilepsy due to folate deficiency. Brit. Med. J. *2*, 759-761.
NOELL, W. K. *et al.* 1960. Cerebral effects of folic acid, pyrimidines, aminoacids and their antimetabolites. Electroenceph. Clin. Neurophysiol. *12*, 238.
PERRY, J., and CHANARIN, I. 1972. Observations on folate absorption with particular reference to folate, polyglutamate, and possible inhibitors to its absorption. Gut *13*, 544-550.
REYNOLDS, E. H. 1967. Effects of folic acid on the mental state and fit frequency of drug-treated epileptic patients. Lancet. *1*, 1086-1088.

REYNOLDS, E. H. 1972. Diphenylhydantoin. Hematologic Aspects of Toxicity in Antiepileptic Drugs, D. M. Woodbury, J. Kiffin Penry, and R. P. Schmidt (Editors). Raven Press Publishers, New York.

REYNOLDS, E. H., HALLPIKE, J. F., PHILLIPS, B. M., and MATTHEWS, D. M. 1965. Reversible absorptive defects in anticonvulsant megaloblastic anaemia. J. Clin. Path. 18, 593–598.

REYNOLDS, E. H., MILNER, G., MATTHEWS, D. M., and CHANARIN, I. 1966. Anticonvulsant therapy, megaloblastic haemopoiesis and folic acid metabolism. Quart. J. Med. N.S. 35, 521–537.

REYNOLDS, E. H., ROTHFELD, P., and PINCUS, J. H. 1973. Neurological disease associated with folate deficiency. Brit. Med. J. 2, 398–400.

RICHENS, A. 1972. Enzyme induction and folate deficiency. Brit. Med. J. 1, 567.

RICHENS, A., and WATERS, A. H. 1971. Acute effect of phenytoin on serum folate concentration. Brit. J. Pharm. 41, 414P–415P.

WELLS, D. G. 1968. Folic acid and neuropathy in epilepsy. Lancet 1, 146.

CHAPTER 11

Nutritional Effects of Oral Contraceptives

Oral contraceptives (OCA) have been available since the early 1960s and at the present time (1974) it has been estimated that approximately 50 million women in developing and developed countries are taking these medications for fertility control (Population Report 1974). The oral contraceptives fall into two general categories, the combination type and the sequential. The combination types are mixtures of an estrogen and a progestin, administered daily, over a period of 20–22 days of each menstrual cycle. With the sequential type the estrogen alone is administered during the first part of the cycle and the estrogen in combination with the progestin is used only during the later portions of the cycle. Estrogens used in oral contraceptives consist in either ethinyl estradiol or its methylester, mestranol. There are two classes of steroids used as progestins in the oral contraceptives: those that are structurally related to 19-nortestosterone, and those which are related to progesterone. The progestational agents which have been used in contraceptive steroids have the advantage that they are active when given by mouth. A comprehensive review of the functions of these antifertility drugs has been published by Saunders (1970).

It is generally agreed that contraceptive steroids cause an inhibition of ovulation and that this effect is via control of pituitary gonadotropin secretion. Oral contraceptives, both of the combination and sequential types, suppress gonadotropin secretion or release from the pituitary gland. The estrogenic component is mainly responsible for the suppression of follicle-stimulating hormone secretion. With the reduction in follicle-stimulating hormone levels, the maturation of the ovarian follicles is impaired so that ovulation does not occur. The progestins can affect luteinizing hormone levels which are necessary to precipitate ovulation. There is now a large body of information showing that contraceptive steroids exert both metabolic and nutritional effects. A review written by Theuer (1972) emphasized that oral contraceptive agents may alter the requirements of women for a number of vitamins and minerals.

FOLIC ACID

It was first reported by Shojania *et al.* (1968) that one of the long-term side effects produced by oral contraceptives was a reduction in serum folate levels. In the following year (1969), these same authors produced data showing that folate metabolism was impaired in women taking oral contraceptives as indicated not only by depressed serum folate levels, but also by decreased red blood cell folate levels and alterations in urinary FIGLU excretion. In another study, Shojania *et al.* (1971) determined serum folate, red cell folate, and the urinary excretion of formiminoglutamic acid (FIGLU) in 176 women receiving combination type oral contraceptives, and in 140 normal control subjects. The group taking OCA had significantly lower serum and red cell folate, and higher urinary FIGLU excretion. There was a rise in serum and red cell folate and a fall in urinary FIGLU excretion within three months after the experimental group stopped taking these drugs. In this study there were no significant differences between hemoglobin and hematocrit values between those on OCA and the control subjects.

A certain number of investigators who have studied the folate status of women taking oral contraceptives have failed to find evidence of folate depletion. Spray (1968) compared the serum and red cell folate of 19 women taking the Pill who were attending a family planning clinic, with those of 34 healthy control subjects, and could not find any difference between the mean serum and red cell folate of the two groups. McLean *et al.* (1969) determined serum folate levels of 39 women receiving two different oral contraceptives and serum folate values of 17 control subjects from a rural north-central Florida clinic population. They could not find any difference between serum folate levels of the two groups. Borderline folate deficiency was noted by these investigators in one-quarter of the subjects receiving the higher estrogen oral contraceptives, but a similar incidence of low folate levels was found in the control group.

Castren and Rossi (1970) studied 30 healthy women before and after three months treatment with oral contraceptives, and they found no significant difference in serum folate levels between the before and after treatment values. The mean levels before treatment were 6.0 ± 2.4 ng/ml and after treatment 5.5 ± 2.2 ng/ml. After treatment, lasting an average of 7.1 cycles, the serum folic acid level was the same as in the control period. These authors give no details at all about the dietary intake of folate among their subjects.

Streiff (1970) reported on seven women between the ages of 21 and 39 years, taking oral contraceptives for at least one and one-half years, who developed folate deficiency with anemia. It was stated by this author that the dietary histories indicated good diets, but no details again are given. Two of Streiff's patients with megaloblastic anemia had a hematologic response when oral contraceptives were discontinued. Another of his patients was treated orally with a daily oral dose of 250 μg of folic acid in the monoglutamic form, and on the fourth day of treatment showed a brisk reticulocyte response, and thereafter there was a rapid remission of her anemia. We are told that four of the other patients did not respond to dietary folate but showed hematologic responses following the administration of 250 μg folic acid/day, even while oral contraceptives were continued. On the basis of simple absorption tests in which either 200 μg monoglutamic folate or the molecular equivalent of polyglutamic folate were administered to 18 normal volunteers, nine of whom had been taking oral contraceptives for at least a year, and the other nine of whom had never taken these drugs, there were differences in the uptake of monoglutamic and polyglutamic folate between the two groups. Absorption of monoglutamic folate was not affected by the administered contraceptives, but according to the tests performed, the absorption of the polyglutamic folate was decreased approximately 50% in the volunteers taking contraceptive steroids. Streiff postulated that the oral contraceptives may interfere with the deconjugation of polyglutamic folate which is necessary to absorption.

Necheles and Snyder (1970) reported two cases of megaloblastic anemia in women taking oral contraceptives and they also studied the absorption of monoglutamate and polyglutamate folate in four women before and two months after starting oral contraceptives. Their results were similar to those of Streiff. Stephens et al. (1972) have reported that the absorption of polyglutamic folate in women on oral contraceptives is similar to that of control subjects if the absorption tests are performed after tissue saturation with a loading dose of folic acid prior to the test. These authors also failed to show any inhibitory effect of individual contraceptive steroid hormones on the hydrolysis of polyglutamic folate by human jejunal mucosal homogenates or guinea pig jejunal lysosomal preparations.

Shojania and Hornady (1973) carried out more exhaustive studies of polyglutamate absorption in women taking oral contraceptives and in a control group. They found that there was a distinctive population of women who showed polyglutamate malabsorption whether or not they were receiving oral contraceptives, and that these women were those who showed low serum folate levels before tissue saturation. There was no evidence of malabsorption for monoglutamic folate either in those on oral contraceptives or in the control subjects. The authors offered two possible explanations of their findings: that perhaps oral contraceptives have an inhibitory effect on polyglutamic folate absorption in only some women, or that those who have low serum folate and folate polyglutamate malabsorptions have had a mild form of malabsorption unrelated to the use of these drugs. They favor the latter possibility because there have been several studies in which megaloblastic anemia developed in contraceptive steroid users who previously had had various forms of recognizable malabsorption.

Toghill and Smith (1971) reported the case of a twenty-one-year-old housewife who had taken oral contraceptives for 13 months and developed megaloblastic anemia. She was given therapeutic doses of folic acid and contraceptive steroid therapy was discontinued. Although there was a hematologic response, jejunal biopsy taken two weeks after starting folic acid showed partial villus atrophy. Xylose malabsorption was not only present while the patient was receiving oral contraceptives, but also at the time of the intestinal biopsy.

Wood et al. (1972) described three cases of folate deficiency anemia in women receiving combined oral contraceptives. The first of these women was found to have celiac disease which the authors believed had been precipitated clinically by administration of the drugs. Their second case of megaloblastic anemia was in a woman who had been taking a marginally folate-deficient diet for a long time, and she became anemic only after taking oral contraceptives for a year. On investigation, she also was found to have evidence of malabsorption. Their third patient showed no evidence of malabsorption, but had a poor diet with marginal or low intake of iron, folic acid, and ascorbic acid. She had also had a past history of anemia which had required parenteral iron and blood transfusions. In this last case the bone marrow remained megaloblastic over a prolonged period after the woman had discontinued intake of oral contraceptives, and it was not until after four months following discontinuance of the oral contraceptives that her serum folate levels entered the normal range, at which time her red cell folate values were still low.

Johnson et al. (1973) described two women without obvious symptoms of small intestinal disease who developed severe folate deficiency anemia while on oral contraceptives. Their anemia developed again after these drugs had been discontinued. One patient was found to have the sprue syndrome and the other regional enteritis. The authors suggest that patients who develop folate deficiency while taking oral contraceptives may have prior disease of the small intestine, or that they may have a poor dietary intake of folic acid.

Information derived from animal and human studies suggests that endocrine effects of oral contraceptives per se on folate metabolism are insufficient to cause folate deficiency. Boots et al. (1975) treated normally cycling female baboons with daily doses of 0.25 mg ethynodiol diacetate and 0.025 mg mestranol for 9 months. Over this period, there was no significant reduction of serum folate over pretreatment levels. Unfortunately the authors did not measure the folate content of the baboon's diet.

Studies by Prasad *et al.* (1975A) have indicated that serum and erythrocyte folate levels in female subjects show wide variability whether or not they are receiving oral contraceptives. They could only find a significant reduction in erythrocyte folate levels in OCA users from an upper socioeconomic level. No significant effects of OCA intake on serum folate were reported. Although it is not clear from this investigation that blood folate levels were related to folate intake, in our own studies of healthy college women, we have shown that whether or not these women are taking oral contraceptives their serum and erythrocyte folate levels are highly correlated with their dietary and supplemental intakes of folate (Kelley and Roe, unpublished). In normal women it appears that the risk of folate deficiency in association with OCA intake is largely determined by diets low in folate which cause prior folate depletion.

There is recent evidence that the minor effects of oral contraceptives on folate metabolism may be recognized by examination of the cytology of the cervical epithelium (Whitehead *et al.* 1973).

Lindenbaum *et al.* (1975) examined Papanicolaou-stained cervicovaginal smears from the 115 middle class women taking oral contraceptives and 50 control subjects for megaloblastic changes. They based their definition of "megaloblastic" alterations in cell morphology in smears as being present when at least 10% of the nuclei of intermediate squamous cells were enlarged (greater than 10 μ in diameter) with or without an increase in nuclear-cytoplasmic ratio and frequent multinuclear cells. Using these criteria, 22 (19%) of the smears from women on OCA and none of the controls were megaloblastic. The authors comment that the cellular changes observed were similar to those found in megaloblastic anemia associated with folate deficiency. It is of interest that four of the women showing megaloblastic changes were on progestational agents only. The women in the experimental group showed no evidence of anemia or of leukocyte abnormalities suggestive of folate deficiency. Serum folate levels were similar in OCA users who exhibited or did not exhibit megaloblastic changes in the cervicovaginal smears and were not depressed in many of the women from either group. Eight patients with megaloblastic cervical smears were re-examined six months after continued OCA intake and again 21 days after folic acid supplementation (10 mg per day). Whereas their cervical smears were unchanged with continued use of the drug, folic acid (PGA) reversed the changes. Four of these women were examined again 3.5 years later without further folic acid administration and the cervical cell morphology had reverted to the megaloblastic type. It is suggested that OCA causes a local depletion of folate coenzymes leading to abnormalities in DNA synthesis by the cervicovaginal cells and resulting in the characteristic megaloblastosis.

Confirmation that folate deficiency, resulting from oral contraceptive use, is multifactorial has been obtained from some recent studies carried out in our laboratory (Martinez and Roe 1974). Erythrocyte and plasma folate assays were obtained from women during the first trimester of pregnancy, either recruited during the summer, that is, May to July (Group 1) or in the winter, that is, October to January (Group 2). The women studied during the summer had significantly higher erythrocyte folate values than those studied in the winter, whether or not they had received oral contraceptives prior to pregnancy. Those women who had received oral contraceptives within six months of becoming pregnant had significantly lower red cell folate and plasma folate levels than the control subjects who had not received these drugs. The lowest values for red cell folate were obtained in women studied in the winter who had also received oral contraceptives. The frequency of intake of rich folate sources in the diet was compared between the subjects studied in the summer and those studied in the winter, and it was found by food frequency records and by estimation of free folate intake that there were significant differences between the intake of free folate in the summer and the winter, in that intake during the summer was increased by the women eating a substantially larger amount of raw vegetables. In other words, seasonal and oral contraceptive-dependent differences in folate levels (red cell) were related to variations in folate source intake. Whether folic acid requirements due to pregnancy and oral contraceptive effects can be supplied by the diet depends on the availability of high folate foods.

Speidel (1973) has pointed out that folate deficiency induced by oral contraceptives and persisting into pregnancy may be a hazard to the fetus. Folic acid deficiency is teratogenic to laboratory animals, though presently there is no direct evidence that this is so in woman. It is suggested that consideration should be given to monitoring the folate levels of women at risk; i.e.: those who have taken oral contraceptives immediately or within six months before becoming pregnant. Further, folate replacement therapy is urged before pregnancy occurs.

Whereas the author highly endorses Speidel's recommendation that women, and particularly women taking oral contraceptives, should be screened with respect to their blood levels of folate, both plasma and erythrocyte, the practical problem remains that there are still insufficient laboratories capable of carrying our microbiological assays for folate, and the newer radioassay methods have still not been fully developed.

Several studies have indicated that the distribution and binding of folate is altered by sex steroids. Markkanen *et al.* (1973) studied the binding of serum folic acid during pregnancy and found that in the last trimester the binding of folic acid to serum proteins increases, particularly the binding to transferrin. According to these authors, similar changes in the binding of folic acid to serum proteins occurs with prolonged use of steroids, though definitive data are given.

Studies by Doctor *et al.* (1963) indicate that ethinyl estradiol increases the urinary excretion of folate metabolites in human subjects. The significance of these findings with respect to the mode of action of oral contraceptives on folate metabolism have yet to be elucidated.

VITAMIN B$_{12}$

It has been shown by Shojania (1971) that serum vitamin B$_{12}$ is lowered by chronic intake of oral contraceptives. In women who were studied by this author with respect to their vitamin B$_{12}$ status, normal Schilling tests were found indicating that vitamin B$_{12}$ absorption was not impaired. Whether or not a defect in vitamin B$_{12}$ metabolism in women on oral contraceptives is related to differences in folate metabolism in these women has not been determined.

ASCORBIC ACID

Briggs and Briggs (1972) showed that the ascorbic acid content of leukocytes and platelets is significantly lowered in women taking oral contraceptives as contrasted with control subjects. Rivers and Devine (1972) reported that the concentration of plasma ascorbic acid is decreased by ingestion of oral contraceptives. These authors later showed that subjects taking oral contraceptives containing an estrogen component and a progestational compound had both lower and non-cyclic plasma ascorbic levels.

McLeroy and Schendel (1973) investigated the ascorbic acid levels in the leukocytes of 126 healthy female subjects. Sixty-three of these subjects served as controls, and the other 63 had received various oral contraceptives for at least a year. The mean dietary intake of ascorbic acid was similar within the persons in the group, and was above the vitamin C requirements for the age group studied. The mean concentration of ascorbic acid in the leukocytes of women who had received oral contraceptives was significantly lower than that of the control subjects. Changes in ascorbic levels in the plasma and leukocytes have not been found to be due to increased urinary excretion of the vitamin. It is suggested that oral contraceptives may either increase the catabolism of ascorbic acid or change tissue distribution. The contraceptive steroids may increase the breakdown of ascorbic acid, by stimulating the liver to release ceruloplasmin, a copper-containing protein with ascorbate oxidase activity.

RIBOFLAVIN

It has been indicated by the work of Rose and McGinty (1968) that the requirement for riboflavin is increased by oral contraceptives. Theoretically, in any situation when increased amounts of pyridoxine are required for normal tryptophan metabolism, the need for riboflavin would be elevated. Wada and Snell (1961) showed that riboflavin is involved in the enzyme system oxidizing pyridoxine phosphate, which is the metabolically active form of this vitamin.

Administration of oral contraceptives results in increased plasma cortisol level (Pulkkinen and Pekkarinen 1967). When Rose and McGinty (1968) administered cortisol to subjects there was an increased excretion of abnormal tryptophan metabolites following a tryptophan load test. According to the work of these authors, niacin and riboflavin given together partially normalized the excretion of abnormal tryptophan metabolites in three of the four subjects who were given cortisol. Niacin alone was without effect, but these authors did not administer riboflavin alone. These studies are briefly discussed by Theuer (1972).

A more direct study of the effects of oral contraceptives on riboflavin status was carried out by Sanpitak and Chayutimonkul (1974). Their experimental sample population consisted of 42 women receiving oral contraceptives who were attending the family planning clinic of Chiang Mai Hospital in Thailand. These women had taken oral contraceptives of various types for periods from three to 96 months. None of them showed any signs of vitamin deficiency, nor had they taken any vitamin supplements for at least two months before the study. The control group consisted of 31 women of similar age and social status who had not taken either oral contraceptives or vitamin supplements for at least two months. Erythrocyte glutathione reductase activity has been widely used in recent years as an index of riboflavin nutrition. This test was used to determine the riboflavin status of the women in this population. Erythrocyte glutathione reductase activity was found to be significantly lower in the women taking oral contraceptives than in those who were control subjects. Further, when erythrocyte glutathione reductase activity was stimulated by the addition of flavin adenine dinucleotide, the experimental group showed values nearly twice as high as those obtained when a similar manipulation was carried out in the control group. The authors did not consider that the lowering of erythrocyte glutathione reductase activity in the oral contraceptive users was such as to interfere with the life span of normal erythrocytes. They postulate that, however, if abnormal erythrocytes were present as would be the case in subjects with glucose-6-phosphate dehydrogenase deficiency (G-6-PD) the moderate riboflavin depletion might be of more serious import.

Recently Briggs and Briggs (1974) reported on the vitamin status of three groups of African women living in the Republic of Zambia. All of these women were said to have been in good health, and none of them showed any clinical signs of vitamin deficiency. The first group were control subjects not receiving any drug therapy; the second were receiving oral contraceptives of the combined type; and the third group were receiving medroxy-progesterone acetate (Depo-Provera, Upjohn), a long-acting contraceptive. All of the women in the treatment groups were in the second or third month of treatment. Women taking the combined type of oral contraceptives showed highly significant decreases in the urinary excretion of riboflavin measured as $\mu g/mol$ creatinine, but this decreased excretion of riboflavin was not found in those who were taking Depo-Provera. Decreases in the plasma levels of ascorbate, vitamin B_{12}, were also found by these authors to be present in the women taking the oral contraceptives of the combined type.

VITAMIN B_6

Rose (1966) reported that estrogen, as well as estrogen-progestagen preparations, caused the increased excretion of 3-hydroxykynurenine and xanthurenic acid following a tryptophan load test. This author further showed that administration of vitamin B_6 (pyridoxine) in large doses caused the reversal of these urinary changes. The finding of these metabolites of tryptophan to excess in the urine of women taking these steroids was accepted as an indication of a subclinical deficiency of vitamin B_6. Measurement of the urinary excretion of xanthurenic acid after administration of an oral load of tryptophan has been accepted as a technique for the detection of vitamin B_6 deficiency. Several changes in the excretion of tryptophan metabolites are said to occur in subclinical and clinical vitamin B_6 deficiency. Not only is there an increased excretion of xanthurenic acid, but also an increased excretion of 3-hydroxykynurenine in relation to the excretion of 3-hydroxyanthranilic acid. In the pathway of tryptophan metabolism, the biosynthesis of several metabolites is dependent on vitamin B_6; including the conversion of 3-hydroxykynurenine to xanthurenic acid and the conversion of 3-hydroxykynurenine to 3-hydroxyanthranilic acid; also, the conversion of kynurenine to anthranilic acid and of kynurenine to kynurenic acid. The paradoxical increase in the urinary excretion of xanthurenic acid in persons believed to be vitamin B_6-deficient has not been adequately explained, though it has been proposed that in subclinical deficiency of this vitamin there is a primary block in the activity of the enzyme kynureninase, and that therefore there are abnormalities in tryptophan metabolism distal to this point. In a recent editorial (Nutrition Reviews 1973) it was pointed out that in many dissimilar human diseases perhaps associated with vitamin B_6 deficiency, increased activity of tryptophan pyrrolase rather than vitamin B_6 deficiency was the cause of the increased excretion of certain metabolites of tryptophan.

The urinary excretion of various metabolites of tryptophan along the kynurenine pathway was measured by Brown et al. (1969) in subjects following a 2 gm load of L-tryptophan. Subjects receiving combination estrogen-progestagen as oral contraceptives excreted elevated levels of kynurenine, hydroxykynurenine, kynurenic acid, and xanthurenic acid. The authors ascribe these changes to an enhanced efficiency in the conversion of tryptophan to niacin metabolites. Since these authors also had shown that both men and women receiving estrogens alone showed similar effects, the changes in tryptophan metabolism were thought to be mainly due to the estrogen component of the oral contraceptive mixtures.

Coon and Nagler (1969) have pointed out that the tryptophan load test as a test for pyridoxine deficiency is fraught with difficulties. Increased production of, or release of, glucocorticoids may bring about increased activity of tryptophan pyrrolase so that there is a shunting of a larger fraction of free tryptophan via the kynurenine pathway resulting in increased urinary excretion of kynurenine and hydroxykynurenine. Several other variables affect the results of the tryptophan load test. These include changes in the patients' protein intake and general state of protein metabolism. Both of these variables influence the amount of free tryptophan available for metabolism via the kynurenine pathway. When there is more free tryptophan available, this brings about adaptive increases in tryptophan pyrrolase activity. Wood et al. (1966) have shown that tryptophan pyrrolase activity increases in mice in the last phases of cancer as protein catabolism increases.

Certain drugs interfered with the tryptophan test, due to actual technical problems with the analytical technique. Such drugs include diphenylhydantoin and reserpine (Price *et al.* 1965).

Miller *et al.* (1974) studied the effect of oral contraceptives on pyridoxine metabolism. Three women on OCA and two control subjects were fed a constant diet containing 1.9 mg pyridoxine for 11 days. Blood and urinary levels of vitamin B_6 and the urinary excretion of 4-pyridoxic acid were determined; also tryptophan load tests were performed. The OCA users excreted less vitamin B_6 in the urine than control subjects, but the urinary excretion of 4-pyridoxic acid was similar in the two groups. The level of B_6 in the blood of the OCA users was slightly lower than that of controls. The tryptophan load tests on the OCA users showed the "abnormalities" found by other authors, though in addition diurnal changes were observed, i.e. differences in the excretion of tryptophan metabolites according to the time of the day the test was carried out.

Aly *et al.* (1971) did not find that oral contraceptives affect the excretion of vitamin B_6 in the urine of their subjects, but it has been suggested that this may have been due to the assay method employed.

Depression occurs rather frequently in women taking oral contraceptives, and the question has arisen whether it is a clinical manifestation of pyridoxine deficiency. Adams *et al.* (1973) have stated the theoretical reasons why abnormal tryptophan metabolism might lead to depression; i.e., increased metabolism of tryptophan via the nicotinic acid-ribonucleotide pathway could result in less tryptophan being available for serotonin synthesis; perhaps kynurenine and 3-hydroxykynurenine inhibit the transport of tryptophan across the blood-brain barrier; or pyridoxine depletion may affect 5-hydroxytryptophan activity in the brain.

Winston (1969) made the original suggestion that administration of vitamin B_6 might relieve the oral contraceptive-induced depression by relieving a deficiency of the vitamin. Baumblatt and Winston (1970) found that administration of vitamin B_6 to 58 women on oral contraceptives who had been complaining of pre-menstrual depression relieved the symptoms in 18 and caused some improvement in 26 persons in the group.

Adams *et al.* (1973) studied 22 women with symptoms of depression which were believed to be due to the effects of oral contraceptives. Only 11 of these women showed biochemical evidence of a real deficiency of vitamin B_6. In the group of women whose depression was believed from clinical grounds to be due to oral contraceptive administration, only half were found to have a biochemical deficiency of the vitamin, and only this group responded to therapeutic administration of vitamin B_6. Whether or not women receiving oral contraceptives should be taking prophylactic vitamin B_6 as a means of preventing depression cannot be defined from this paper, due to the small size of the sample. But in view of the risk of relative vitamin B_6 deficiency, there are many who presently advocate such a step.

OTHER NUTRITIONAL EFFECTS OF ORAL CONTRACEPTIVES

Vitamin A

Increased plasma vitamin A levels have been found in women taking oral contraceptives (Gall *et al.* 1971). Briggs *et al.* (1972) also showed that women taking combination type oral contraceptives had a significantly higher plasma vitamin A level than persons not receiving these drugs, but that the vitamin A levels of persons receiving a long-acting, parenterally administered progestin contraceptive did not show these changes.

Wild *et al.* (1974) confirmed that there was a significant increase in vitamin A levels in women taking oral contraceptives. These workers were concerned that high vitamin A levels induced by oral contraceptives might persist when oral contraceptives were discontinued and pregnancy supervened, thus conferring a teratogenic hazard. However, they found that during early pregnancy there was no significant difference in vitamin A levels between those who had recently been taking oral contraceptives and those who had not.

Vitamin E

In rats, some of the side effects of oral contraceptives resemble those of vitamin E deficiency. For this reason, Aftergood and Alfin-Slater (1974) considered the possibility that there might be an increased requirement for vitamin E in these animals. Slight but significant lowering of plasma tocopherol levels was found in animals receiving 0.002 mg mestranol and 0.05 mg norethynodrel per day for 4 or 28 days with vitamin E.

It was suggested that lowering of the alpha-tocopherol levels in the plasma could be the result of an effect of oral contraceptives on lipoprotein distribution and that it may reflect a redistribution of α-tocopherol due to decreased availability of the protein carrier. There was no evidence in these rats that the contraceptive drug mixture induced overt vitamin E deficiency, nor has there been any report that oral contraceptives impair vitamin E status in human subjects.

Vitamin K

A number of studies have been directed towards elucidation of the risk of thromboembolic phenomena, occurring as a side effect of oral contraceptive intake (Vessey and Doll 1968; 1969). The risk of thromboses is dose-related to the estrogen content of the oral contraceptives (Inman *et al.* 1970). In the laboratory rat, estrogens diminish the requirement for vitamin K (Mellette 1961). Increased serum levels of vitamin K-dependent clotting factors as well as other clotting factors have been found in women taking oral contraceptives (Egeberg and Owren 1963; Rutherford *et al.* 1964; D'Arcy and Griffin 1972). Mink *et al.* (1974) monitored the effects of sequential oral contraceptives on serum clotting factors in a group of women that they had under observation for two years. Vitamin K-dependent factor activity was elevated in women after a three months intake of OCA, and remained elevated for the period of study. Factor V and plasminogen activity were also elevated at three months but not thereafter.

These observations suggest that the need for vitamin K is reduced by oral contraceptives. In further support of this theory, it has been shown that women on OCA exhibit a subnormal response to coumarin anticoagulants (Scrogie *et al.* 1967).

Zinc

Halsted *et al.* (1968) reported that women taking oral contraceptives have significantly lower plasma zinc levels than control subjects. There has been some concern that OCA may increase zinc requirements.

However, Prasad *et al.* (1975B), while confirming the earlier reports of lowered plasma zinc as a result of OCA intake, found that women receiving Norinyl (1 mg norethindrone and 50 μg mestranol) had slightly elevated erythrocyte zinc levels. They consider the possibility that OCA may cause a redistribution of zinc between red cells and plasma rather than an actual zinc depletion.

Copper

Increases in blood copper levels and in ceruloplasmin levels have been found in women taking OCA, and it has been suggested that these drugs may increase the absorption of dietary copper (O'Leary and Spellacy 1968; Tovey and Lathe 1968).

Calcium

Caniggia *et al.* (1970) administered a combined type oral contraceptive to 15 post-menopausal women for six months. They then compared the intestinal absorption of radiocalcium before and after drug treatment and found that there was an increased calcium absorption in the OCA users. It was suggested by these authors that the estrogen component of the oral contraceptives improved the intestinal absorption of calcium.

Iron

It has been suggested that dietary iron requirements of women on OCA are slightly less than those of other women during the reproductive period of life (Theuer 1972). Observations that these drugs decrease menstrual blood loss would support this contention (Larsson-Cohn 1966).

Certain investigators have found that both serum iron and iron-binding capacity are increased in women on OCA (Jacobi *et al.* 1969; Mardell *et al.* 1969). However, in a recent study of female college students, while elevated total iron-binding capacity was related to OCA use, there was no significant association between serum iron levels and intake of these drugs. A significant number of these young women had iron intakes below recommended daily levels (Halstead and Roe, unpublished).

BIBLIOGRAPHY

ADAMS, P. W. *et al.* 1973. Effect of pyridoxine hydrochloride (vitamin B_6) upon depression associated with oral contraception. Lancet *1*, 897–904.

AFTERGOOD, L., and ALFIN-SLATER, R. B. 1974. Oral contraceptive-α-tocopherol interrelationships. Lipids *9*, 91–96.

ALY, H. E., DONALD, E. A., and SIMPSON, M. H. W. 1971. Oral contraceptives and vitamin B_6 metabolism. Am. J. Clin. Nutr. *24*, 297–303.

BAUMBLATT, M. J., and WINSTON, F. 1970. Pyridoxine and the Pill. Lancet *1*, 832–833.

BOOTS, L., CORNWELL, P. E., and BECK, L. R. 1975. Effect of ethynodiol diacetate and mestranol on serum folic acid and vitamin B_{12} levels and on tryptophan metabolism in baboons. Am. J. Clin. Nutr. *28*, 354–362.

BRIGGS, M. and BRIGGS, M. 1972. Vitamin C requirements and oral contraceptives. Nature *238*, 277.

BRIGGS, M., and BRIGGS, M. 1974. Oral contraceptives and vitamin nutrition. Lancet *1*, 1234–1235.

BRIGGS, M., BRIGGS, M., and BENNUN, M. 1972. Steroid contraceptives and plasma carotenoids. Contraception Internat. J. *6*, 275–288.

BROWN, R. R., ROSE, D. P., PRICE, J. M., and WOLF, H. 1969. Tryptophan metabolism as affected by anovulatory agents in vitamin B_6 in metabolism of the nervous system. Ann. N.Y. Acad. Sci. *166*, 44–56.

CANIGGIA, A. *et al.* 1970. Intestinal absorption of calcium 47 after treatment with oral oestrogen, gestagens in senile osteoporosis. Brit. Med. J. *4*, 30–32.

CASTREN, O. M., and ROSSI, R. R. 1970. Effect of oral contraceptives on serum folic acid content. J. Obstet. Gynaecol. Brit. Commonwealth *77*, 548–550.

COON, W. W., and NAGLER, E. 1969. The tryptophan load as a test for pyridoxine deficiency in hospitalized patients in vitamin B_6 in metabolism of the nervous system. Ann. N.Y. Acad. Sci. *166*, 30–43.

D'ARCY, P. F. and GRIFFIN, J. P. 1972. Iatrogenic Diseases. Oxford Univ. Press, New York, Toronto.

DOCTOR, V. M., SUTOW, W. W., and TRUNNELL, J. B. 1963. Effect of steroid hormones on urinary excretion of citrovorum factor by patients with prostatic cancer or leukemia. Proc. Soc. Exp. Biol. Med. *113*, 737-740.

EGEBERG, O. and OWREN, P. A. 1963. Contraception and blood coagulability. Brit. Med. J. *1*, 220-221.

GALL, I., PARKINSON, C., and CRAFT, I. 1971. Effect of oral contraceptives on human plasma vitamin A levels. Brit. Med. J. *2*, 436-438.

HALSTED, J. A., HACKLEY, B. M., and SMITH, J. C. JR. 1968. Plasma-zinc and copper in pregnancy and after oral contraceptives. Lancet *2*, 278-279.

INMAN, W. H. W., VESSEY, M. P., WESTERHOLM, B., and ENGELUND, A. 1970. Thromboembolic disease and the steroidal content of oral contraceptives. A report to the committee on safety of drugs. Brit. Med. J. *2*, 203-209.

JACOBI, J. M., POWELL, L. W., and GAFFNEY, T. J. 1969. Immunochemical quantitation of human transferrin in pregnancy and during the administration of oral contraceptives. Brit. J. Haemat. *17*, 503-509.

JOHNSON, C. K., GEENEN, J. E., HENSLEY, G. T., and SOERGEL, K. H. 1973. Small intestinal disease, folate deficiency anemia, and oral contraceptive agents. Digest. Dis. *18*, 185-190.

LARSSON-COHN, U. 1966. An appraisal of the clinical effect of three different oral contraceptive agents and their influence on transaminase activity. Acta Obstet. Gynecol. Scand. *45*, 499-514.

LINDENBAUM, J., WHITEHEAD, N., and REYNER, F. 1975. Oral contraceptive hormones, folate metabolism, and the cervical epithelium. Am. J. Clin. Nutr. *28*, 346-353.

MARDELL, M., SYMMONS, C., and ZILVA, J. F. 1969. A comparison of the effect of oral contraceptives, pregnancy and sex on iron metabolism. J. Clin. Endocrinol. *29*, 1489-1495.

MARKKANEN, T. *et al.* 1973. Binding of folic acid to serum proteins. I. The effect of pregnancy. Acta Haemat. *50*, 85-91.

MARTINEZ, O., and ROE, D. A. 1974. Diet and contraceptive steroids (OCA) as determinants of folate status in pregnancy. Fed. Proc. *33*, 715.

McLEAN, F. W., HEINE, M. W., HEALD, R., and STREIFF, R. R. 1969. Relationship between the oral contraceptive and folic acid metabolism. Am. J. Obstet. Gynecol. *104*, 745-767.

McLEROY, V. J., and SCHENDEL, H. E. 1973. Influence of oral contraceptives on ascorbic acid concentrations in healthy, sexually mature women. Am. J. Clin. Nutr. *26*, 191-196.

MELLETTE, S. J. 1961. Interrelationships between vitamin K and estrogenic hormones. Am. J. Clin. Nutr. *9*, suppl. 109-116.

MILLER, L. T., BENSON, E. M., EDWARDS, M. A., and YOUNG, J. 1974. Vitamin B_6 metabolism in women using oral contraceptives. Am. J. Clin. Nutr. *27*, 797-805.

MINK, I. B., CONNEY, N. G., NISWANDER, K. R., MOORE, R. H., *et al.* 1974. Progestational agents and blood coagulation. V. Changes induced by sequential oral contraceptive therapy. Am. J. Obstet. Gynecol. *119*, 401-405.

NECHELES, T. F., and SNYDER, L. M. 1970. Malabsorption of folate polyglutamate associated with oral contraceptives therapy. New Eng. J. Med. *282*, 858-859.

O'LEARY, J. A., and SPELLACY, W. N. 1968. Serum copper alterations after ingestion of an oral contraceptive. Science *162*, 682.

POPULATION REPORT. 1974. Oral contraceptives—fifty million users. Series A, No. 1, Dept. Med. and Public Affairs, George Washington Univ. Medical Center, Washington, D.C.

PRASAD, A. S. *et al.* 1975A. Effect of oral contraceptive agents on nutrients: II. Vitamins. Am. J. Clin. Nutr. *28*, 385-391.

PRASAD, A. S. *et al.* 1975B. Effect of oral contraceptive agents on nutrients: I. Minerals. Am. J. Clin. Nutr. *28*, 377-384.

PRICE, J. M., BROWN, R. R., and YESS, M. 1965. Testing the functional capacity of the tryptophan-niacin pathway in man by analysis of urinary metabolites. Adv. Metab. Dis. *2*, 159-225.

PULKKINEN, M. O., and PEKKARINEN, A. 1967. The levels of 17-hydroxy-corticosteroids in the plasma of users of oral contraceptives. Acta Endocr. (Kobenhaven) Suppl. *119*, 156.

RIVERS, J. M., and DEVINE, M. M. 1972. Plasma ascorbic acid concentrations and oral contraceptives. Am. J. Clin. Nutr. *25*, 684-689.

ROSE, D. P. 1966. The influence of oestrogens on tryptophan metabolism in man. Clin. Sci. *31*, 265-272.

ROSE, D. P., and McGINTY, F. 1968. The influence of adenocortical hormones and vitamins upon tryptophan metabolism in man. Clin. Sci. *35*, 1-9.

RUTHERFORD, R. N., HOUGIE, C., BANKES, A. L., and COBURN, W. A. 1964. The effects of sex steroids and pregnancy on blood coagulation factors. Comparative study. Obstet. Gynecol. *24*, 886-892.

SANPITAK, N., and CHAYUTIMONKUL, L. 1974. Oral contraceptives and riboflavin nutrition. Lancet *1*, 836-837.

SAUNDERS, F. J. 1970. Endocrine properties and mechanism of action of oral contraceptives. Fed. Proc. *29*, 1211-1219.

SCROGIE, J. J., SOLOMON, H. M., and ZIEVE, P. D. 1967. Effect of oral contraceptives on vitamin K-dependent clotting activity. Clin. Pharmacol. Therap. *8*, 670-675.

SHOJANIA, A. M. 1971. Effect of oral contraceptives on vitamin-B_{12} metabolism. Lancet *2*, 932.

SHOJANIA, A. M., and HORNADY, G. J. 1973. Oral contraceptives and folate absorption. J. Lab. Clin. Med. *82*, 869-875.

SHOJANIA, A. M., HORNADY, G., and BARNES, P. H. 1968. Oral contraceptives and serum-folate levels. Lancet *1*, 1376-1377.

SHOJANIA, A. M., HORNADY, G., and BARNES, P. H. 1969. Oral contraceptives and folate metabolism. Lancet *1*, 886.

SHOJANIA, A. M., HORNADY, G., and BARNES, P. H. 1971. The effect of oral contraceptives on folate metabolism. Am. J. Obstet. Gynecol. *111*, 782-791.

SPEIDEL, B. D. 1973. Folic acid deficiency and congenital malformation. Develop. Med. Child Neurol. *15*, 81-83.

SPRAY, G. H. 1968. Oral contraceptives and serum folate levels. Lancet *2*, 110-111.

STEPHENS, M. E. M. *et al.* 1972. Oral contraceptives and folate metabolism. Clin. Sci. *42*, 405-414.

STREIFF, R. R. 1970. Folate deficiency and oral contraceptives. J. Am. Med. Assoc. *214*, 105-108.

THEUER, R. C. 1972. Effect of oral contraceptive agents on vitamin and mineral needs: A review. J. Reprod. Med. *8*, 13-19.

TOGHILL, P. J., and SMITH, P. G. 1971. Folate deficiency and the pill. Brit. Med. J. *1*, 608-609.

TOVEY, L. A. D., and LATHE, G. H. 1968. Caeruloplasmin and green plasma in women taking oral contraceptives, in pregnant women and in patients with rheumatoid arthritis. Lancet *2*, 596-600.

VESSEY, M. P., and DOLL, R. 1968. Investigations of relation between use of oral contraceptives and thromboembolic disease. Brit. Med. J. *2*, 199-205.

VESSEY, M. P., and DOLL, R. 1969. Investigation of relation between use of oral contraceptives and thromboembolic disease. A further report. Brit. Med. J. *2*, 651-657.

WADA, H., and SNELL, E. E. 1961. The enzymatic oxidation of pyridoxine and pyridoxamine phosphate. J. Biol. Chem. 236, 2089-2095.

WHITEHEAD, N., REYNER, F., and LINDENBAUM, J. 1973. Megaloblastic changes in the cervical epithelium. J. Am. Med. Assoc. 226, 1421-1424.

WILD, J., SCHORAH, C. J., and SMITHELLS, R. W. 1974. Vitamin A, pregnancy, and oral contraceptives. Brit. Med. J. 1, 57-59.

WINSTON, F. 1969. Oral contraceptives and depression. Lancet 2, 377.

WOOD, J. K., GOLDSTONE, A. H., and ALLAN, N. C. 1972. Folic acid and the pill. Scand. J. Haemat. 9, 539-544.

WOOD, S. JR., RIVLIN, R. S., and KNOW, W. E. 1966. Biphasic changes of tryptophan pyridoxase level in tumor-bearing mice and in mice subjected to growth hormone and stress. Cancer Res. 16, 1053-1058.

CHAPTER 12

Nutritional Effects of Antituberculous Drugs

ISONICOTINIC ACID HYDRAZIDE (ISONIAZID, INH)

The early trials with isoniazid as a drug for the treatment of tuberculosis suggested that side effects were of minor importance and that little acute or chronic toxicity was shown. In the 1952 report of the Tuberculosis Chemotherapy Trials Committee of the Medical Research Council of Great Britain, 173 patients with pulmonary tuberculosis were treated with isoniazid, and among these, 107 were reported to have had no toxic manifestations throughout a 3 mo. period of treatment. Among the side effects of patients included in this study there was mention in the report of drowsiness, tremor and twitching of the limbs, disturbances of micturition, constipation, flushing, itching, and dermatitis. Probably very few of these reactions pertain to drug-nutrient interrelationships which will be the subject of the following discussion (British Medical Journal 1952).

At about the same time as the Medical Research Council's first report on the use of the drug in pulmonary tuberculosis, several authors (Dowling *et al.* 1953) reported cases of tuberculosis in which neurological side effects appeared and there was one case published in which a patient developed acute pellagra (McConnell and Chetham 1952). Pegum (1952) described the "burning feet" syndrome in a patient receiving 150 mg isoniazid for 1 wk only, and he suggested that this condition was caused by competitive inhibition of niacin by the isoniazid. Jones and Jones (1953) described two patients who had a peripheral neuropathy associated with isoniazid intake. In the first case there were also signs of pellagra. Although there were several cases of pellagra among the early cases of tuberculosis treated with the drug, it soon became clear to clinicians that a much more common side effect was a peripheral neuritis or neuropathy. Both of these toxic reactions are examples of the inhibitory effect of the drug on vitamin metabolism and/or utilization. It first occurred to Biehl and Vilter (1954A) that the neuritis which developed or might develop in patients receiving isoniazid was a metabolic defect induced by the drug. These workers noted the similarity of this neuritis with that produced by the vitamin B_6 antagonist, deoxypyridoxine, which led them to study vitamin B_6 metabolism in patients receiving isoniazid in various doses. Seventy-four previously untreated patients, under the direction of Drs. Biehl and Vilter, received daily doses of isoniazid ranging from 6–24 mg/kg body weight. This treatment was continued for 2–12 mo. unless toxicity occurred. Peripheral neuritis appeared in 19 of these patients, this side effect being related directly to the daily dose level of the drug. In their first report, they gave an excellent description of the INH neuritis which they stated is bilateral and peripheral consisting of paresthesia, numbness, burning pain and weakness. Physical findings included hyposthesia and exaggerated or absent tendon reflexes, though in the earlier stages objective findings were usually absent. They noted that if the drug was discontinued, the symptoms would disappear within a few weeks, although residual neuropathy might persist for a year at least, if the drug was continued for more than a few weeks after the beginning of symptoms. They collected 24-hr urine subsamples from some of their patients, and analyzed the samples for excretion of the vitamin B_6 metabolite, pyridoxic acid, and also for the major excretion metabolite of nicotinic acid, N^1-methylnicotinamide. They also measured the vitamin B_6 excretion. They found that after the initiation of isoniazid therapy, there was a marked increase in excretion of vitamin B_6 but the excretion of the pyridoxic acid and the nicotinic acid metabolite were normal in all patients studied. Test doses of tryptophan were given to these same patients and the excretion of xanthurenic acid was measured. Some patients showed an increased xanthurenic acid excretion during the test with tryptophan. Twenty of their previously untreated patients were given 20 mg/kg body weight of isoniazid with 50–450 mg of vitamin B_6 daily. None of these patients developed a neuropathy over a 10-wk observation period. This latter report seems rather inconclusive, though the authors state that in their experience, neuritis develops in 40% of patients on isoniazid, usually within eight weeks of the beginning of treatment. A few of their patients who received pyridoxine as a treatment for isoniazid neuritis did not show substantial benefit. Additional experiments are cited, that isoniazid depletes the tissues of vitamin B_6 through the formation and excretion of the isonicotinylhydrazone of pyridoxal. The *in vitro* formation of this complex and its properties had been described by Sah (1954) shortly before the publications by Biehl and Vilter (1954B).

Many investigators have confirmed the protective effect of vitamin B_6 against the development of the peripheral neuropathy during intake of isoniazid (Carlson *et al.* 1956). These authors found that 50 mg pyridoxine/day was sufficient to protect against neuritis in patients receiving 16 mg isoniazid/kg body weight. Although Ungar *et al.* (1954) showed that vitamin B_6 does not interfere with the antituberculous effect of isoniazid *in vitro* or *in vivo*, and Hawkins and Steenken (1963) demonstrated that the vitamin B_6 in ordinary doses does not lower the isoniazid concentrations in the serum of laboratory animals, it has been shown that very large doses of the vitamin will inhibit the effectiveness of the drug in tuberculous mice (McCune et al. 1957).

Although Biehl and Vilter originally subscribed to the theory that the principal cause of vitamin B_6 deficiency in patients on isoniazid was through the production of the INH pyridoxal hydrazone which could be excreted in the urine, subsequent work has shown that this may be a subsidiary mechanism and that the major way in which isoniazid produces a vitamin B_6 deficiency is by its inhibition of various vitamin B_6 dependent enzymatic reactions (Vilter 1964).

According to the work of Levy et al. (1967), in tuberculous patients on isoniazid who do not show clinical evidence of vitamin B_6 deficiency, the urinary excretion of vitamin B_6 is not greatly increased by the drug.   These authors suggest that there may be another explanation for isoniazid-induced peripheral neuropathy. In a later study that was carried out by Levy (1969), vitamin B_6 balance was investigated in two slow, and one rapid, inactivator of isoniazid and also the effect of high dosage isoniazid treatment on vitamin B_6 balance was studied.   There was an increase in the urinary excretion of vitamin B_6 in all three subjects, but changes in vitamin B_6 balance were different in the different subjects, such that a positive balance was observed in all three subjects prior to isoniazid administration, but during the time the drug was given the balance became somewhat less positive in one of the slow inactivators and increased slightly in the other two subjects.   As a result of these findings Levy suggests that the loss of vitamin B_6 from the body during high dosage isoniazid administration is not great enough to support the theory that isoniazid produces vitamin B_6 deficiency through vitamin depletion.   It has been noted by Standall et al. (1974) that, whereas 50 mg vitamin B_6 is a sufficient daily supplement to maintain a satisfactory pyridoxine status in patients taking a high dosage of INH, diets which are not supplemented with vitamin B_6 are usually inadequate to maintain patients on low doses of the drug in adequate pyridoxine status.   Supplementation with pyridoxine is recommended for patients receiving isoniazid.

People who are genetically predisposed to pyridoxine-responsive anemia may develop overt signs of the anemia after taking isoniazid. McCurdy and Donohoe (1966) described three patients who had hypochromic anemias which developed while they were receiving isoniazid.   Their anemia responded in part to the administration of pyridoxine. While these patients are described as having a pyridoxine-responsive anemia which, according to the authors, was influenced by the intake of INH, it is difficult to interpret the report fully because two of the patients had a glucose-6-phosphate dehydrogenase deficiency and the patients were on multiple drug regimens.

Isoniazid is inactivated by acetylation. Individual variation in the rate of isoniazid acetylation in man was first noted by Hughes et al. in 1956, and this trait was studied in families by Knight et al. (1959). Blood levels of isoniazid, when determined 6 hr after a standard oral dose of the drug, show a bimodal distribution within populations. Price Evans et al. (1960), who originally made this discovery, proposed that isoniazid metabolism is determined by two allelic genes at a single locus and that those persons who are slow inactivators or acetylators of the drug are homozygous for an autosomal recessive gene. This hypothesis has been supported by subsequent studies. The frequency of the gene for slow acetylation varies with populations and is relatively low in Asiatic peoples. A full discussion of this subject is given by La Du (1972). The slow acetylation phenomenon which determines the rate of activation of isoniazid, as well as related drugs, results from a reduced level of liver acetyltransferase (Peters et al. 1965; Genne 1965).

There is now quite extensive evidence that the incidence and severity of peripheral neuropathy due to interference with vitamin B_6 status is much more frequent in slow acetylators of the drug (Devadatta et al. 1960). The story of the effect of isoniazid on pyridoxine status provides an excellent example of acquired pyridoxine dependency. Vitamin B_6 requirement for patients on isoniazid has to be increased above the recommended dietary allowances by perhaps 40–50 mg/day (Carlson et al. 1956).

There have been a number of instances in which very large doses of isoniazid have been ingested for suicidal purposes. Cases who have attempted suicide in this manner have been successfully treated by administration of intravenous pyridoxine. It has been recommended that 1 gm of pyridoxine be administered for each gram of isoniazid ingested. Acute isoniazid intoxication is associated with convulsions simulating status epilepticus. It has been seen that when intravenous pyridoxine is given there is a marked lessening and earlier termination of seizure activity. It has also been suggested that if peritoneal dialysis is used to treat isoniazid poisoning, pyridoxine be added to each liter of fluid used in dialysis. This procedure is justified in that maximal clearance of isoniazid might thus be obtained while reducing the loss from the body of pyridoxine. No toxicity has been detected from administration of intravenous pyridoxine (Katz and Jobin 1970; Lemercier et al. 1963).

As mentioned previously, cases of pellagra have been reported in patients on isoniazid therapy. DiLorenzo (1967), described a pellagra-like syndrome associated with isoniazid treatment which responded to combined medication with niacin and vitamin B_6. He explained the isoniazid-induced niacin deficiency, by postulating that since pyridoxine is a necessary coenzyme in the metabolism of tryptophan, and in its conversion to niacin, the pyridoxine antagonist isoniazid could cause pellagra by interfering with niacin synthesis.

Although pellagra is a rare complication of isoniazid therapy among well nourished patients, persons with tuberculosis who are also debilitated by the effects of the disease or from the combined effects of the disease and a poor diet, are prone to develop pellagra during antituberculous treatment with this drug. Shankar (1955) has given us reliable evidence that isoniazid may play a substantial role in precipitating the development of endemic pellagra in undernourished Indian people. He described 50 cases of pellagra seen during a period of one year, of whom 90% described their diet as consisting of millet with a small amount of dahl (a bean paste) and occasional vegetables and chilis. Of these individuals, 76% did not consume any milk, and 70% did not eat any foods made with wheat. Ten percent of these patients had coexisting tuberculosis for which they were receiving isoniazid, and the author assumed that the drug may have been the final straw which caused them to develop pellagra. Pellagra has been also seen to develop among Bantu subjects with tuberculosis who were receiving isoniazid. These patients were on a very poor diet prior to the initiation of treatment and during drug treatment (Wood 1955).

CYCLOSERINE

Cycloserine has been used quite extensively in the treatment of tuberculosis, usually in a multiple drug regimen in combination with isoniazid and para-aminosalicylic acid. Like isoniazid, cycloserine has been identified as a pyridoxine antagonist. When both isoniazid and cycloserine are given together to experimental animals, it has been shown that a hypochromic anemia may develop which is characteristic of a vitamin B_6 deficiency (Harriss et al. 1965). A few patients who have received isoniazid and cycloserine combined as therapy have developed a sideroblastic anemia and this anemia has responded to withdrawal of the drug and treatment with pyridoxine. However, the hematologic responses to treatment have not been uniform (Verwilghen et al. 1965).

Klipstein et al. (1967), described two patients who developed megaloblastic anemia during combined therapy of tuberculosis with isoniazid and cycloserine. In both cases it was found that the anemia was due to folate deficiency. These workers made serum folate determinations in 120 patients with pulmonary tuberculosis and in 40 control subjects. Serum folate concentrations were subnormal in 36% of patients with untreated pulmonary tuberculosis who were investigated, and levels were subnormal in 7% of patients receiving isoniazid, but were subnormal in 52% of patients receiving combined treatment with isoniazid and cycloserine. The authors are of the opinion that cycloserine can induce folate deficiency, though the mechanism whereby this drug exerts such an effect is unknown. No evidence was obtained that a vitamin B_{12} deficiency had been induced by cycloserine.

PARA-AMINOSALICYLIC ACID (PAS)

This antituberculous drug has been shown to cause malabsorption, particularly malabsorption of vitamin B_{12}. This subject has already been discussed in relation to drug-induced malabsorption. While other antituberculous drugs may impair the vitamin status of patients, the commonest drug-induced vitamin deficiencies associated with intake of tuberculostatic agents are pyridoxine deficiency and vitamin B_{12} depletion. Emphasis is placed on the need to monitor tuberculous patients with respect to their vitamin status while they are on therapy, and to insure optimal intake of vitamins which are likely to be depleted by the various drugs they are likely to be taking. Intake of other drugs for the treatment of intercurrent disease should be limited as far as possible in tuberculous patients to those pharmacologic agents which do not interfere with vitamin absorption or utilization. Whenever necessary vitamin supplementation should be given to prevent or correct avitaminosis, this being uniformly the case with respect to pyridoxine (Roe 1971).

The antituberculous drug, pyrazinamide, is also a pyridoxine antagonist and as such is capable of producing a vitamin B_6 deficiency with sideroblastic anemia. Such an anemia is reversible when the drug is withdrawn (McCurdy et al. 1966).

BIBLIOGRAPHY

BIEHL, J. P., and VILTER, R. W. 1954A. Effects of isoniazid on pyridoxine metabolism. J. Am. Med. Assoc. 156, 1549–1552.
BIEHL, J. P., and VILTER, R. W. 1954B. Effect of isoniazid on vitamin B_6 metabolism: Its possible significance in producing isoniazid neuritis. Proc. Soc. Exp. Biol. Med. 85, 389–392.
CARLSON, H. B., ANTHONY, E. M., RUSSELL, W. F., JR., and MIDDLE-BROOK, G. 1956. Prophylaxis of isoniazid neuropathy with pyridoxine. New Eng. J. Med. 255, 118–122.

DEVADATTA, S. *et al.* 1960. Peripheral neuritis due to isoniazid. Bull. World Health Organization *23*, 587-598.
DiLORENZO, P. A. 1967. Pellagra-like syndrome associated with isoniazid therapy. Acta Dermat.-Venereol. *47*, 318-322.
DOWLING, G. B., WADDINGTON, E., HOWELL, R. G., and REES, D. L. 1953. Six cases of *lupus vulgaris* treated with isoniazid. Proc. Royal Soc. Med. *46*, 163-164.
GENNE, J. W. 1965. Partial purification and properties of the isoniazid transacetylase in human liver. Its relationship to the acetylation of p-aminosalicylic acid. J. Clin. Invest. *44*, 1992-2002.
HARRISS, E. B., MacGIBBON, B. H., and MOLLIN, D. L. 1965. Experimental sideroblastic anaemia. Brit. J. Hemat. *11*, 99-106.
HAWKINS, J. E., and STEENKEN, W., JR. 1963. Effect of chemical adjuvants on high doses of Streptomycin and of isoniazid in laboratory animals. Am. Rev. Resp. Dis. *87*, 717-725.
HUGHES, H. B., SCHMIDT, L. H., and BIEHL, J. P. 1956. The metabolism of isoniazid; its implications in therapeutic use. Trans. Conf. Chemotherap. Tuberc. St. Louis *14*, 217-222.
JONES, W. A., and JONES, G. P. 1953. Peripheral neuropathy due to isoniazid. Lancet *1*, 1073-1074.
KATZ, G. A., and JOBIN, G. C. 1970. Correspondence. Large doses of pyridoxine in the treatment of massive ingestion of isoniazid. Am. Rev. Resp. Dis. *101*, 991-992.
KLIPSTEIN, F. A., BERLINGER, F. G., and JUDEN REED, L. 1967. Folate deficiency associated with drug therapy for tuberculosis. Blood *29*, 697-711.
KNIGHT, R. A., SELIN, M. J., and HARRIS, H. W. 1959. Genetic factors influencing isoniazid blood levels in humans. Trans. Conf. Chemotherap. Tuberc. St. Louis. *18*, 52-58.
LA DU, B. M. 1972. Isoniazid and pseudocholinesterase polymorphisms. Fed. Proc. *31*, 1276-1285.
LEMERCIER, J. P., DORDAIN, M., and LANGLOIS, M. 1963. Acute toxicity from isoniazid. Rev. Tuberc. (Paris) *27*, 1137-1144.
LEVY, L. 1969. Mechanism of drug-induced vitamin B$_6$ deficiency. Ann. N.Y. Acad. Sci. *166*, 184-190.
LEVY, L., HIGGINS, L. J., and BURBRIDGE, T. N. 1967. Isoniazid-induced vitamin B$_6$ deficiency. Metabolic studies and preliminary vitamin B$_6$ excretion studies. Am. Rev. Resp. Dis. *96*, 910-917.
McCONNELL, R. B., and CHETHAM, H. D. 1952. Acute pellagra during isoniazid therapy. Lancet *2*, 959-960.
McCUNE, R., DEUSCHLE, K., and McDERMOTT, W. 1957. The delayed appearance of isoniazid antagonism by pyridoxine *in vivo*. Amer. Rev. Tuberc. *76*, 1100-1105.
McCURDY, P. R., and DONOHOE, R. F. 1966. Pyridoxine-responsive anemia conditioned by isonicotinic acid hydrazide. Blood *27*, 352-362.
McCURDY, P. R., DONOHOE, R. F., and MAGOVERN, M. 1966. Reversible sideroblastic anemia caused by pyrazinoic acid (pyrazinamide). Ann. Intern. Med. *64*, 1280-1284.
PEGUM, J. S. 1952. Nicotinic acid and burning feet. Lancet *2*, 536.
PETERS, J. H., MILLER, K. S., and BROWN, P. 1965. Studies on the metabolic basis for the genetically determined capacities for isoniazid inactivation in man. J. Pharmacol. Exp. Therap. *150*, 298-304.
PRICE EVANS, D. A., MANLEY, K. A., and McKUSICK, V. A. 1960. Genetic control of isoniazid metabolism in man. Brit. Med. J. *2*, 485-491.
ROE, D. A. 1971. Drug induced deficiency of B vitamins. N.Y. State J. Med. *71*, 2770-2777.
SAH, P. P. T. 1954. Nicotinyl and isonicotinyl hydrazones of pyridoxal. J. Am. Chem. Soc. *76*, 300.

SHANKAR, P. S. 1955. Pellagra in Gulbarga. J. Ind. Med. Soc. *54*, 73–75.

STANDALL, B. R., KAO-CHEN, S. M., YANG, G-Y., and CHAR, D. F. B. 1974. Early changes in pyridoxine status of patients receiving isoniazid therapy. Am. J. Clin. Nutr. *27*, 479–484.

TUBERCULOSIS-CHEMOTHERAPY TRIALS COMMITTEE, MEDICAL RESEARCH COUNCIL. 1952. The treatment of pulmonary tuberculosis with isoniazid. Brit. Med. J. *2*, 735–746.

UNGAR, J., PARKIN, K. R., TOMICH, E. G., and MUGGLETON, P. W. 1954. Effect of pyridoxine on the action of isoniazid. Lancet *2*, 220–221.

VERWILGHEN, R., REYBROUCK, G., CALLENS, L., and COSEMANS, J. 1965. Antituberculous drugs and sideroblastic anaemia. Brit. J. Hemat. *11*, 92–98.

VILTER, R. W. 1965. The vitamin B_6-hydrazide relationship. *In* Vitamins and Hormones, R. S. Harris, J. A. Loraine, and I. G. Wool (Editors). Academic Press, New York and London.

WOOD, M. M. 1955. Central nervous system complications during INH treatment of pulmonary tuberculosis. Brit. J. Tuberc. *49*, 20–29.

CHAPTER 13

Nutritional Effects of Anti-Parkinson Drugs: L-dopa

Patients with Parkinson's disease have a marked to extreme reduction in 3-hydroxytyramine (dopamine) in the neostriatum and in the substantia nigra regions of the brain (Hornykiewicz 1966). Parkinsonism has been explained at least in part by Andén et al. (1964) and Bertler et al. (1958) as an impairment of the nigra-neostriatal dopamine neuronal transmitter systems. Since dopamine cannot enter the central nervous system, it cannot be used as a replacement therapy in Parkinsonism. However, the amino acid 3,4,dihydroxyphenylalanine (dopa) can pass into the brain where it is decarboxylated to dopamine (Gey and Pletscher 1964). Conversion of dopa to dopamine within the brain forms the theoretical basis for the use of dopa or L-dopa in Parkinsonism.

The first observations of the effects of dopa on Parkinsonism were made by Birkmayer and Hornykiewicz (1961), who gave DL-dopa intravenously. Cotzias et al. (1967) showed that the L-isomer of this amino acid, when given orally, gave more effective clinical results in Parkinsonism with fewer toxic side effects than the DL-form. Although L-dopa is now a standard treatment modality for the control or partial control of Parkinson's disease, the drug exhibits a number of important side-effects. Wanger et al. (1971) studied 154 patients receiving L-dopa, and they found that 25% of these patients had one side effect; 50% had two or more side effects, and in 10% of their patients the disease was uncontrollable by the drug. According to Cotzias (1971), the most common side effect is the development of involuntary movements which are distinguishable from the Parkinsonian tremor. This side effect is the usual reason for reduction in the dosage of L-dopa. When L-dopa is given, the dose often has to be very large because much of the drug may not reach the brain, since it is rapidly metabolized peripherally with the formation of degradation products including dopamine, which as previously mentioned, do not cross the blood-brain barrier. Such drug wastage can be limited by pretreating the patient with an inhibitor of dopa decarboxylase that is only active peripherally (Sourkes 1971). Levodopa in combination with L-alpha-methyldopa hydrazine has been found to be a combination causing inhibition of drug metabolism (Vesell 1971).

Knowing that the decarboxylation of dopa to form dopamine is dependent upon the presence of pyridoxal phosphate, Duvoisin et al.

(1969) thought that pyridoxine might increase the therapeutic effects of L-dopa. They gave pyridoxine hydrochloride to some patients with Parkinsonism who were receiving maintenance doses of L-dopa, and found that large doses of the vitamin completely eliminated the clinical effect of the drug, while smaller doses reduced or abolished its therapeutic activity, or reduced the dyskinetic side effects. When pyridoxine was given there was a lower plasma level of L-dopa following its administration. Similar pyridoxine-induced effects were obtained by Wanger (1972), who found that doses of this vitamin as low as 50 mg/day produced partial reversal of drug effects within 24 hours and complete abolition of benefits in 3 to 4 days. Doses of pyridoxine as low as 5 mg/day significantly decreased the beneficial effects of the drug. Dyskinetic movements were again reduced by the vitamin in 50% of cases studied. Leon et al. (1971) studied three men and a woman with Parkinsonism who had achieved stable improvement of their disease while receiving L-dopa. Their maintenance levels of L-dopa range from 3.5 to 6.0 grams daily in divided doses. These patients were maintained on their prior dosage schedules of L-dopa during a control period of 1–2 weeks before pyridoxine was given, and during an 8–10 day period while receiving the vitamin. Clinical observations were made daily on these patients. Blood was collected from the subjects while they were fasting before and 1-½ and 2-½ hours after their initial morning doses of L-dopa. The test dose of L-dopa was 1.0 gm/3 subjects and 0.5 gm/4th subject. After the morning test dose of L-dopa the subjects resumed their usual dose of the drug following collection of the 2-½ hour blood specimen. Urine samples were collected for 8 hours following the initial dose of L-dopa for determination of dopa, dopamine, dihydroxyphenylacetic acid, and homovanillic acid. During the time that the patients were receiving pyridoxine hydrochloride, 50 mg of this vitamin was given orally with the initial dose of L-dopa on the days of specimen collection. On other days 25 mg of the vitamin was given twice daily. Three of the four subjects experienced an increase in their symptoms and signs of Parkinsonism when pyridoxine was given along with the L-dopa. In one of these subjects it was necessary to increase the patient's daily dose of L-dopa from 6 to 8 grams in order to maintain the previous level of clinical improvement. The fourth patient did not show any reversal in clinical improvement from L-dopa when the vitamin was given, but previous symptoms of nausea and involuntary movements attributable to L-dopa disappeared. When L-dopa was given alone there was a rapid increase in plasma dopa levels in all subjects 1-½ and 2-½ hours after administration of the drug. However, when pyridoxine was given with the drug, there was a smaller rise in plasma dopa concentrations. The 8-hour urinary excretion levels of dopa and dopamine decreased over 60% during the time that the vitamin was given. These changes in the urinary levels of these substances were evident on the first day the patients were given pyridoxine. The authors' comment that their findings of reduced plasma and urinary levels of dopa when pyridoxine is given with L-dopa suggest this interference in the amount of L-dopa available to enter the brain. It is further postulated that pyridoxine accelerates the peripheral decarboxylation of dopa to dopamine (Leon et al. 1971). It was found by Hsu et al. (1973) that co-administration of L-dopa and pyridoxine to Parkinson patients produced significant decreases of dopa in the urine, and at the same time increased urinary excretion of dopamine and dihydroxyphenylacetic acid. Changes in the urinary excretion of dopa and dopamine and dihydroxyphenolacetic acid were not significantly changed in control subjects.

It is unclear why the urinary changes brought about by the simultaneous administration of L-dopa and pyridoxine in Leon's studies differ from those of Hsu and his co-workers.

Several writers have discussed the mechanism whereby pyridoxine neutralizes the effects of L-dopa. Evered (1971) put forth the hypothesis that a Schiff base would be formed between the L-dopa and pyridoxal-5'-phosphate, the biologically active form of vitamin B_6. In order to substantiate his theory, he carried out experiments and found that L-dopa does combine with pyridoxal-5'-phosphate at pH 7.4. He raised the question whether vitamin B_6 could be classed as an amino acid antagonist, believing in the case of L-dopa this is true. Friedman (1970) was the first author to be concerned with the possibility that chronic L-dopa administration could induce pyridoxine deficiency, particularly in persons who have a high requirement for this vitamin. Among such persons he cites diabetics, alcoholics, those suffering from malnutrition or malignancies, patients exposed to industrial hydrazine fuels, and those receiving such drugs as INH, cycloserine or penicillamine which are known to be vitamin B_6 antagonists. Van Woert (1972) draws our attention to the fact that some pharmaceutical companies have suggested that low pyridoxine diets should be used with L-dopa in the treatment of Parkinsonism. Although a low pyridoxine diet might be expected to increase the amount of L-dopa reaching the brain, there are other considerations which suggest that this might be an unwise or dangerous procedure. Not only does L-dopa form a Schiff base with pyridoxal phosphate, but also it is known that L-dopa inhibits pyridoxal kinase, the enzyme which converts pyridoxal to the active coenzyme pyridoxal-5'-phosphate (Ebadi et al. 1968). A significant reduction in the levels of pyridoxal-5'-phosphate has been found to occur in the brains of animals given L-dopa in doses comparable to those given to patients with Parkinsonism (Kurtz and Kanfer 1971). A low plasma pyridoxine value was found by Golden *et al.* (1970) in a patient with Parkinsonism who developed a burning sensation of his feet when he was receiving L-dopa. A middle-aged male patient was referred to the author because he had developed seborrheic dermatitis while receiving L-dopa therapy for Parkinsonism. Examination revealed extensive scaling dermatitis of the scalp and face, and similar lesions not as extensive on the forearms. He had a confusional psychosis, hypochromic anemia and evidence of a marked peripheral neuropathy. On questioning his wife it was established that he had been taking L-dopa at a dose of 20 gm/day over a period of 10 months. When he was given vitamin B_6 the symptoms of pyridoxine deficiency disappeared and it was possible to stabilize his Parkinsonism by giving a reduced dose of L-dopa.

It is now possible to maintain the clinical effectiveness of L-dopa without recourse to pyridoxine restriction. The introduction of systemic decarboxylase inhibitors such as carbidopa has enabled greater delivery of L-dopa to the brain at much lower doses. The combination of L-dopa and carbidopa not only decreases the requirement for L-dopa, but prevents the loss of the drug effect produced by dietary pyridoxine (Mars 1974).

Evidence that L-dopa depresses the absorption of amino acids has been presented by several authors. Granerus *et al.* (1971) studied the effect of L-dopa on the absorption of L-phenylalanine in nine patients with Parkinsonism. They found that L-dopa only depressed the absorption of L-phenylalanine when the two substances were given simultaneously. It has been shown also that absorption of L-dopa is affected by concurrent administration of other amino acids. The observed inhibitory effect of a high protein intake on the therapeutic efficacy of L-dopa has been attributed to competitive absorption of dietary amino acids and L-dopa in the G.I. tract (Cotzias *et al.* 1968).

Lehmann (1973) demonstrated that six patients with Parkinson's disease receiving L-dopa showed low serum tryptophan levels after tryptophan loading as compared to similar post-loading levels of tryptophan when the drug was excluded. It is not clear from this report that this effect of L-dopa is actually due to drug-induced amino acid malabsorption. Although in a few patients with low serum tryptophan levels after test doses of the amino acid, the urinary excretion of tryptophan was also extremely low, the significance of this finding is in doubt because of the co-existence of bacilluria which may have caused degradation of the excreted tryptophan. In this same report, as also in an earlier communication by the same author (Lehmann 1971), theory and case documentation were set forth suggesting that mental depression and even dementia in the Parkinson patients on L-dopa could be relieved by giving tryptophan in a dosage of 1 g three times daily. It is not only suggested by Lehmann that L-dopa may lower the gastrointestinal uptake of tryptophan during L-dopa administration, but also that there may be a decreased influx of tryptophan into the brain and a consequent decreased synthesis of serotonin (5-HT). This could conceivably account for the observed mental symptoms in those receiving L-dopa though proof that this is so would require further investigation using appropriate animal models. The literature carries conflicting reports of the effects of tryptophan in people receiving L-dopa whereas, earlier studies either suggest that tryptophan administration during L-dopa therapy diminishes the effectiveness of the drug, or that tryptophan has no effect on pharmacologic function. Later investigations have tended to support Lehmann's finding that tryptophan treatment has a beneficial effect on the psychiatric side effects induced by L-dopa (Papavasiliou et al. 1969; Birkmayer and Neumayer 1972; Coppen and Metcalfe 1972; and Sano and Taniguchi 1972).

Studies in rats by Ordonez and Wurtman (1974) have shown that folate-deficient animals demonstrate significant decreases in brain S-adenosyl-methionine when treated with L-dopa in doses comparable to those used to treat Parkinson's disease. Their investigations have shown that, whereas in folate deficiency per se, altered methyl group metabolism occurs in other organs than the brain, L-dopa increases transmethylation in this tissue and impairs the brain's capacity to maintain methionine levels. It is suggested that during chronic L-dopa treatment of patients, excessive utilization of the de novo pathway for methyl group synthesis could increase nutritional requirements for folic acid and for vitamin B_{12}. Whether or not relative or absolute deficiency of folic acid or vitamin B_{12} contribute to cerebral side effects of L-dopa has not been established.

BIBLIOGRAPHY

ANDÉN, N. E. et al. 1964. Demonstration and mapping out of nigroneostriatal dopamine neurons. Life Sciences 3, 523–530.

BERTLER, A., CARLSSON, A., and ROSENGREN, E. 1958. A method for the fluorometric determination of adrenaline and nonadrenaline in tissues. Acta Physiol. Scand. 44, 273–292.

BIRKMAYER, W., and HORNYKIEWICZ, O. 1961. Dihydroxyphenylalanine (DOPA)—Effect on the akinesis of Parkinsonism. Wein Klin. Wochenschr. 73, 787–788.

BIRKMAYER, W., and NEUMAYER, F. 1972. The treatment of the DOPA-psychosis with L-tryptophan. Nervenarzt 43, 76–78.

COPPEN, A., and METCALFE, M. 1972. Levodopa and L-tryptophan therapy in Parkinsonism. Lancet 1, 654–658.

COTZIAS, G. C. 1971. Levodopa in the treatment of Parkinsonism. J. Am. Med. Assoc. 218, 1903–1908.

COTZIAS, G. C., VAN WOERT, M. H., and SCHIFFER, L. M. 1967. Aromatic amino acids and modification of Parkinsonism. New Eng. J. Med. 276, 374–379.

COTZIAS, G. C. et al. 1968. Parkinsonism and dopa. Trans. Assoc. Am. Phys. 81, 171–183.

DUVOISIN, R. C., YAHR, M. D., and COTE, L. D. 1969. Reversal of "dopa effect" in Parkinsonism by pyridoxine. Trans. Am. Neurol. Assoc. 94, 81–84.

EBADI, M. S., RUSSELL, R. L., and McCOY, E. E. 1968. The inverse relationship between the activity of pyridoxal kinase and the level of biogenic amines in rabbit brain. J. Neurochem. 15, 659–665.

EVERED, D. F. 1971. L-dopa as a vitamin-B_6 antagonist. Lancet 1, 914.

FRIEDMAN, S. A. 1970. Levodopa and pyridoxine-deficient states. J. Am. Med. Assoc. 214, 1563.

GEY, K. F., and PLETSCHER, A. 1964. Distribution and metabolism of DL-3,4-dihydroxy[2-^{14}C]phenylalanine in rat tissues. Biochem. J. 92, 300–308.

GOLDEN, R. L., MORTATI, F. S., and SCHROETER, G. A. 1970. Levodopa, pyridoxine and the burning feet syndrome. J. Am. Med. Assoc. 213, 628.

GRANERUS, A.-K. et al. 1971. Inhibition of L-phenylalanine absorption by L-dopa in patients with Parkinsonism. Proc. Soc. Exp. Biol. Med. 137, 942–944.

HORNYKIEWICZ, O. 1966. Dopamine (3-hydroxytyramine) and brain function. Pharmacol. Rev. 18, 925–964.

HSU, T. H., BIANCHINE, J. R., PREZIOSI, T. J., and MESSIHA, F. S. 1973. Effect of pyridoxine on levodopa metabolism in normal and Parkinsonian subjects. Proc. Soc. Exp. Biol. Med. 143, 578–581.

KURTZ, D. J., and KANFER, J. N. 1971. L-dopa: Effect on cerebral pyridoxal phosphate content and coenzyme activity. J. Neurochem. 18, 2235–2236.

LEHMANN, J. 1973. Tryptophan metabolism in levo-dopa-treated Parkinsonism patients. Acta Med. Scand. 194, 181–189.

LEHMANN, J. 1971. Levodopa and depression in Parkinsonism. Lancet 1, 140.

LEON, A. S., SPIEGEL, H. E., THOMAS, G., and ABRAMS, W. B. 1971. Pyridoxine antagonism of levo-dopa in Parkinsonism. J. Am. Med. Assoc. 218, 1924–1927.

MARS, H. 1974. Levodopa, carbidopa and pyridoxine in Parkinson's disease. Metabolic interactions. Arch. Neurol. 30, 444–447.

ORDONEZ, L. A., and WURTMAN, R. J. 1974. Folic acid deficiency and methyl group metabolism in rat brain: Effects of L-dopa. Arch. Biochem. Biophys. 160, 372–376.

PAPAVASILIOU, P. S., GELLENE, R., and COTZIAS, G. C. 1969. Modification Dyskinesias accompanying treatment with dopa. In Psychotropic Drugs and Dysfunctions of the Basal Ganglia. A Multidisciplinary Workshop. G. E. Crane and R. Gardener (Editors). Govt. Printing Off., Washington, D.C.

SANO, J., and TANIGUCHI, K. 1972. L-Hydroxytryptophan (L-5-HTP)-treatment of Parkinson's disease. Munch. Med. Wschr. 114, 1717.

SOURKES, T. L. 1971. Actions of Levo-dopa and dopamine in the central nervous system. J. Am. Med. Assoc. 218, 1901–1911.

VAN WOERT, M. H. 1972. Low pyridoxine diet in Parkinsonism. J. Am. Med. Assoc. 219, 1211.

VESELL, E. S., NG., L., PASSANANTI, G. T., and CHASE, T. N. 1971. Inhibition of drug metabolism by levodopa in combination with a dopa-decarboxylase inhibitor. Lancet 2, 370.

WANGER, S. L. 1972. The management of Parkinson's disease. Med. Clin. N. Am. 56, 693–707.

WANGER, S. L., KOTT, H. S., and FAGER, C. A. 1971. Parkinson's disease: Treatment with L-dopa. Lahey Clin. Found. Bull. 20, 1–9.

CHAPTER 14

Safety and Prevention

RISKS THAT DRUGS MAY PRODUCE NUTRIENT DEPLETION

In order to be able to discuss adequately the measures that should be taken to control, minimize or prevent drug-induced malnutrition, it is necessary to recapitulate the reasons why such side effects of drugs occur. More drugs are available than ever before, that have the capacity or may be found to carry the risk of inducing nutrient depletion. Such drugs are increasingly available, not only to well nourished persons and populations, but also to those who are constantly in a suboptimal nutritional status, as for example in many developing countries. Drugs are frequently administered to those who are malnourished through primary disease processes. Anticonvulsants, drugs used in the control of tuberculosis and malaria, as well as oral contraceptives, are prescribed for chronic usage which may result in a slow but constant nutrient drain.

Habitual self-medication may be associated with excessive intakes of over-the-counter drugs, such as antacids and laxatives which are then capable of causing malnutrition. These drugs, as well as prescription medications, may be used other than in the clinical situations for which they were first intended, and may be taken in dosages far exceeding therapeutic indications.

The nutritional side effects of drugs may be a necessary concomitant of therapeutic drug usage. This is true in the case of antivitamins used in the treatment of neoplastic disease, antibiotics such as neomycin, and anticoagulants.

Certain people receiving drugs may be particularly susceptible to nutritional side effects. Such high risk individuals or groups have not been sufficiently identified. Physicians have not been made sufficiently aware that their patients may be predisposed to the development of drug-induced malnutrition through genetic or pharmacogenetic characteristics, faulty diet, malabsorption, renal or hepatic dysfunction, or alcoholism. The additive or synergistic effects of drugs, diet and disease in the production of malnutrition have not been adequately presented in widely read medical journals. Thus, the medical profession is often unaware of the nutritional hazards brought about by the long-term administration of drugs.

Recommended nutrient intakes are seldom planned to overcome the nutrient drain imposed by drug intake. Indeed, very little attention has been given to the adequacy of the diet consumed by those receiving drugs. While multivitamin and megavitamin preparations are advertised and prescribed for the treatment of a host of symptoms unrelated to nutritional deficiency, nutrient supplements tailored to the needs of specific drug users are not easily obtained.

Inadequate laboratory facilities exist at a regional or local level for the biochemical evaluation of nutritional status. It is therefore difficult for physicians, even if they realize the risk of drug-induced malnutrition, to study their patients with respect to functional impairment in nutritional status.

EVALUATION OF RISK IN EXPERIMENTAL ANIMALS

Drug-induced nutritional deficiencies which occur as a side effect of drug usage have been identified in individual patients or patient groups, and have seldom been predicted from animal studies performed prior to drug release. Following the documentation of specific drug-induced malnutrition in man, attempts have been made to explain the mechanism by studies using experimental animals or animal models. Routine screening of drugs for their nutritional side effects has not been a conventional procedure in the establishment of drug safety either by pharmaceutical companies or government testing laboratories.

The design of animal experiments which can be used to evaluate the risk of adverse nutritional effects of drugs is a much needed endeavor requiring the expertise of nutritionists and pharmacologists alike. If such studies are to be relied upon as a predictive tool for the assessment of nutritional effects of pharmacological agents in man, certain criteria must be met as follows:

1) The experimental animal must have the same qualitative nutritional requirements as those of man.

2) Metabolism of the drug under investigation must be similar in the experimental animal and in human subjects.

3) It should be possible to create nutrient depletion in the experimental animal in a period not exceeding the duration of subacute toxicity tests (approximately 3 months).

4) If the drug is to be given orally, mixed with the animal's diet, it must be ascertained that the drug does not cause a marked decrease in food intake. Decreased food intake alone will, of course, lead to growth failure and/or signs of malnutrition in the animal.

5) The stress induced by drug administration must not cause a significant change in the animal's nutrient requirements.

6) Sufficient animals should be used to overcome intergroup differences in growth characteristics and state of nutrition.

7) In studies of the nutritional effects of drugs on the fetus, it must be possible to show that the drug effect is identical with the effects of nutrient depletion by diet, and that the drug effects can be prevented by appropriate nutritional intervention.

Animal models can be used in several ways to determine the risks of malnutrition due to drugs. Provided that an appropriate species and strain is used, animals can be employed to screen drugs for specific nutritional effects. It should be remembered, however, that in coprophagous rodents, such as the laboratory rat, resistance to nutrient depletion may occur because nutrients synthesized in their guts are consumed. Thus, experimental drug-induced folate deficiency in the rat may only be produced with coprophagy prevention. Caution should be exercised in extrapolating data from experimental animals to man with respect to the nutritional effects of drugs. Certain animal species may be much more sensitive to the nutritional effects of foreign chemicals than others, and it is usually appropriate to use several species. Drugs in subacute experiments should usually be administered by the same route by which they are given in man, though in prolonged studies with lipid-soluble drugs it may be appropriate to introduce the drug subcutaneously as a silastic implant.

Animals can be used to study variables that condition drug-induced malnutrition including drug dosage, duration of drug administration, diet, age, sex, maturity and visceral pathology. While animal models have been and are being used to study mechanisms whereby drugs exert their nutritional effects, no concerted effort has been made up to this time to use animals to screen drugs for multiple nutritional effects. Development of such screening procedures and their implementation should be an integral part of drug safety testing.

RESTRICTIONS ON HUMAN STUDIES

Constraints on the use of human research subjects are necessarily limiting studies of drug-induced malnutrition. For example, among geriatric patients informed consent may be impossible due to mental disability, and this restricts the use of such populations who are, in fact, the principal drug users. For the same reason, it may be difficult to study epileptics or others confined within institutions such as mental hospitals.

Another major barrier to the performance of studies of patient groups is the limited availability of funds. Whereas all research needs money and most research funds are in short supply, the problem of funding becomes even more acute when related to nutritional research in human subjects. Granted that it may be possible to obtain financial support to cover studies of selected nutritional parameters, in particular diseases, it is far more expensive to set up an investigation of drug-induced or drug-associated malnutrition. Major costs include the establishment of a laboratory for the biochemical evaluation of nutritional status, personnel costs and the costs of data handling. At the present time there are so few laboratories where nutritional status can be adequately evaluated, that it becomes expedient for the investigator to set up his or her own laboratory. A more economical system would be regional laboratories for nutritional status determinations which would be able to offer services to many investigators.

Those readers who share with the author the experience of having set up surveys and studies of the nutritional status of drug users, and have attempted to establish causal relationships, know that a major problem to be overcome is that of adequate staffing. Whether the study is to be carried out in an institution or in one or more communities, it is necessary to include one or more clinical nutritionists, a dietitian, research technicians to carry out the laboratory studies, as well as various kinds of paramedical personnel. The few major studies that have been carried out of nutritional status among those receiving medications have either been conducted by physicians or by physician-nutritionists. While it is desirable to physician-nutritionists to direct studies in the field under consideration, there are few people qualified in both professions and fewer who are interested in drug-nutrient relationships.

In order to examine relationships between drug intake and change in nutritional status, accurate dietary and drug intake records must be obtained. It is curious that while, for many years, dietitians have been trained to obtain information on food consumed by their patients or clients, there is no comparable professional group who has acquired the expertise to be able to obtain information on drug intake. Such information is usually picked up by the physician and is notoriously inaccurate. Dietitians, and particularly therapeutic dietitians, have the facility to obtain accurate records of food, and hence nutrient intake of patients in hospitals or other institutions. Outside of institutions it is extremely difficult to obtain accurate diet history by recall or by any other established method. This means that if one is studying the relative roles of drug and diet as causative factors in malnutrition, gross inaccuracies and misconceptions may arise because dietary factors are either over or under-estimated as risk factors. Drug histories of people outside institutions are frequently inaccurate, major omissions pertaining to non-prescription drugs which are not mentioned by subjects and not called for the interrogating physician.

Basic studies which succeed in identifying drugs as causal agents in nutrient depletion are easier to design and carry out than surveys which are aimed at identifying the nutritional impact of drugs in defined populations.

When patients receiving medications are surveyed with respect to their nutritional status and an attempt is made to establish relationships between particular drugs and particular forms of nutrient depletion, an immediate difficulty arises because in many instances the people are receiving multiple drug regimens. Even if through previous studies in man or in experimental animals it is suspected that one drug or drug group is responsible for the nutrient depletion, it is often not medically feasible to withdraw that drug in order to observe whether there is an improvement in nutritional status of a specific kind. For example, if a person were taking diphenylhydantoin and developed vitamin D deficiency, a causal relationship might be suspected on the basic of previous experience. On the other hand, if a patient were taking six drugs at the same time, one of which was glutethimide, and he also developed vitamin D deficiency, it might be difficult to establish a drug relationship. Multiple drug regimens pose a whole variety of problems. Patients are often given several drugs for the treatment of one disease, and several of these drugs may be capable of causing nutritional deficiency. The problem is to define which drug is responsible for which deficiency. If investigation and intervention are to be through a single drug withdrawal, the physician must be alert to the risk that control of the disease process may thereby be diminished or lost.

HUMAN STUDIES

Information on the incidence, etiology and risk of drug-induced malnutrition will come from prospective studies in human subjects. All of the following types of investigations are required, information from one supplementing that from another.

Comprehensive Drug Surveillance

It would be possible to obtain statistical information on the relationships between laboratory indices of nutritional status and drug intake in hospital populations from a rather moderate extension of the Boston Drug Surveillance Program (Jick et al. 1970). Food frequency data and simple biochemical parameters of nutritional status could be added to this information retrieval system. It should be emphasized, however, that without any change in the present Boston Drug Surveillance Program forms, it is possible to obtain important information with respect to drug-induced malnutrition. For example, it would be possible to establish the incidence of hypocalcemia among hospital patients receiving different drugs or drug groups. Another kind of information that could currently be obtained would be the relationship between intake of specific vitamin preparations or otherwise, and the incidence of certain drug associated anemias.

Nutritional Status of Conspicuous Drug Users

Perhaps the most central need at the present time is to investigate the nutritional status of those populations who are on long-term medications.   Such a study is presently being developed by the author with respect to geriatric populations. The aims of these investigations are as follows: a) to evaluate the health and nutritional status of defined populations of drug users; b) to obtain records of their nutrient and drug intake; c) to examine the relative importance of diet, drugs and disease as factors determining the nutritional status of persons within the sample; d) to examine the effects of drug withdrawal and/or nutritional intervention as modalities which further show causal relationships between drugs and nutritional status; e) based on the outcome of these studies, to examine the nutritional effects of drugs in animal models; and f) to examine the feasibility of expanding the current drug surveillance program to include dietary and nutritional status information so that factors determining the nutritional side effects of drugs can be identified.

Sample populations may consist in hospital patients within acute care or extended care facilities, as well as persons attending specialized or family practice clinics. For studies of the nutritional effects of oral contraceptives, it is advised that women attending family planning clinics or gynecology clinics be studied. In the case of any one sample population, demographic data must initially be obtained. Further data collection would be in six separate areas. These would include 1) food intake; 2) drug intake; 3) disease categories; 4) clinical assessment; 5) psychosocial behavior; and 6) biochemical, hematological and radiological parameters of nutritional status.

In order to obtain an accurate record of habitual food intake, a complete index of all foods consumed over a specific period should be obtained. In the case of hospital populations, this will mean determination of actual food consumed. This includes records of all foods presented or given to the patients as well as weighing back of uneaten foods and beverages. On the assumption that meals are prepared from standardized recipes and that there is a rotation of the standard diet, nutrient intake can be determined through use of the USDA Handbook No. 8 (Watt and Merrill 1963).

Through analysis of these data it will be possible to obtain a measure of the variability of nutrient intake per day, and to assess the minimal number of days necessary to obtain a realistic measure of the habitual nutrient intake.

A drug profile must be obtained from patient records which should include the drug or drugs received by generic and proprietary names according to drug groups, dosages, duration of intake and therapeutic indications. Additionally, a record should be kept of the intakes of all drugs and nutrient supplements taken over a period similar to that of the food intake records.

A general medical history should be obtained in all cases, and a listing of all medical and psychiatric illnesses present at the time when each subject is investigated.

The nutrition examination should follow the procedures adopted in the HANES Study (1972).

Initial laboratory studies should include screening procedures for the evaluation of nutritional status, as well as a biochemical profile. Blood and urine samples should be obtained from all subjects at the time they enter the study. Blood should be analyzed for glucose, urea nitrogen, uric acid, creatinine, thyroxine (T-3 and T-4), bilirubin, alkaline phosphatase, transaminases (GOT and GPT), cholesterol, calcium and phosphorus, total protein, albumin, globulin, amylase, lipase, sodium, potassium, CO_2, chloride, hemoglobin, packed cell volume, red blood cell count, total and differential white blood cell count. An oral glucose tolerance test should be routinely performed as well as urinalysis. Some of these determinations are indicators of nutritional status, while others related more specifically to physiological abnormalities which may contribute to malnutrition. Screening procedures for the evaluation of vitamin and mineral status should follow the guidelines laid down under the earlier discussion of the diagnosis of drug induced malnutrition. The requirement for further nutritional studies will be indicated by the characteristics of the population and more particularly by the drug history and the results of screening procedures. Whether or not particular biochemical determinations relevant to nutritional status are carried out will also depend upon the research protocol.

Data analysis and follow-up must be individualized to the needs of particular investigations. However, the following recommendations are made for the assessment of association between drug intake and nutritional status. Each illness of each subject should be tabulated by diagnosis according to the International Classification of Diseases (1967). Diagnostic groupings can also be made according to the systems of the body. Thus, subjects can be grouped according to whether physical or mental disease is present and if, for example, physical disease exists, in what category, e.g. cardiovascular, gastrointestinal, etc. Similarly patients can be grouped according to actual diagnostic classifications. Intake of specific nutrients for each subject should be classified as to whether they are equal to or above Recommended Dietary Allowances or below that level. The drugs taken by subjects should be grouped into categories according to therapeutic use and mode of action. Since multiple drug regimens are common, the first step in analysis should be a series of multiple regressions with the biochemical and hematological parameters relating to nutritional status as the dependent variables. The independent variables should be of the (0,1) variety, each one given a value according to whether the patient is or is not taking a drug in that category. Interaction effects between drugs can also be added to the equation when there is an *a priori* reason for supposing that a synergistic or additive effect may be present. Correlations between clinical diagnosis, nutrient intake, and nutritional status should be examined.

From this preliminary series of analyses, certain drug categories and nutritional parameters may prove to be substantially related to the sample population. More detailed studies of these particular drug categories can then be undertaken to see 1) which of the drugs in the categories are implicated; and 2) how the nutrient intake and the drug intake interact.

Finally, intervention studies can be carried out. In those instances where it is medically acceptable to attempt drug withdrawal, there should be a division of subjects into four groups. The individuals in these groups can be matched according to the original state of the nutritional parameter involved, then randomly assigned to groups allowing factorial design. The four groups in intervention studies would be: 1) no intervention; 2) nutrient supplementation; 3) drug withdrawal; and 4) both nutrient supplementation and drug withdrawal. If it proves impossible to match patients in groups of four according to the original state of the nutritional parameter, this may be used instead as a covariate in the analysis.

Such investigations will offer opportunities to study the importance of specific drug intake as a determinant of impaired nutritional status. They will also allow identification of common or less common drugs which impair nutritional status and the nutritional deficiencies, both clinical and subclinical, which are thus produced. Data obtained can be used to generate recommendations for nutrient supplementation of the diets of sample populations who are receiving certain drugs or drug groups found to have nutritional side effects.

PUBLIC HEALTH ASPECTS

The most controversial issue pertaining to the effects of drugs on nutritional status relates to measures that might be taken to minimize the risk of drug-induced malnutrition within any community or population. In those instances in which a drug is being taken by very large population groups, as for example in the case of oral contraceptives, nutrient supplementation of common foods is being suggested as a viable method for reducing the risk of vitamin depletion which may be brought about by the drug. It is necessary that the food to be supplemented be in common usage and that it does not require any preparation which might reduce the level of the added nutrient. For example, in order to diminish the risk of folic acid or vitamin B_6 depletion in women on oral contraceptives, these vitamins could be added in appropriate amounts to breakfast cereals. It would seem an appropriate measure to examine the feasibility and usefulness of this procedure in defined sample populations in whom nutritional status could be monitored from a biochemical and hematologic standpoint. Caution would have to be exercised in regulating the level of nutrients, such as vitamins added to food items, in order to avoid counteraction of desired drug effects and in the case of folic acid to avoid masking the presence of pernicious anemia.

Another measure which is currently being considered is the formulation of special nutrient supplements in pill form which could be given in conjunction with specific medications as required. One such formulation might be for children or adults receiving anticonvulsant drugs; another for persons on oral contraceptives and yet another for those receiving drugs for the treatment of tuberculosis. The number of such preparations that it would be feasible and useful to produce can largely be assessed by determination of the size of the population at risk. In general, dietary counseling for people taking drugs known to affect nutritional status is unlikely to be an effective means of reducing the risk, because food intake is dictated by ingrown habit as well as economic considerations. In individual patients, however, it may be possible to obviate the risk of drug-induced deficiency conditions by prescribing appropriate diets.

As is the original intention of this book, physicians and medical students should be made more aware of the risks of drug-nutrient interaction. They should not only be informed about the risks of drug-induced malnutrition, but should be encouraged to support measures to reduce its incidence. Such measures would include avoidance of unnecessary prescriptions, limitations of multiple drug regimens, support for the control of over-the-counter drug sales and the dissemination of information on the nutritional effect of drugs to nurses, paraprofessional personnel and their patients themselves.

BIBLIOGRAPHY

HEALTH AND NUTRITION EXAMINATION SURVEY, U.S. (HANES) 1972. Examination staff procedures manual for the health and nutrition examination survey, 1971–73. Instruction manual part 15a. PHS/USDHEW, National Center for Health Statistics, U.S. Govt. Printing Off., Washington, D.C.

INTERNATIONAL CLASSIFICATION OF DISEASES, 8th rev., adapted for use in the USPHS Publ. 1693, 1–45, National Center for Health Statistics, 1967.

JICK, H. et al. 1970. Comprehensive drug surveillance. J. Am. Med. Assoc. 213, 1455–1460.

NATL. RES. COUNCIL, NATL. ACAD. SCI. 1974. Recommended Dietary Allowances, 8th Ed. Natl. Res. Council, Natl. Acad. Sci., Washington, D.C.

WATT, B. K., and MERRILL, A. L. 1963. Composition of foods, raw, processed, prepared. Agric. Handbook No. 8, U.S. Dept. Agr., Washington, D.C.

Index

Abetalipoproteinemia, 43
Abortions, 189
Acetaldehyde, 19
Acetylation, 242
ACTH, 23, 26
Actinomycin D, 85
Activity coefficient, 124. *See also* Erythrocyte glutathione reductase assay
ADH, 40. *See also* Alcohol dehydrogenase
African trypanosomiasis, 166
Albumin, 9, 48, 118, 126, 259
Alcohol, 17, 78-79, 119, 203-207
Alcohol dehydrogenase, 19, 40, 47-48, 205
Alcoholic(s), 23, 25, 41, 48, 50, 195-196, 202-207
Alcoholism, 83, 202-210
Aldehyde dehydrogenase, 19
Alkaline phosphatase, 34, 118, 126, 137-138, 146, 217, 259
Alkalosis, 50
Allopurinol, 46
Alpha-ketoglutaric acid, 25
Alpha-2-macroglobulin, 9, 48
Aluminum hydroxide, 27, 145
Amethopterin, 156. *See also* Methotrexate
Amino acids, 147, 169
4-Amino-4-dioxy-10-methyl-folic acid, 157. *See also* Methotrexate
Δ-Aminolevulinic acid, 6-7, 172
Aminopterin, 156, 158-159, 190, 192
4-Aminopteroylglutamic acid, 156. *See also* Aminopterin
Ammonium chloride, 51
Amphetamines, 196. *See also* Dextroamphetamine; Stimulants
Ampicillin, 168
Amprolium, 25
Amylase, 259
Amyloidosis, 78
Analgesics, 150-152, 187, 194
Anemia, 7, 12, 14, 23, 43, 46, 48, 72-74, 76, 78-80, 119, 121, 123, 133-134, 161-162, 164-168, 171-172, 176, 217, 225, 241-244, 261
Anorectic agents, 76, 85-86, 148-149, 195
Antacids, 95, 145-147, 187-188
Anthranilic acid, 231
Antiarthritics, 99
Antibacterial agents, 132-133

Antibiotics, 38, 44, 120, 132, 178, 188, 253
Anticoagulants, 99, 155, 177-180, 234, 253
Anticonvulsants, 27, 54, 94, 125-136, 137-138, 191-192, 211-221, 253
Antidepressants, 32, 188
Antiemetics, 187
Antihemorrhagic factor, 36
Anti-inflammatory agents, 134-135
Antimetabolites, 20, 57, 154-155. *See also* Antivitamins
Anti-Parkinson drugs, 247-252
Antirachitic, 31
Antituberculous drug(s), 15, 165, 172, 239-246
Antivitamins, 53, 57, 154-186
Apoenzyme, 74, 154, 170
Appetite suppressants, 195, 197. *See also* Dextroamphetamine
Ariboflavinosis, 207
Arterial occlusion, 78
Ascorbic acid, 26-27, 44, 81-82, 85, 151-152, 228-229
Aspirin, 16, 45, 121, 151, 160, 194. *See also* Salicylates
Asthma, 198
ATP, 3-4, 22
ATPase, 50
Atromid S, 134. *See also* Clofibrate
Avitaminoses, 77, 79, 86
Azaribine, 168
Azathioprin, 168
6-Azauridine triacetate, 168
Azulfidine, 135. *See also* Salicylazosulfapyridine

Bacilluria, 250
Bacitracin, 132
Bacteria, 167
Balanitis, 161
Barbiturates, 51, 179, 187, 196
Beri-beri, 25
Beta-carotene, 39
Biguanides, 17, 78, 135
Bile acids, 8, 31, 133, 135
Bile salts, 39, 52, 132-133
Bilirubin, 259
Biogenic amines, 11
Bisacodyl, 131
Bishydroxycoumarin, 58

Biuret method, 118
Blind loop(s), 78
Bone disease, 125-126
Bone marrow, 12, 119-120, 165-167, 171, 204, 225
Bone mineral content (BMC), 138
Borate, 52, 150. See also Boric Acid
Boric acid, 21, 52, 134, 150, 257
Boston Drug Surveillance Program, 257
Brain development, 189
"Burning Feet" syndrome, 122, 239
Burns, protein requirements, 81

Cachexia, malignant disease, 86
Calciferol, 218
Calciferol-25-hydroxylase, 29
Calcinosis Universalis, 139
Calcitonin, 31
Calcium, 27, 30-31; 34-35; 83-85, 118, 125-126, 132, 136-139, 145-147, 177, 207, 217, 234-235, 259
Canadian Nutrition Survey, 2
Cancer, 85-86, 176
Carbidopa, 250
Carbonic anhydrase, 47
Carcinogenesis, 86
Carcinoma, 158, 160
Carotene, 39, 52, 118, 131. See also Beta-carotene
Carotenoids, 118
Catecholamines, 154
Cathartics, 57, 129, 131-132
Ca X P, 118
Celiac sprue syndrome, 76, 132, 225. See also Gluten-sensitive enteropathy
Cerebellar degeneration, 206
Ceruloplasmin, 46, 229, 234
Cervical epithelium, OCA effect, 226
Cervico-vaginal smears, 226-227
Cheilosis, 171
Chelating agents, 149-150
Chemotherapeutic agents, 85
Children, hyperactive, 196-199
Chloral hydrate, coumarin-albumin binding, 178
Chloramphenicol, 176, 178-179
Chlordiazepoxide, 212
Chloride, 259
Chloro-ethylthiamine, 24
Chloroquine phosphate, 165

Chlorthalidone, 148
Chlorthiazide, 51, 148
Cholecalciferol, 28, 31, 219
Cholesterol, 132-133, 135, 259
Cholestyramine, 17, 38, 41, 44, 78-79, 133-134, 179
Cholic acid, 134
Choline, synthesis of, 10
Chondroitin, 193
Chondrosarcomata, 86
Choriocarcinoma, 158, 160
Chorioretinitis, 165
Christmas factor, 37. See also clotting factor (IX)
Chromium, radiolabeled (^{51} Cr), 121
Cirrhosis, 23, 25, 41, 48-49, 83, 163, 167, 195
Citrovorum factor, 157. See also Folinic acid; 5-Formyltetrahydrofolate; 5-Formyltetrahydrofolic acid; Leucovorin
Cleft lip, 191
Cleft palate, 191
Clofibrate, 42, 134, 178-179
Clotting factors, 37, 178. See also Prothrombin (II)
Cobalamin(s), 11, 74
Coccidiosis, prophylaxis, 25
Coenzyme(s), 57, 71, 154
Coenzyme A, 50
Colchicine, 78-79, 134-135
Collagen biosynthesis, 174
Colon, spastic, 145
Congestive heart failure, malabsorption syndrome, 78
Conjugase, 8, 214
Convulsions, 72, 74, 173
Copper, 52, 149, 173-175, 234
Coproporphyrinogen III, 7
Corneal vascularization, 124
Corticosteroids, 78, 159, 198
Cortisol, 229
Cortisone, 26
Coumarin, 178-179, 234
Craniotabes, 33
Creatinine, 259
2-^{14} C-Riboflavin, 150
Cyclophosphamide, 168
Cycloserine, 15, 169, 171-172, 143-244
Cystathionuria, 74

Cysteine, 48
Cystic fibrosis, 48, 78
Cystine, 174
Cystinuria, 78, 149, 174
Cytosine arabinoside, 168
Cytochromes, 46
Cytotoxic agents, 155
Cytoxan, 168

Dahl, 243
Daraprim, 165. *See also* Pyrimethamine
Dark adaptation, 48
Data analysis, 259-260
Dehydroretinol, 38
Delirium tremens, 51, 206
Delta-aminolevulinic acid, 6-7, 74, 172
Delta-aminolevulinic acid synthetase, 7, 74
Demineralization, 145
5'-Deoxyadenosyl cobalamin, 13
Deoxycholic acid, 134
Deoxypyridine, 168-169, 171, 239
Deoxyribonucleic acid (DNA), 157
Deoxyuridine, 157, 164
Deoxyuridylate, 11
Deoxyuridylic acid, 157
Depo-provera, 230
Depression, 232-233
Dermatitis, 23, 78, 124, 171, 174, 198, 250
Dermatoses, 81
Desoxyribonucleic acid. *See* DNA
Dextroamphetamine, 178-179, 197-198
D-glucaric acid, 216
1,25-DHCC, 30. *See also* 1,25-Dihydro-xycholecalciferol
Diabetes mellitus, 78, 135
Diagnosis, 259-260
Dialysis, 242
2,4-Diaminopyrimidine, 164. *See also* Pyrimethamine
Diarrhea, 131, 133
Dibothriocephalus latus, 78
Dicumarol, 38, 177
Diet, 85, 97, 110-117, 243
Digitalis, 25
Digoxin, 51, 148
7-Dihydrocholesterol, 28
Dihydrocortisone, 26
Dihydrofolate, 11

Dihydrofolate reductase, 11-12, 164-167, 215
1,25-Dihydroxycholecalciferol, 29-30, 75, 139
24,25-Dihydroxycholecalciferol, 30
Dihydroxyphenylacetic acid, 248-249
3,4-Dihydroxyphenylalanine, 247. *See also* Dopa
1,1-Dimethylhydrazine, 173
Diphenylhydantoin, 16, 32, 58, 137-139, 179, 191-192, 211, 213-215, 219, 232, 257
Diphosphonates, 27, 32-33, 139-140
Disaccharidase, 78, 85, 134
Disease(s), 70-75, 78, 80-83, 86, 92
Disodium ethane-1-hydroxy-1, 1-diphos-phonate. *See* Diphosphonates
Disodium etidronate, 139-140. *See* Diphos-phonates
Disulfiram, 19
Diuresis, 148
Diuretics, 51, 147-149
DNA, 10-11, 15, 96, 157, 164, 166-167
DNA-thymine, 147, 167
DOP, 171
Dopa, 6, 247-250
Dopamine, 6, 247-249
Doxycycline, 44
D-penicillamine, 49, 149, 174-175. *See also* Penicillamine
DPH, 95, 99. *See also* Diphenylhydantoin
Drug addicts, 27
Drug(s), 15, 52-53, 56, 92-100, 106-110, 121, 155, 176, 187-196, 222, 253-261
Drug metabolism, 19, 22, 27, 52-58, 93-95
Drug-nutrient interactions, 52-58
dTMP, 157
dU, 167
dUMP, 157
Dwarfism, 48
D-xylose test, 117-118. *See also* Xylose
Dysfunction, testicular, 48
Dysgeusia, 49
Dysmaturity, 195
Dysosmia, 49

Ecchymoses, 37, 42
EDTA, 149
EGOT, 123

EGPT, 123
Egypt, 47
Elderly, 98-99
Embryogenesis, 75, 188-189
Encephalopathy, 161
Endotoxin, 82
Enteritis, 78, 85
Enzymes, 154
Epileptic(s), 95, 137-138, 191-192, 211-214, 216-218
Epinephrine, 6
Ergosterol, 28
Erythrocyte, 25, 43, 119-120, 123-124, 126, 174, 229-230
Erythroderma, 80
Erythroid hypoplasia, 23
Erythropoiesis, 23, 80, 162, 167
Erythropoietin, 23-24, 84
Estrogen(s), 45, 222-223, 231, 234-235
Ethacrynic acid, 147-148
Ethambutol, 149-150
Ethanol, 19, 40, 204, 208. *See also* Alcohol
Ethinyl estradiol, 228
Ethionamide, 169
Ethynodiol diacetate, 225-226
Experimental drug, 42

Factor V, 234
Factor X, 37
FAD, 20, 22
FAD pyrophosphorylase, 22
Fanconi syndrome, 147
Fatty acids, 43, 133
Fecal analysis, 118, 126, 134
Ferritin, 46
Ferrochelatase, 46
Ferroxidases, 46
Fetal, 75-76, 188-196
Fetus, 75-76, 188, 191-192, 194
FIGLU, 120, 223. *See also* Formimino-glutamic acid
Fistulae, 78
Flavin adenine dinucleotide, 20, 124. *See also* FAD
Flavin coenzymes, 20
Flavin mononucleotide, 20-22, 46
Flavokinase, 22
Flavoprotein, 22
5-Fluorouracil, 20, 162
FMN, 20-22, 46
Folacin, 7-9

Folate, 8-12, 14, 16-17, 72-73, 76, 78, 80-81, 83, 85, 89, 96-97, 99, 118-120, 126, 133, 135-136, 150-151, 160-162, 164-167, 211-216, 223-228, 244, 255
Folic acid, 7-11, 22, 75-76, 79, 96, 156-158, 161-162, 164-167, 188-189, 204-205, 212-217, 222-228, 251, 161
Folic acid antagonists, 156-157, 164
Folinic acid, 96-97, 157, 160-161, 165-167, 191
Follicular hyperkeratosis, 27
Food, 97, 111-116, 258, 261
Formiminoglutamic acid, 12, 120, 223
10-Formiminotetrahydrofolate, 11
Formiminotransferase, 73
5-Formyltetrahydrofolic acid, 72, 214
FT-9045, 176-177
Furfural hydrazide, 173
Furosemide, 147-148

Galactoflavin, 23, 86
Gantrisin, 165
Gastric resection, 78
Giardia lamblia, 78
Glossitis, 124, 171
Glucocorticoids, 18, 24, 31-32, 136, 198, 231
Glucose, 135, 259
Glucose-6-phosphate dehydrogenase deficiency, 230, 242
Glucosuria, 147
Glucuronides, 31
Glutamic acid, 6
Glutamic acid decarboxylase, 6
Gluten-sensitive enteropathy, 78-79, 168. *See also* Celiac sprue syndrome
Glutethimide, 27, 32, 139, 257
G-6-PD, 230
Gonadotropin, suppression, OCA, 222
GOT, 259. *See also* Transaminases
Gout, 134
GPT, 259. *See also* Transaminases
Growth, 75-76, 86, 195-199
Guiac test, 121

HANES Study, 259
Harrison's sulcus, 33
25-HCC, 29. *See also* 25-Hydroxy-cholecalciferol
25-HEC, 29
Hematocrit, 223

Heme, 6, 44, 46, 74, 79
Hemodialysis, 81
Hemoglobin, 222, 259
Hemolysis, 46
Hemopoiesis, 205, 212
Hemoproteins, 7
Hemorrhagic diathesis, 38
Hepatic fibrosis, 162
Hepatocytes, 24, 83
Hepatolenticular degeneration, 173
Hepatotoxicity, 163
Heroin, 196
Histidine, 10, 48
Hodgkin's disease, 86
Homocysteine, 11, 13
Homocystinuria, 74
Homovanillic acid, 213, 248
Hookworm, 78
Hormone, 51, 99, 154, 196, 198-199, 222
5-HT. See Serotonin
Hydralazine, 15, 169, 172
Hydrazide(s), 52, 150, 169, 172
Hydrazines, 173
Hydrazones, 169-170, 173
Hydrochlorthiazide, 51, 148
Hydrogen peroxide hemolysis test, 43
3-Hydroxyanthranilic acid, 231
25-Hydroxycholecalciferol, 29, 32, 75, 99-100, 125, 138, 218-219
25-Hydroxycholecalciferol-1-hydroxylase, 75
25-Hydroxyergocalciferol, 29
5-Hydroxyindoleacetic acid, 213
3-Hydroxykynurenine, 230-232
11β-Hydroxylation, 19
25-Hydroxylation system, 29
Hydroxyproline, 199
3-Hydroxytyramine, 247. See also Dopamine
Hypercalcemia, 30
Hypercalciuria, 84, 145, 206
Hyperlipoproteinemia, 42
Hypermetabolic states, 82-83
Hyperparathyroidism, 148
Hypoalbuminemia, 49, 195
Hypocalcemia, 34, 85, 131, 137-139, 147, 206
Hypogammaglobulinemia, 166
Hypogeusia, 49
Hypoglycemic agents, 135, 192-193
Hypokalemia, 85, 147

Hypolipidemic agents, 133-134
Hypomagnesemia, 50-51, 85
Hypoparathyroidism, 78
Hypophosphatemia, 34, 145-147
Hypoprothrombinemia, 37, 178
Hyposmia, 49
Hyposthesia, 240
Hypovitaminemia, 2
Hypovitaminosis(es), 81, 98

Immaturity, 48, 194
Imuran, 168. See also azathioprin
Indole, 194
Indomethacin, 179
Infant(s), 33, 43, 195-196
Infection, 82
Inflammatory bowel disease, 135
INH, 46, 93, 123, 150, 169-173, 239-241
Injury, radiation, 78, 85
International Classification of Diseases, 259
Intestinal, 78, 147
Intoxication, 174
Intrinsic factor, 13, 72, 121, 134-135
Iran, 47
Iron, 23, 43-46, 81, 85, 121, 134, 187-188, 235
Isoniazid, 99, 240-242. See also Isonicotinic acid hydrazide; INH
Isonicotinic acid hydrazide, 15, 20, 93-94, 165, 169. See also INH; Isoniazid

Jejuno-ileal bypass, 85

Kanamycin, 132
King-Armstrong units, 34
Korsakoff's syndrome, 206
Kwashiorkor, 23, 78
Kynurenic acid, 175, 231
Kynureninase, 231
Kynurenine, 174, 231-232
Kyphoscoliosis, 33, 35

Lactase deficiency, 117
Lactation, 75-76
Lactose intolerance, 117
Laennec's cirrhosis, 205
L-alpha-methyldopa hydrazine, 247
Lamina propria, 132
Laxatives, 27, 95, 118, 147
L-dopa, 16, 122, 124, 169, 176, 247-251

Leishmaniasis, 166
Leucovorin, 214. *See also* Citrovorum factor; Folinic acid; 5-Formyltetrahydrofolic acid
Leukemia, 158
Leukopenia, 119, 159-160, 165
Lipase, 259
Lipid peroxides, 42
Lipoprotein, 43, 233
Looser's zones, 35, 146
L-phenylalanine, 250
Lymphangiectasia, 78, 85
Lymphoma, 78
Lymphosarcoma, 86

Macrocytosis, 161, 167-168, 204, 212
Macroglobulin, 174-175
Macroglobulinemia, 174
Macro-ovalocytes, 166
Macrophages, 132
Magnesium, 49-51, 85, 145, 148, 206
Malabsorption, 56, 77, 85, 117-119, 129-144, 205, 225
Malaria, 164-165
Maldigestion, 52, 56, 76, 133, 205
Malformations, 188-191, 193-195, 216
Malnutrition, 85-86, 95-99, 102-105, 117-126, 188, 202, 253
Marasmus, 23
Marchiafava-Bignami's disease, 206
Mean corpuscular volume, 12, 119. *See also* Erythrocyte
Measurements, radiotelemetric, 136
Medroxy-progesterone acetate, 230
Mefenamic acid, 178
Megaloblastosis, 15, 79, 168
Menaquinone, 36. *See also* Vitamin K_2
Meningoencephalocele, 190
6-Mercaptopurine, 20, 168
Mercury poisoning, 147
Mersalyl, 148
Mestranol, 222-233, 234
Metabolites, nutrient, 154
Metalloenzymes, 47
Metaphase, 135
Metformin, 17, 135. *See also* Biguanides
Methacycline, 44. *See also* Antibiotics
5,10-Methyltetrahydrofolate, 11
Methionine, 10, 13, 251
Methotrexate, 12, 16, 56, 80, 96, 150, 158-164. *See also* Amethopterin

Methyl-cyanocobalamin, 13
5,10-Methylenetetrahydrofolate, 11, 215
N^5,N^{10}-Methylenetetrahydrofolic acid, 11, 157
Methylmalonic acid, 15, 120
Methyl-malonyl-coenzyme A, 13, 15
Methylphenidate, 196-198
Methylprednisolone, 198
9-Methyl-pteroylglutamic acid, 190
Methyltetrahydrofolate, 9-11, 14-15
5-Methyltetrahydrofolate, 11
5-Methyltetrahydrofolic acid, 72, 213-214. *See also* N^5-Methyltetrahydrofolic acid
Micelle, 131
Microsomal enzyme inducer(s), 32, 58, 94, 138-139, 179, 215-216
Microvilli, 129
Mineral oil, 27, 33, 38, 78, 130-131
Mitochondrial enzymes, 74, 170-172
Mitochondrion, 7
Mitosis, counting, 159
MMH, 100, 173
Monomethyl hydrazine, 100, 173
Morel's corticoid sclerosis, 206
Mortality, 195
MTX, 158. *See also* Methotrexate
Mucopolysaccharide(s), 40, 193
Myelofibrosis, 80
Myoglobin, 46
Myositis ossificans, 139

N-acetylpenicillamine, 174
N-acetyl transferase, 93-94
NAD, 18-20, 40
NADH, 46. *See also* Nicotinamide adenine dinucleotide
NADP, 4, 18-19
NADPH, 19
Natriuresis, 148
N-dichloroacetyl-DL-serine, 176
Neomycin, 39, 78, 130, 132-133, 178-179
Neostriatum, 247
Neuritis, 122-123, 171, 240
Neuromyopathy, 43
Neuropathy, 7, 25, 122, 172, 202, 206, 239, 241-242, 250
Neutrophil, 12, 119, 165-166
N-formyl kynurenine, 18
N^5-formyltetrahydrofolic acid, 72, 214
Niacin, 5, 17-20, 85, 239, 243

Nicotinamide, 18-19
Nicotinamide adenine dinucleotide, 18
Nicotinamide adenine dinucleotide phosphate, 18
Nicotinic acid-ribonucleotide pathway, 232
Night blindness, 41
N-isopropyl-α-(2-methylhydrazino)-p-toluamide, 173
Nitrogen, 84, 86, 132, 134
N^1-Methylnicotinamide, 18, 240
N^5-Methyltetrahydrofolate transferase, 73
N,N^1-Diisopropylethylene diamine, 149. See also Ethambutol
Norepinephrine, 6
Norethindrone, 234
Norethynodrel, 233
Norinyl, 234
19-Nortestosterone, 222
Nucleic acid, 75
Nutrient, 2, 52-56, 75-87, 92-93, 114, 116, 132, 134, 253-254, 260
Nutritional deficiency, 70, 119
Nutritional status, drug users, 258-261

Obesity, 85, 202
Oral contraceptives, 16, 18, 26, 43, 45, 72, 97, 123, 136, 222-238, 253, 258, 261
Organogenesis, 190
Osteoid, 33, 36, 139-140
Osteopenia, 31
Osteoporosis, 139, 207
Ouabain, 212
Ovarian follicles, 222
Ovulation, 222
Oxford Record Linkage Study, 191, 216
Oxyphenbutazone, 179
Oxytetracycline, 44. See also Antibiotics

Paget's disease, 139-140
Pancreatic lipase, 39, 56, 132-133
Pancreatitis, 43, 78, 206
Paraaminobenzoic acid, 57
Paraaminosalicylic acid, 17, 133, 165, 171, 244. See also PAS
Parahydroxylation, 95
Parathyroid, 31, 83
Parenteral alimentation, 86
Paresthesia, 240
Parkinson's disease, 16, 247, 251
Parrot's nodes, 33

PAS, 78, 122, 133, 172, 244. See also Paraaminosalicylic acid
PBG, 7
Pellagra, 18-20, 78, 171, 202, 207, 239, 243
Pellagrous, 7
Penicillamine, 16, 169, 173-176
Pentamidine isethionate, 17, 96, 166
pH, 132, 135-136
Pharmacogenetics, 93
Phenformin, 17, 135. See also Biguanides
Phenobarbital, 16, 32, 137-139, 191-192, 211, 213
Phenolphthalein, 130-132
Phenylbutazone, 179
5- Phenyl-5'- parahydroxyphenylhydantoin, 95
Phenyramidol, 179
Phosphate, 44, 137
Phosphorus, 31, 34-35, 118, 125-126, 137-138, 145-146, 259
Photon absorptiometry, 34, 138, 217
Phylloquinone, 36-37
Physician's Desk Reference, 110
Phytate(s), 44, 47
Pill, 223. See also Oral contraceptives (OCA)
Pityriasis rubra pilaris, 80, 158
Placental transfer, 76, 188-189
Plasminogen activity, 234
Pneumocystis carinii pneumonia, 166
Pneumoencephalograms, 73
Polycythemia rubra vera, 164
Polyglutamate hydrolase, 214. See also Conjugase
Polyglutamate(s), 8, 215
Polymyxin, 132
Polyneuritis, 173
Porphobilinogen, 7
Porphyria, 51
Porphyrins, 154
Post-gastrectomy, 85
Potassium, 17, 84, 118, 132, 134-136, 259
Prednisone, 23, 136, 165, 198
Pregnancy, 75-76, 98, 187, 195-196, 227
Primidone, 16, 32, 137, 191-192, 211
Procarbazine, 173
Proconvertin, 37. See also Clotting factor
Progestational agents, 222, 226
Progesterone, 222
Progestin, 222
Promyelocytes, 203

Pronormoblasts, 23
Protein, 85, 126, 174, 259
Protein-losing enteropathy, 81, 85, 118, 131
Prothrombin, 37, 126, 177. *See also* Clotting factor
Protocollagens, 26
Protoporphyrin, 7, 46
Provitamin D, 28
Psoriasis, 80, 158-160, 163
Psychosis, 250
Pteridine ring, 156-157
Pteridines, 22
Pteroyldiglutamic acid, 72
Pteroylglutamic acid, 215
Pteroylmonoglutamic acid, 10, 215. *See also* Folic acid
Pteroylpolyglutamic acid, 72
Pteroyltriglutamic acid, 72
Purine, 164
Pyrazinamide, 169, 171-172, 244
Pyridine nucleotides, 18
Pyridoxal, 3-4, 52, 171, 173, 240, 249
Pyridoxal kinase, 3-4, 169, 249
Pyridoxal phosphate, 3-6, 18, 22, 96, 123, 150, 169, 170, 172-173, 247, 249-250
Pyridoxamine, 3-4, 171, 176, 180
4-Pyridoxic acid, 232, 240
Pyridoxine phosphate, 4, 17-18, 22, 74-75, 169, 171-172, 175, 177, 189, 232, 241-244, 248-249
Pyrimethamine, 16, 80, 96, 164-166, 191
Pyrithiamine, 24

Quinidine, 179

Radiation enteritis, 85
Radioimmunoassay, 199
Red blood cell hypoplasia, 23. *See also* Erythrocyte
Regional enteritis, 168, 225
Regional ileitis, 78
Renal defect, 146-148
Resection, gastrointestinal, 79
Reserpine, 232
Reticulocyte(s), 46, 224
Reticulocytopenia, 23
Retinal, 40-41, 205
Retinol, 38-41, 48, 205. *See also* Vitamin A

Retinol-binding protein, 39
Retinyl ester(s), 38-39
Retinyl oleate, 39
Retinyl palmitate, 39
Retinyl stearate, 39
Rheumatoid arthritis, 76, 80-81, 149-151, 174
Rheumatoid factor, 174
Riboflavin, 18, 21-24, 52, 81-82, 85-86, 124, 150, 189, 229-230
Roboflavin 5'-phosphate, 20-22, 46
Ribonucleic acid, 188
Ribulose-5-phosphate, 25
Rickets, 27, 31-34, 97, 100, 118, 125, 137-139, 211, 217-219
Rickety rosary, 33
Risks, nutrient, 253
Rodents, 255

S-adenosyl-methionine, 251
Salicylamide, 194-195
Salicylates, 38, 45, 179, 194
Salicylazosulfapyridine, 16, 135
Salicylic acid, 194
Sarcoma, 176, 179
Schiff base(s), 5, 52, 96, 150, 249
Schilling test, 120-121, 136, 228
Schizophrenia, 175
Scleroderma, 78, 174
Screening tests, 126
Scurvy, 27, 207
Seasonal factors, 97
Sedatives, 188
Se-GSH, 42
Selenium-glutathione peroxidase system, 42
Serotonin, 6, 11, 232, 251
Serum, 12, 34-35, 46, 118, 120-121, 123, 125-126, 128, 136-137, 217-218
Sickle cell disease, 76, 79-80
Sideroblasts, 171
Siderocytes, 171
Silastic implant, 254
Slow acetylation, 93-94
[35]S-Methionine, 193
Sodium, 118, 132, 134, 215, 259
[35]S-Sulfate, 193
Stanford Binet score, 190
Status epilepticus, 213, 242

Steatorrhea, 43, 51, 77, 85, 117-118, 132-133, 162
Steroidogenesis, 19
Steroid(s), 40, 43, 45, 49, 176, 179, 222
Stimulants, 188
Stomatitis, 12, 124, 161, 171
Strictures, 78
Strongyloides, 78
Strophanthin, 148
Strychnine, 212
Stuart-Prower factor, 37
Subacute combined degeneration, 14
Substantia nigra, 247
Succinyl-coenzyme A, 6, 13, 15
Succinyl-sulfathiazole, 189
Sucrase, 132
Sucrose, 132
Sulfa drugs, 57
Sulfamethoxazole, 168
Sulfate, 189, 194-195
Sulfisoxazole, 165, 179
Sulfolipids, 195
Sulfomucopolysaccharides, 195
Sulfonamides, 167, 179, 188
Sulfonylureas, 192-193
Surgery, 84-85
Syndromes, 76-79, 132
Systemic sclerosis, 174. *See also* Scleroderma

TCA cycle, 19
Teratogenic factors, 118-195, 227, 233
Tetany, 34-35, 206-207
Tetracycline, 27, 44, 132
Tetrahydrofolate, 10-11, 156, 215
Thiamin, 24-25, 82, 123, 204
Thiazides, 148
Thiosemicarbizide, 169-170, 173
Thiosemicarbizones, 169
Thrombocytopenia, 159
Thromboembolic phenomena, 233-234
Thymidine-^{3}H-methyl (^{3}HTdR), 166
Thymidylate synthetase, 15
Thymidylic acid, 157
Thymine, 11, 164
Thyrotoxicosis, 82
Thyroxine (T-3, T-4), 259
Tocopherols, 41, 43, 233
Tolbutamide, 179, 192-193
Toxoplasmosis, 164, 191

Tranquilizers, 188
Transaminases, 169, 259
Transcobalamin I, 13
Transcobalamin II, 13, 73
Transferrin, 9, 45-46, 48-49
Triamterene, 16, 96, 147, 166-167
1,24,25-Trihydroxycholecalciferol, 30
Triiodothyronine, 41
Trimethoprim, 167-168
Triple lumen perfusion system, 215
Tropical sprue, 78-79
Tryptophan, 6, 18, 22, 122-123, 169, 174-176, 229-232, 240, 243, 250-251
Tuberculosis, 76, 133, 172, 239, 243-244
Tyrosine, 6

UDMH, 173
Ulcer, peptic, 45
Ulceration, intestinal, 12
Ultraviolet light, 28, 31, 52, 137
UMDH, 100
Unsymmetrical dimethylhydrazine, 100
Urea nitrogen, 259
Uremia, 83-84, 146
Uric acid, 259
Uroporphyrinogen, 7, 111
USDA Handbook No. 8, 258

Villi, 85, 132
Vitamin(s), 52, 71-75, 131, 133, 150, 154, 187-188, 205
Vitamin A, 38-41, 47-48, 82, 85-86, 118, 131, 133, 189, 205, 233
Vitamin A$_1$ alcohol, 38. *See also* Retinol
Vitamin A$_2$ alcohol, 38
Vitamin B$_6$, 3-8, 74, 121-123, 168-177, 230-233, 239-241
Vitamin B$_{12}$, 11, 13-15, 72-74, 78-80, 83, 85, 120-122, 135, 214, 216-217, 228, 251
Vitamin C, 26. *See also* Ascorbic acid
Vitamin D, 27-35, 50, 52, 75, 83, 85, 118, 125, 131, 133, 136-138, 140, 145, 189, 211, 218
Vitamin D$_2$, 28-29, 31, 137-138, 218
Vitamin D$_3$, 28-29, 31, 136-137, 139
Vitamin E, 41-43, 233
Vitamin K, 36-37, 42, 54, 85, 131, 133, 177, 179, 192, 233-234
Vitamin K$_1$, 36-37, 177-178

Vitamin K2, 36, 52
Vitamin K3, 36

Warfarin, 42, 177-179
Weight loss, 85, 197
Wernicke's encephalopathy, 25, 206
Whipple's disease, 43
Wilson's disease, 149, 174-176. *See also*
     Hepatolenticular degeneration
Wound healing, 49, 84-85

X intermediates, 7
Xanthine oxidase, 46
Xanthurenic acid, 122, 174-175, 177, 230,
     240
Xanthurenic aciduria, 74
X-Methyl-pteroylglutamic acid, 189
X-ray, 135
Xylose, 131

Zinc, 46-49, 52, 84-85, 148-149, 206, 234
Zoxazolamine, 27